Paramedic Case Studies

35 Prehospital Emergencies Explored and Explained

Richard Pilbery

Disclaimer

Class Professional Publishing have made every effort to ensure that the information, tables, drawings and diagrams contained in this book are accurate at the time of publication. The book cannot always contain all the information necessary for determining appropriate care and cannot address all individual situations; therefore, individuals using the book must ensure they have the appropriate knowledge and skills to enable suitable interpretation. Class Professional Publishing does not guarantee, and accepts no legal liability of whatever nature arising from or connected to, the accuracy, reliability, currency or completeness of the content of *Paramedic Case Studies: 35 Prehospital Emergencies Explored and Explained*. Users must always be aware that such innovations or alterations after the date of publication may not be incorporated in the content. Please note, however, that Class Professional Publishing assumes no responsibility whatsoever for the content of external resources in the text or accompanying online materials.

Text © Richard Pilbery 2021

All rights reserved. Without limiting the rights under copyright reserved above, no part of this publication may be reproduced, stored in or introduced into a retrieval system, or transmitted, in any form or by any means (electronic, mechanical, photocopying, recording or otherwise) without the prior written permission of the publisher of this book. The information presented in this book is accurate and current to the best of the authors' knowledge. The authors and publisher, however, make no guarantee as to, and assume no responsibility for, the correctness, sufficiency or completeness of such information or recommendation.

Printing history

This edition first published 2021

The authors and publisher welcome feedback from the users of this book. Please contact the publisher:

Class Professional Publishing,
The Exchange, Express Park, Bristol Road, Bridgwater TA6 4RR
Telephone: 01278 427 826
Email: post@class.co.uk
www.classprofessional.co.uk

Class Professional Publishing is an imprint of Class Publishing Ltd

A CIP catalogue record for this book is available from the British Library

Paperback ISBN: 9781859599532
eBook ISBN: 9781859599679
Cover design by Richard Stone, UK
Artwork by Nigel Downing
Designed and typeset by PHi Business Solutions

Contents

About the Authors — v
Foreword — vii
List of Abbreviations and Acronyms — ix

Chapter 1: Airway and Breathing — 1
    Severe Airway Contamination in Cardiac Arrest — 1
    Tracheostomies — 9
    Pneumothorax — 17
    Chronic Obstructive Pulmonary Disease — 25

Chapter 2: Circulation — 37
    Chest Pain — 37
    Pacemakers and ICDs — 45
    Sickle Cell Disease — 54
    Tachyarrhythmias — 62

Chapter 3: Disability — 75
    Brain Attack — 75
    Transient Loss of Consciousness — 83
    Headache — 91
    Autonomic Dysreflexia — 99

Chapter 4: Exposure — 111
    Drowning — 111
    Heat-Related Illness — 118
    Carbon Monoxide Poisoning — 126

Chapter 5: Medical Emergencies — 135
    Anaphylaxis — 135
    Hypoglycaemia — 141
    Pulmonary Embolism — 148
    Addison's Disease — 155

Chapter 6: Trauma — 167
    Thermal Burns — 167
    Conducted Electrical Devices — 175
    Ankle Injuries — 181
    Pelvic Trauma — 188

Contents

Chapter 7: Obstetrics and Gynaecology — **199**
 Care of the Newborn — 199
 Childbirth Complications — 207
 Postpartum Haemorrhage — 220
 Female Genital Mutilation — 229

Chapter 8: Paediatrics — **237**
 Croup — 237
 Feverish Illness in Children — 244
 Meningococcal Disease — 252

Chapter 9: Mental Health — **263**
 Mental Disorders and the Mental Health Act — 263
 Eating Disorders — 272

Chapter 10: Older People — **281**
 Frailty — 281
 Dementia — 288
 End-of-Life Care — 296

Assessment — **307**
 Airway and Breathing — 307
 Circulation — 311
 Disability — 315
 Exposure — 319
 Medical Emergencies — 322
 Trauma — 326
 Obstetrics and Gynaecology — 330
 Paediatrics — 334
 Mental Health — 337
 Older People — 339

Index — **343**

About the Authors

Richard Pilbery FCPara is a Research Paramedic employed by Yorkshire Ambulance Service NHS Trust and Associate Lecturer at Sheffield Hallam University. He is an editor for the College of Paramedics' *British Paramedic Journal* and co-author of *Ambulance Care Practice*, *Ambulance Care Essentials* and *First Responder Care Essentials*.

Contributors

Katie Duncan is a Paramedic and Teaching Fellow in Paramedic Science at the University of Greenwich. She joined the University in 2020 and previously worked at South East Coast Ambulance Service as an Operational Paramedic. She commenced her Paramedic Science BSc (Hons) degree in 2011 at Canterbury Christchurch University and completed her degree in 2014, at which point she began employment at South East Coast Ambulance Service. Katie has a keen interest in education, simulation and trauma. She also works as a Bank Paramedic at Lydden Hill Race Circuit alongside Critical Care Paramedics and Doctors.

Sid Fletcher is a Senior Practitioner for the Sheffield out-of-hours mental health team. He qualified as a Social Worker in 1994 and has been approved under the Mental Health Act since 1997. As part of his role, he undertakes formal mental health assessments that may or may not result in a client getting sectioned. However, most of his work is predominantly focused on assessing clients in crisis, usually with some other attendant emergency professional in tow.

Melinda (Dolly) McPherson is an Advanced Clinical Practitioner at the University Hospital Southampton and a HEMS Paramedic with the Hampshire and Isle of Wight Air Ambulance. She is a degree paramedic with an MSc in Advanced Practice working towards her prescribing qualification. She has experience in the NHS across a number of environments including the ambulance service, minor injuries, the emergency department and within GP practices. She has an interest in reading and writing academic literature with previous publications in the *Journal of Paramedic Practice* and *Standby CPD*.

Aimee Yarrington has been a qualified Midwife since 2003. She has worked in all areas of midwifery practice, from the high-risk consultant led units to the low-risk stand-alone midwife-led units. She left full-time midwifery practice to join the ambulance service, starting as an Emergency Care Assistant and working her way up to Paramedic while always keeping her midwifery practice up to date. She has worked in several areas within the ambulance service including the emergency operations centre and the education and training department. Her work towards improving the education of pre-hospital maternity care has led to her being awarded a fellowship award from the College of Paramedics. She strives to improve the teaching and education for clinicians in dealing with pre-hospital maternity care.

Foreword

I don't know about you, but I've found keeping up-to-date with paramedic practice challenging throughout my career. To try and solve this thorny problem, I had an idea to collate resources relating to a topic, including relevant research, guidelines and the like, to make it easier for me to refresh my memory about various patient presentations and how to recognise and appropriately manage them. However, it was only when my good friend Lorna Downing from Class Professional Publishing got involved that I actually did something about it ... and *Standby CPD* was born.

I wrote a monthly CPD article for SIX years ... that's 72 issues, and had a lot of fun (and a lot of frustration) doing so. Since I cannot see myself ever writing a memoir, this compendium of case studies is the next best thing. If I've learnt one thing from the past 20+ years in clinical practice, it is that you simply cannot make up the patients, colleagues and situations you find yourself in when working for an ambulance service.

These case studies are mostly written by me, but always with the help and advice of others. However, there were definitely topics that I was not an expert in and, to resolve this issue, I have been fortunate to have the support of other authors.

I am a great believer in 'Education by Stealth': engaging the reader with an engrossing, tongue-in-cheek and humorous case study, before hitting them with science, knowledge and guidance. I hope you enjoy it!

Richard

List of Abbreviations and Acronyms

ABG	Arterial blood gas
AF	Atrial fibrillation
AMHP	Approved mental health professional
APC	Anterior-posterior compression
AVNRT	AV-nodal re-entry tachycardia
AVRT	AV re-entry tachycardia
BASH	British Association for the Study of Headaches
BBB	Bundle branch block
BLS/ALS	Basic/advanced life support
BMI	Body mass index
BP	Blood pressure
BVM	Bag-valve-mask
CED	Conducted electrical device
CIED	Cardiovascular implanted electronic devices
CM	Combined mechanical
CNS	Central nervous system
COPD	Chronic obstructive pulmonary disease
CPD	Continuing professional development
CPR	Cardiopulmonary resuscitation
CRH	Corticotropin releasing hormone
CT	Computed tomography
CT	Computerised tomography
CWI	Cold-water immersion
DIC	Disseminated intravascular coagulation
DVT	Deep vein thrombosis
ECG	Electrocardiograph
ED	Emergency department
EOC	Emergency operations centre

List of Abbreviations and Acronyms

ETA	Estimated time of arrival
FAST	Face Arm Speech Test
FGM	Female genital mutilation
GCA	Giant cell arteritis
GCS	Glasgow Coma Scale
GP	General practitioner
GTN	Glyceryl trinitrate
HART	Hazardous area response team
HASU	Hyper acute stroke unit
HIV	Human immunodeficiency virus
HPV	Hypoxic pulmonary vasoconstriction
HSP	Heat-shock proteins
ICD	Internal cardio-defibrillator
ICS	Intercostal space
ICU	Intensive care units
IHS	International Headache Society
IM	Intramuscular
IV	Intravenous
IVC	Inferior vena cava
JVD	Jugular venous distension
LAD	Left anterior descending
LBBB	Left bundle branch block
LBP	Lipopolysaccharide binding protein
LC	Lateral compression
LCA	Left coronary artery
LMA	Laryngeal mask airway
LOS	Lower oesophageal sphincter
LVEF	left ventricular ejection fraction
MDT	Multidisciplinary team
MHA	Mental Health Act
MI	Myocardial infarction

List of Abbreviations and Acronyms

MOH	Medication overuse headache
MTC	Major trauma centre
NBG	NASPE/BPEG generic
NCT	Narrow complex tachycardia
NIV	Non-invasive ventilation
NO	Nitric oxide
OCD	Obsessive compulsive disorder
OH	Orthostatic hypotension
OHCA	Out-of-hospital cardiac arrests
OPA	Oropharyngeal airway
PAC	Premature atrial complex
PD	Personality disorder
PDA	Posterior descending artery
PE	Pulmonary embolism
PEA	Pulseless electrical activity
PGD	Patient group direction
PICU	Paediatric intensive care unit
PNES	Psychogenic non-epileptic seizures
PPCI	Primary percutaneous coronary intervention
PPE	Personal protective equipment
PPH	Primary postpartum haemorrhage
PPS	Psychogenic pseudo-syncope
PPV	Positive-pressure ventilation
PSP	Primary spontaneous pneumothorax
PSVT	Paroxysmal supraventricular tachycardia
PTSD	Post-traumatic stress disorder
RBBB	Right bundle branch block
RBC	Red blood cell
RCA	Right coronary artery
RNLI	Royal National Lifeboat Institution
ROS	Reactive oxygen species

List of Abbreviations and Acronyms

ROSC	Return of spontaneous circulation
RRV	Rapid response vehicle
RSV	Respiratory syncytial virus
RTC	Road traffic collision
RVI	Right ventricular infarction
SALAD	Suction-assisted laryngoscopy airway decontamination
SCD	Sickle cell disease
SCI	Spinal cord injury
SIRS	Systemic inflammatory response syndrome
SMACC	Social Media and Critical Care Conference
SVC	Superior vena cava
SVT	Supraventricular tachycardia
TBSA	Total body surface area
TEP	Tracheo-oesophageal puncture
TIA	Transient ischaemic attack
TLoC	Transient loss of consciousness
TLR	Toll-like receptors
TTH	Tension-type headache
UOS	Upper oesophageal sphincter
VF	Ventricular fibrillation
VS	Vertical shear
VT	Ventricular tachycardias
WHO	World Health Organization

1   Airway and Breathing

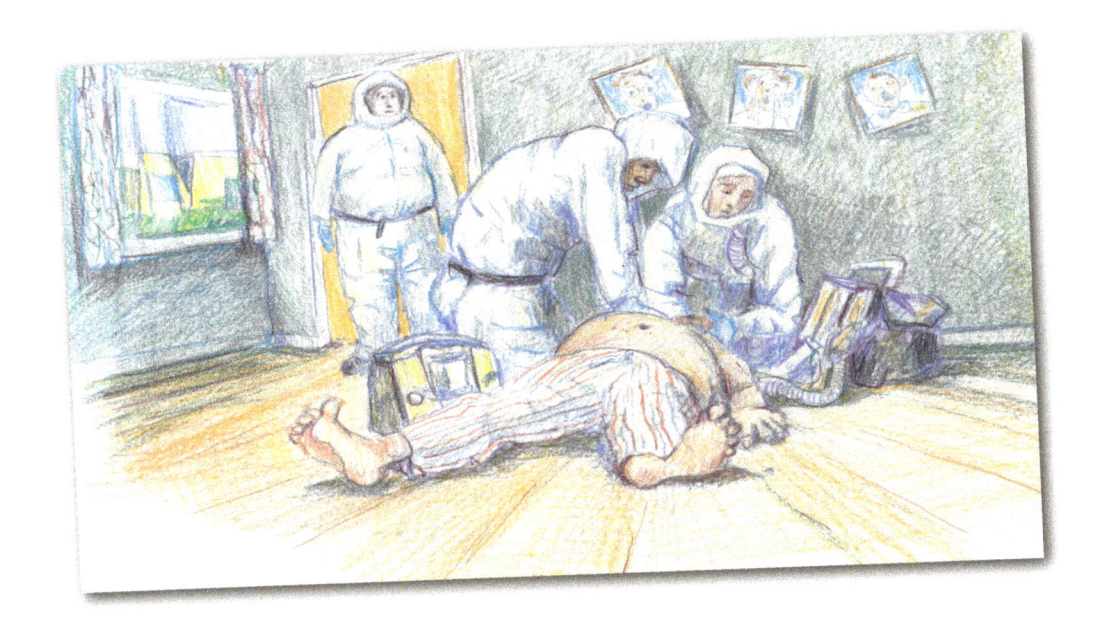

Severe Airway Contamination in Cardiac Arrest

You are on standby watching with morbid fascination as your colleague, Dave, devours his breakfast, a BLT from his favourite greasy spoon café. He mumbles something incoherent with a mouthful of bacon, lettuce and tomato and smiles. You resist the temptation to chide him for talking with his mouth full as you have been getting increasingly worried that you are turning into your parents. The lettuce stuck in his teeth is a bit off-putting, but before you can say anything you're passed details of your next job; backing up another crew for a 52-year-old cardiac arrest with cardiopulmonary resuscitation (CPR) in progress.

It's only 8 minutes away, so you elect to grab your personal protective equipment (PPE) while your colleague tries to swallow the remaining half of his (unchewed) BLT. You don the gown and place the powered respirator and hood in the passenger-side footwell. By the time you arrive outside the address, you just need to don the hood and turn on the respirator and are good to go. You pass your colleague a Tyvek coverall and his face drops. "No gowns left, I'm sorry," you say, not sorry.

> What are you going to do now: **Head straight into the house** (read on) or **grab some gear** (skip the next paragraph)?

Chapter 1   Airway and Breathing

Head straight into the house

The best thing about backing up a crew is that they take all the kit required into the address, which saves you from heavy lifting. However, as you pass the side of the other crew's vehicle, something makes you try the side door. It's unlocked and dutifully slides open, revealing the suction unit mounted on the wall. You have a feeling that grabbing some additional gear might be a good idea.

Grab some gear

You know the crew ahead will have taken most kit they require for the cardiac arrest, but you've found from personal experience that with only two pairs of hands, crews often cannot grab the suction unit and it ends up staying in the ambulance. You retrieve the unit from the wall bracket and locate a straight bougie for good measure.

The door of the address is ajar and you announce your presence before pushing the door open and entering. You hear a call from one of the other crew members and follow the sound of her voice into the living room. The paramedic, Sarah, acknowledges your presence before returning her attention back to her fingers, which are on the patient's carotid artery. "We've got ROSC," she says matter-of-factly, before completing an A to E assessment of the patient. You survey the scene and see that Sarah and her colleague have already done all of the hard work, with good 360° access to the patient and kit dumped in appropriate places.

As Sarah completes her assessment, your colleague puffs his way into the room, looking quite ridiculous in the coverall, although Sarah doesn't miss a beat and remains professional while giving you a sitrep. The patient, Brian, had been complaining of chest pain for 30 minutes prior to the call but wouldn't let his wife, Karen, call for help. Once he'd collapsed, she called 999 straight away and was coached in telephone CPR. Sarah and her colleague had literally come clear from a job on the same estate at the time of the call, and were by the Brian's side within 4 minutes of the call. Brian was in VF, but a couple of 200 J shocks had re-established a cardiac output. "Still apnoeic though," she notes.

Sarah mulls over the list of tasks that need completing. Karen is understandably upset and is currently smoking a cigarette just outside the kitchen door. However, updating her on Brian's condition means leaving the room. The airway needs addressing, not least because her colleague, a brand-new staff member, is currently ventilating the patient with the entire contents of the bag-valve-mask (BVM) twenty times a minute. "We also need a full set of observations including a 12-lead ECG, and an extrication plan which keeps Brian horizontal, if possible," she thinks to herself.

> What should Sarah ask you to do first: **Attend to the airway** (read on) or **Something else** (skip the next paragraph)?

Attend to the airway

Sarah asks if you could take over airway management so her colleague can obtain a full set of observations including a 12-lead ECG. The new staff member, Erin, hands you the BVM and you commence gentle ventilation at a rate of 10 per minute while preparing a supraglottic airway for insertion.

Something else

Sarah asks if you wouldn't mind getting a full set of observations including a 12-lead ECG, while she updates Karen on Brian's current condition. However, Dave is already one-step ahead having reflexively applied a blood pressure cuff and is currently wrestling with a tangled mess of ECG leads. He catches your eye and directs your attention towards the head of the patient where Sarah's colleague, Erin, is still over-ventilating the patient. You decide to offer to take over the airway and ask Sarah's colleague to prepare a size 4 i-gel for insertion.

With the i-gel sufficiently lubricated and the patient's head in an optimal position, you remove the oropharyngeal airway and pick up the i-gel. As you pull down on the patient's chin to assist the introduction of the i-gel, you notice that Dave's oropharynx is rapidly filling up with a noxious smelling liquid … it looks like Erin's over-ventilating has come back to bite you all.

What are you going to do: **Grab the suction unit** (read on) or **Call for Sarah** (skip the next paragraph)?

Grab the suction unit

You curse under your breath but are thankful that at least you had the presence of mind to bring in the suction unit. You snap at Erin to set up the suction unit. However, getting stroppy with an already nervous colleague does not help at all, and you watch precious seconds go by as she tries to connect the suction tubing and catheter to the unit. You realise that you need more help and call for Sarah.

Call for Sarah

Your heart sinks as you realise that if Brian's airway is not rapidly cleared, the cautious but optimistic picture that Sarah is currently painting for Karen is going down the pan. You call her name in the universally understood urgent tone that indicates something is going very wrong. She promptly appears from the kitchen and immediately moves to the suction unit, swiftly setting it up, switching it on and passing you the suction catheter. You manage to empty Brian's oropharynx but as you put down the suction catheter in order to pick up the i-gel, you can see the oropharynx filling up again. You repeat the suction but every time you stop suctioning, his oropharynx re-fills. You and Sarah are morbidly engrossed at this phenomenon, and it is Dave who points out Brian's bradycardia and pulse oximetry reading of 75% before the monitor complains of poor perfusion. Sarah again feels for a carotid pulse and her face drops; Brian has re-arrested. Dave immediately starts chest compressions and directs Erin to position herself on the opposite side of Brian in order to facilitate a timely exchange of chest compressions once his two minutes are up. Dave's chest compressions are really effective, but have the unfortunate side effect of increasing the flow of effluent from Brian's oropharynx and it starts to spill from the corners of his mouth.

What are you going to do: **Continue suctioning** (read on) or **Something else** (skip the next paragraph)?

Continue suctioning

You plough on trying to clear Brian's oropharynx while Sarah assembles the equipment required for tracheal intubation. However, you cannot keep the oropharynx clear long enough to get a suitable view and then suction unit becomes full, causing a delay while Sarah runs off to the ambulance to fetch a replacement suction liner. You are helpless as the passive regurgitation of Brian's stomach contents overflow into his lungs. Despite a textbook resuscitation attempt, you never gain control of Brian's airway and end up stopping resuscitation after 20 minutes, feeling like a terrible clinician.

Chapter 1 Airway and Breathing

Something else

You eye the suction unit and see it is already half full. In an attempt to regain some situational awareness, you briefly look up from Brian's oropharynx, which has been the sole focus of your attention and see Dave's concerned face. He tries an encouraging smile, revealing the lettuce still stuck in his teeth. This briefly abates your rising stress levels and from the back of your mind, you recall an acronym, SALAD; suction-assisted laryngoscopy airway decontamination.

"We need continuous suction during the intubation attempt," you announce. You recall the technique, and after taping up the vent hole on the suction catheter, invert your grip so that you can use the suction catheter to manipulate Brian's mandible, teasing it forward with the laryngoscope blade following behind. You make it to the top of the oesophagus and the continuous suction enables you to park the tip of the laryngoscope blade in the vallecula. After swapping the catheter over to the left-hand side of the mouth, you are able to get a clear path for the bougie first, followed by the tracheal tube. With the cuff inflated, and placement confirmed both by auscultation and a good capnography waveform, you let out a sigh of relief. You continue a textbook resuscitation attempt, but Brian never recovers and after a team discussion Sarah stops the resuscitation attempt. You can't help feeling like this was an opportunity missed, but are grateful that you managed to get past 'airway' as otherwise, Brian would not have stood a chance.

Scale of the problem

Regurgitation (when stomach contents return to the oropharynx) is common in out-of-hospital cardiac arrests (OHCA), occurring in around 25% of cases.[1] Potentially more serious but less frequent, is aspiration (when oral or gastric contents reach the larynx and beyond), which complicates about 15% of OHCA.[1] Failure to obtain a laryngeal view due to gastric contents and blood (from oesophageal varices for example) are also a common reason why tracheal intubation attempts fail.[2]

Anatomy, physiology and pathophysiology

During cardiac arrest, the ventilations provided to patients will be distributed to the lungs and stomach, with volumes to each dependent mainly on patient-related factors such as lower oesophageal sphincter (LOS) pressure, airway resistance and respiratory system compliance.[3] Together with the LOS, the upper oesophageal sphincter and protective laryngeal reflexes comprise the normal physiological mechanisms to reduce the risk of aspiration.[4] All three of these are severely compromised during cardiac arrest.

Lower Oesophageal Sphincter

The LOS is formed from a section of distal oesophagus and, normally, is at a pressure of approximately 20 cmH$_2$O. This pressure typically exceeds gastric pressure, creating a physiological barrier to prevent gastro-oesophageal reflux. However, this rapidly falls just before (and during) cardiac arrest to around 5 cmH$_2$O, increasing the likelihood of passive regurgitation and air entering the stomach during positive-pressure ventilation (PPV). Gastric distention not only increases the risk of regurgitation, but also elevates the diaphragm, decreasing lung movement and respiratory system compliance, resulting in less effective ventilation.[3]

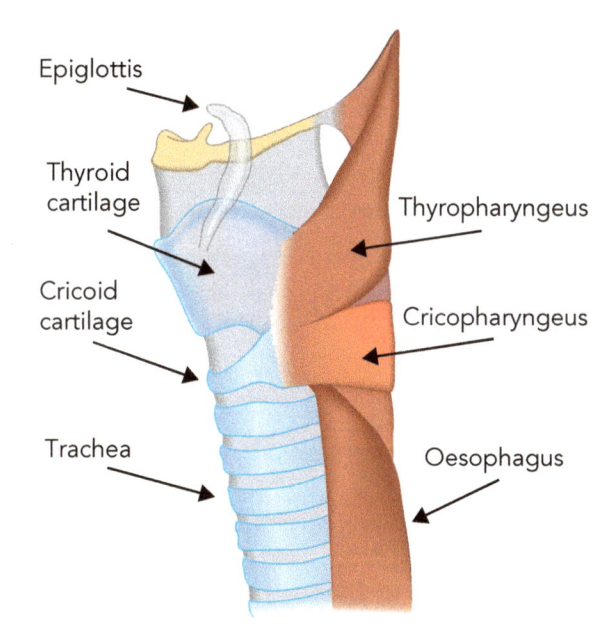

Figure 1.1 The inferior pharyngeal constrictor muscle separates into the thyropharyngeus and cricophyaryngeus.

Upper Oesophageal Sphincter

The upper oesophageal sphincter (UOS) is formed by the two parts of the inferior pharyngeal constrictor muscle (thyropharyngeus and cricopharyngeus) and the cervical oesophagus (Figure 1.1). The movements of these structures (particularly the cricopharyngeus) form an important part of the swallowing reflex.[5] During swallowing, the thyropharyngeus contracts as the cricopharyngeus relaxes, allowing a food bolus to be propelled into the oesophagus. UOS tone reduces as the patient's level of consciousness falls, leading to loss of this important mechanism for preventing oesophageal contents entering the pharynx.[4]

Laryngeal Reflexes

As with UOS, protective upper airway reflexes such as the pharyngeal (gag) reflex, coughing, expiration and laryngospasm are variably affected as level of consciousness reduces. This is not just an important consideration during cardiac arrest, but also following return of spontaneous circulation since airway reflexes are likely to remain impaired.[6]

Risk factors

While all OHCA patients should be treated as having a high-risk for aspiration, there are certain factors that are known to increase the risk:[4,7]

- Obesity – The increased size of the abdomen in obese patients results in a higher intra-abdominal pressure and displacement of the diaphragm. This must be overcome with higher inspiratory pressures, increasing the risk of gastric insufflation (blowing something into a body cavity, in this case, the stomach).
- Pregnancy – The gravid (pregnant) uterus displaces the stomach, altering the angle formed between the oesophagus and stomach, which together with higher concentrations of progesterone, reduce LOS pressure. In addition, a reduced concentration of the motilin hormone leads to delayed gastric emptying.
- Chronic lung disease – Increased airway resistance can make ventilation of patients with asthma and COPD difficult, increasing the risk of hypoventilation and gastric insufflation.
- Drowning – Regurgitation of stomach contents and swallowed water is common following drowning. In addition, significant amounts of foam can be generated as water mixes with plasma in the alveoli. Pulmonary compliance can fall dramatically, making supraglottic airways unfeasible. However, tracheal intubation can be complicated by foam and pulmonary oedema, which will require continuous suctioning to enable visualisation of the cords.[8]

Chapter 1 Airway and Breathing

Management

There are several techniques you can (and one you shouldn't) utilise to manage severe airway contamination in cardiac arrest:

- Patient positioning – This is likely to be limited in a typical OHCA; however, if your patient is on a trolley and you can place them head down, this may be useful in reducing the volume of contaminant that is aspirated while you definitively secure the airway.
- Suction – The mainstay of clearing the airway is aggressive suctioning with a wide-bore rigid-suction catheter, preferably one without a vent hole, since occluding the hole is easily forgotten when clinicians are faced with severe and ongoing airway contamination.[9] In the event of ongoing airway contamination, a strategy for providing continuous suction during tracheal intubation will be required, either utilising an assistant to hold the suction in situ on the left-hand side of the patient's mouth, or by using the SALAD technique.
- Cricoid pressure – This is not recommended routinely as part of airway management in cardiac arrest, and there is no evidence to support (or refute) its use with ongoing airway contamination due to regurgitation of stomach contents.[7] An alternative technique, left paratracheal compression, has been advocated instead, which has the advantage of not compromising laryngeal view during intubation. Again, this has not been tested during severe airway contamination in OHCA.[10]
- Intentional oesophageal intubation – Blind insertion of a tracheal tube will almost certainly enter the oesophagus. On inflating the cuff, in theory, the regurgitated stomach contents will pass via the tube and no longer obstruct the oropharynx.[11]

SALAD Technique

SALAD was developed as a simulation exercise in 2014, by a US anaesthetist Dr. Jim DuCanto. It was subsequently introduced into several US academic emergency medicine departments, culminating in its presentation at the 2015 Social Media and Critical Care Conference (SMACC). This raised the profile of the technique internationally. Following its introduction to the international community at SMACC, multiple medical educators introduced the technique in their own institutions and services across Australasia, Europe and Asia.

No large studies have been conducted on patients, but in simulated severe airway contamination scenarios, paramedics using the SALAD technique were able to intubate on the first attempt more often and faster than conventional suctioning techniques.[12,13]

Take the following steps to perform SALAD:[14,15]

1. Optimally position the patient to maximise the probability of intubation success (for example, external auditory meatus level with sternal notch).

2. Use the largest bore suction catheter you can find. If your suction catheter has a vent hole, cover this with tape.

3. Hold the suction catheter (wide-bore, rigid) in a clenched-fisted right hand, with the distal end of the catheter pointing caudad and posterior, to enable manipulation of the tongue and mandible as required. The curve

Severe Airway Contamination in Cardiac Arrest

of the rigid-suction catheter should mirror the curve of the structures of the upper airway.

4. Lead with suction to enable identification of relevant anatomical structure (posterior portion of tongue, epiglottis, vallecular and laryngeal outlet) (Figure 1.2) and follow with the laryngoscope (particularly important with video laryngoscopes to avoid contaminating the optics).

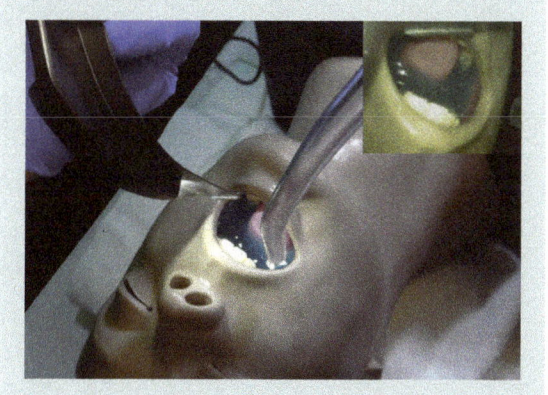

Figure 1.2 Lead with suction to help identify anatomical structures and prevent contamination of video laryngoscope optics.

5. In order to facilitate placement of the tracheal tube, the suction catheter is moved across to the left side of the mouth and the suction catheter 'parked' in the top of the oesophagus to provide continuous suction during the remainder of the intubation attempt (Figure 1.3). This can be achieved either by sliding the catheter under the laryngoscope

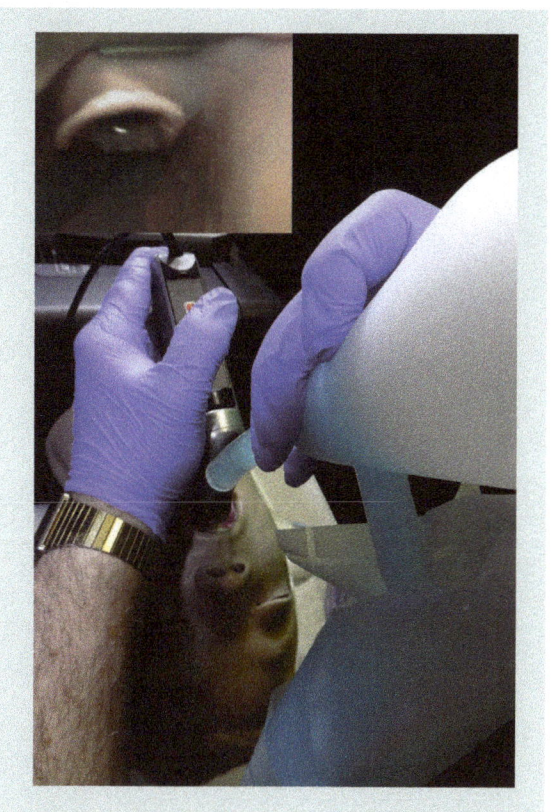

Figure 1.3 Move the suction catheter to the left-hand side of the mouth to facilitate placement of the tracheal tube.

blade, or by briefly removing the catheter and inserting it to the left of the laryngoscope blade.

6. Insert the index finger of the right hand into the right-hand side of the oropharynx to create a 'channel' for tracheal tube delivery (known as the SALAD poke, Figure 1.4).

Chapter 1 Airway and Breathing

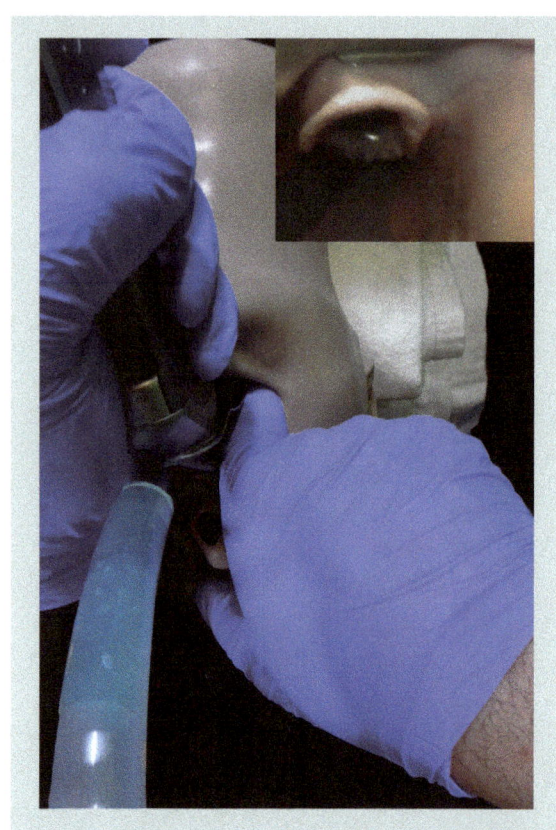

Figure 1.4 Insert your index finger into the oropharynx to create a 'channel' for the tracheal tube (known as the SALAD poke).

7. Intubate with a bougie.
8. Inflate the cuff on the tracheal tube to prevent further contamination of the lower airway.
9. Suction down the tracheal tube with a flexible suction catheter prior to ventilation to remove any residual contaminant prior to ventilation (Figure 1.5).

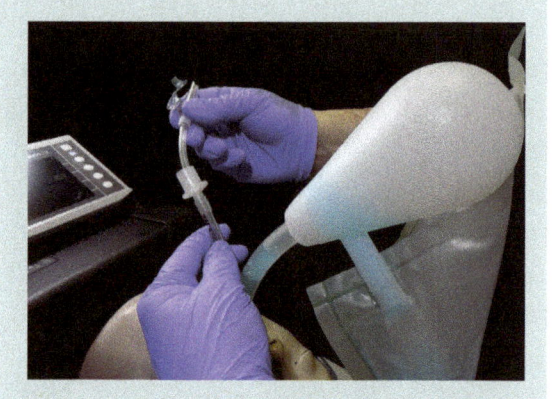

Figure 1.5 Suction down the tracheal tube prior to ventilation.

Source: Images courtesy of Dr. James DuCanto [C BY-SA 4.0 (https://creativecommons.org/licenses/by-sa/4.0)], via Wikimedia Commons.

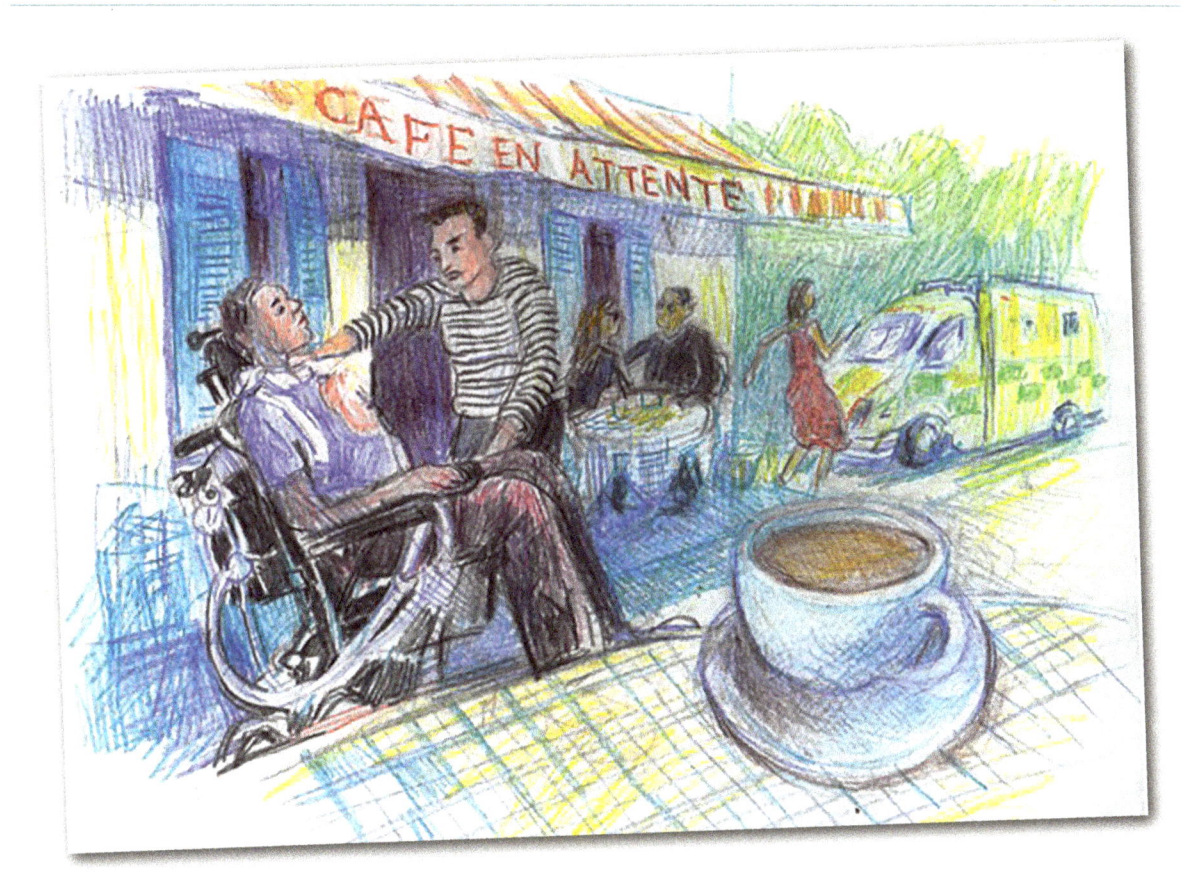

Tracheostomies

You are on standby enjoying the sunshine and rather wishing that you were sitting outside a newly opened French-themed café, sipping your favourite beverage and watching the world go by. The MDT bongs into life and grants part of your wish. The emergency call is located at the newly opened French-themed café and the patient is a 45-year-old man with breathing problems.

It takes you less than a minute to arrive on scene and the patient is easy to spot. He is the one sat in a motorised wheelchair which looks heavy, but comes complete with a box mounted at the back with a tube running to his … neck. It's a ventilator and the patient has a tracheostomy. You turn to your colleague and try to recall when either of you received any training around tracheostomy management. Your colleague gives an impressively authentic Gallic shrug and turns off the engine.

A young woman runs over to the ambulance and introduces herself as the patient's daughter. "It's my dad's ventilator," she blurts out: "it seems to be malfunctioning and my mum's gone off to the shops." You quickly

Chapter 1   Airway and Breathing

exit the ambulance and head over to the patient as she explains that her father suffered a high cervical spinal injury a year ago and now cannot breathe for himself. After a quick introduction, you head around to the back of the chair to look at the ventilator. The daughter, Irma, is right, the ventilator is chirping loudly and there appears to be a high-pressure warning on the touch screen interface. Irma explains that it is a new model and she is still trying to get to grips with it. The manual is in a basket just under the ventilator and runs to 500 pages, but helpfully has been translated into six languages (including French).

> What are you going to do: **Browse a chapter** entitled 'Getting up and running with your EzVent 5000' (read on) or **Do something else** (skip the next paragraph)?

Browse a chapter

You try speed-reading the chapter and tentatively push a few buttons. It makes no difference. The ventilator continues its alarm and the patient's chest does not appear to be moving. You need to do something else.

Do something else

You realise that you have become rather focused on the ventilator and neglected the patient's airway. A should come before B. No one on scene knows how to use the ventilator, so you take it out of the equation, remove the tubing from the patient's tracheostomy and reach for a BVM. You mutter some reassuring words as you connect the BVM (minus the mask) to the patient's tracheostomy tube. The patient's eyes are wide with fear, but at least he still appears conscious.

The tracheostomy tube appears to be sitting correctly, but your attempts to ventilate are unsuccessful. You remove the BVM and check the tube. It looks like a double-cannula design, so you remove the inner cannula, which has something rather unsavoury sticking out of the end. Your colleague has assembled the suction unit and places a suction catheter on the end of some tubing, but it won't pass beyond the end of the tracheostomy tube.

The patient's head is starting to loll about as hypoxia sets in and you realise that time is running out. Irma recalls that her father still has an upper airway, "unlike the man next to him in hospital who had his voice-box removed due to cancer."

> A patent upper airway sounds encouraging, what are you going to do: **Attempt to ventilate with the BVM** (read on) or **Keep looking at the tracheostomy tube** (skip the next paragraph)?

Attempt to ventilate

The patient is now unresponsive and accepts an oropharyngeal airway (OPA) without complaint. You attempt to get his head into a good position, no easy task with him sat up in a wheelchair, and attempt to ventilate. Nothing happens. Frantically searching for a solution, your eyes fall upon a pilot balloon and inflation valve that looks exactly like the sort you see on an endotracheal tube. You realise that the tracheostomy tube has a cuff.

Keep looking

A closer inspection of the tracheostomy tube reveals a pilot balloon and inflation valve, suggesting the tube has a cuff, which is inflated. A 10 ml syringe soon empties the air out of the cuff and you are finally able to make the patient's chest rise with the BVM. However, his habitus (you'd politely call him obese) and seated position are making it difficult to ventilate effectively and you know this is only a short-term solution. You hear yourself mutter the words, "I think we need to take the tube out." Your colleague looks at you aghast, but it is clear that it's not patent and is simply having a negative effect on the flow of air.

After a brief stand-off while you and your colleague have a silent exchange over who is going to remove the tube, which you win since you are still ventilating with the BVM, your colleague tentatively takes hold of the end of the tube and gently extracts it from the stoma. As a reward for his efforts, he gets a long piece of dried phlegm in his face during the next squeeze of the bag. However, like a true professional, he manages to occlude the stoma with his gloved hand while quietly retching.

Just then, the patient's wife returns from shopping and surveys the scene. "I've only been gone 10 minutes," she snaps, "why didn't you call me?" Irma looks down at her feet while her mother deftly extracts a bag from behind the chair and rummages for a replacement tracheostomy tube and inserts it into the stoma. A few button presses to the ventilator later and with the ventilator tubing connected to the tube, the patient is breathing again. The patient's wife borrows your oxygen cylinder for several minutes to increase the oxygen supply to her husband who quickly recovers. They both rebuff your offer of a trip to the local emergency department and head off down the high street, leaving you to clear up the mess you've created outside of the café.

Scale of the problem

A tracheostomy is an artificial opening made into the trachea through the neck (Figure 1.6). There are around 5,000 tracheostomies performed in head and neck surgery each year in England, with around 10,000–15,000 mostly temporary tracheostomies undertaken in intensive care units (ICUs).[16] Most of those will be removed prior to discharge from ICU, but an (unknown) number of patients are managed in the community, leading to more than 750 admissions each year in England when they malfunction.[17]

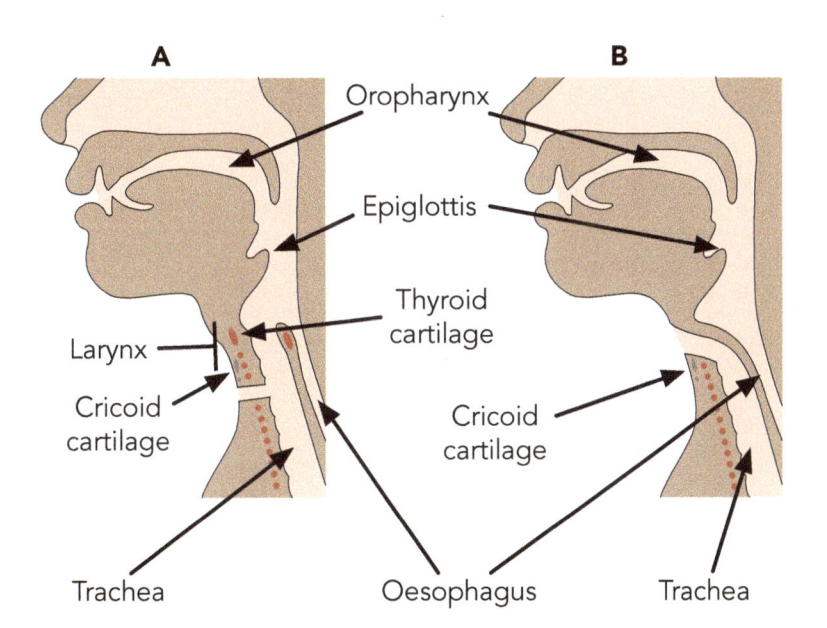

Figure 1.6 The anatomical differences between (A) tracheotomy and (B) laryngectomy.

Chapter 1 Airway and Breathing

There are a number of indications for a tracheostomy, including:[18]

- Prolonged intubation
- Facilitation of ventilation support/ventilator weaning
- More efficient pulmonary hygiene (i.e., managing secretions)
- Upper airway obstruction with any of the following:
  - Stridor, air hunger, retractions
  - Obstructive sleep apnoea with documented arterial desaturation
  - Bilateral vocal cord paralysis
- Inability to intubate
- Adjunct to major head and neck surgery/trauma management
- Airway protection (neurological diseases, traumatic brain injury)

As the name suggests, a laryngectomy is the removal of the larynx. This is typically due to involvement of the larynx in oral, pharyngeal and laryngeal cancers. If the patient requires a total laryngectomy, the larynx is removed and the trachea cut and stitched to the front of the neck.[16] This is important for subsequent management, because these patients cannot be ventilated from the mouth and/or nose (Figure 1.6).

Physiological changes with tracheostomies

In addition to a hole (stoma) in the patient's neck and (in the case of tracheostomy) a tube in the trachea, there are a number of important physiological consequences in a tracheostomy and a laryngectomy:[16]

- Upper airway anatomical dead space is reduced by up to 50% – This can be advantageous when weaning patients off mechanical ventilation.
- Upper airway warming, humidification and filtering is lost – This is a serious problem, leading to thick and dry secretions which can easily block a stoma or tracheostomy tube.
- Ability to swallow is affected – This is a problem with tracheostomies, as the tracheostomy tube and/or cuff interferes with the mechanics of swallowing, including pressing on the oesophagus behind the trachea, leading to a physical obstruction as well as tethering the anterior structures of the neck, limiting the movement of the larynx required for safe swallowing.
- The patient cannot speak – This can cause distress and anxiety for patients and can make communication difficult.
- Sense of taste and smell can be lost – This can lead to reduced appetite and affect the general health of the patient if not addressed.
- Altered body image – This is an important psychological factor.

Tracheostomy tubes

There are a wide variety of tracheostomy tubes, which can seem rather overwhelming. However, tubes are broadly classified into the following categories:[16]

- Cuffed/uncuffed
- With/without inner cannula
- Fenestrated/unfenestrated.

Cuffed/uncuffed tubes

As with adult endotracheal tubes, a cuffed tracheostomy tube has a soft balloon around the distal end, which is inflated by injecting air into the pilot balloon via the injection port (Figure 1.7). These are used when patients require PPV and/or when the patient cannot protect their own airway from secretions. Note that if the cuffed tube is inflated and the lumen becomes blocked or occluded, the patient will not be able to breathe!

Uncuffed tubes tend to be used in longer-term patients, but since they lack the cuff, it is important that these patients have an effective cough and gag reflex to minimise the chance of aspiration. These tubes are not suitable for PPV.

Tracheostomies

Uncuffed, double-cannula tracheostomy tubes are the safest type to use in the community.[16]

Fenestrated tubes

These tracheostomy tubes have an opening on the outer cannula which allows air to pass through the patient's oro- and nasopharynx. This is helpful because it allows the patient to talk and produce an effective cough. However, fenestrations increase the risk of aspiration and prevent PPV unless a non-fenestrated inner cannula is used. Non-fenestrated inner cannulas should also be used if the patient requires suction (Figure 1.8).

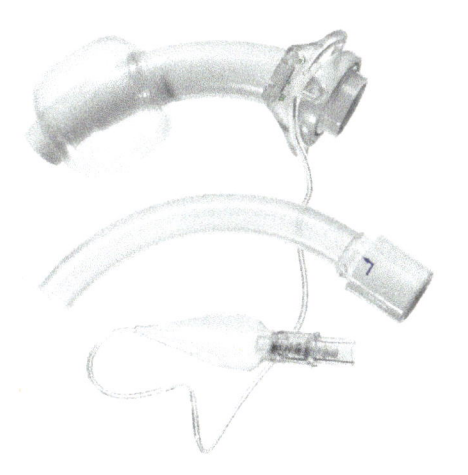

Figure 1.7 A cuffed, unfenestrated tracheostomy tube (top). Inner cannula with no fenestrations (middle). Pilot balloon and inflation valve for tracheostomy cuff (bottom).

Inner cannulas

Tracheostomy tubes with an inner cannula (sometimes called double-cannula or double-lumen tubes) consist of an outer tube or cannula which maintains airway patency, and an inner cannula, which can be removed for cleaning and/or disposed of and replaced (Figure 1.8).

Patient assessment red flags

The assessment of a tracheostomy patient is the same as for any other and begins with A, for airway. The following lists a number of red flag signs and symptoms that should alert you to a complication with the patient's tracheostomy:[16]

Airway flags

- Patients with cuffed tracheostomy tubes should not be able to speak. If they can, air is escaping from around the cuff, placing the patient at risk of aspiration. Grunting, snoring and stridor also indicate an airway problem
- Pain at the tracheostomy site
- Difficulty in passing a suction catheter into the trachea
- An altered or absent capnography trace.

Breathing flags

- Apnoea(!) detected by capnography or clinically
- Increasing ventilator support or oxygen requirements
- Respiratory distress, either reported by the patient or observed clinically due to the presence of:
  o Accessory muscle use

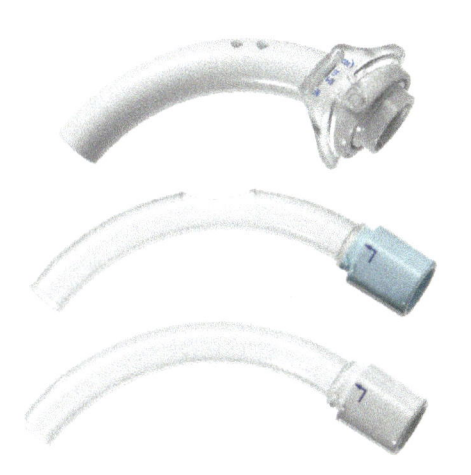

Figure 1.8 An uncuffed, fenestrated tracheostomy tube (top). Inner cannula with opening for fenestrations (middle). Inner cannula with no fenestrations (bottom).

Chapter 1 Airway and Breathing

- o Increased respiratory rate
- o Increased airway pressures
- o Decreased tidal volume
- Surgical emphysema (air in the subcutaneous tissues around the neck, but can expand to other areas)
- Patient complaint about being unable to breathe or having difficulty in breathing.

Specific tracheostomy flags

- Visibly displaced tracheostomy
- Blood or blood-stained secretions around the tube
- Increasing discomfort or pain
- Large volumes of air required to keep a cuff inflated.

General flags

- Alteration in any of the following:
  - o Heart rate
  - o Blood pressure
  - o Level of consciousness including anxiety, restlessness and confusion.

Management of the tracheostomy patient

Patients with tracheostomies have a potentially patent upper airway, since the upper airway and trachea are anatomically connected. However, it is quite possible that the reason the patient had a tracheotomy in the first place is that their upper airway is difficult or impossible to manage. Take the following steps to manage a tracheostomy emergency:[19,20]

Help and equipment

These are not patients to manage on your own. Get assistance from colleagues if possible. If a relative or carer is present, it is quite possible that they know more about tracheostomy management than you do, so listen to their advice and encourage them to help.

Patients may well have equipment to hand such as replacement tubes, but you can manage with the equipment from your vehicle:

- Airway adjuncts such as oro- and naso-pharyngeal airways
- Bag-valve-mask (BVM)
- Supraglottic airway devices
- Laryngoscope and endotracheal tubes
- Catheter mount
- Gum-elastic bougie
- Monitor capable of waveform capnography.

Airway and breathing

Check and open the upper airway as normal. Look, listen and feel for breathing at the face and tracheostomy site for no more than 10 seconds. Apply waveform capnography to the tracheostomy tube as soon as possible.[21]

If the patient is breathing, apply high-flow oxygen (preferably humidified) to both face and tracheostomy. This may require two cylinders, or the addition of a flowmeter into the Schrader valve of the oxygen cylinder. If the patient is not breathing, making agonal gasps or there are no signs of life, start chest compressions and follow the basic/advanced life support (BLS/ALS) algorithms while continuing to troubleshoot the tracheostomy, since this may be the cause of the cardiac arrest.

Tracheostomy patency

Start by checking for and removing the following:

- Decannulation caps (used when removing tracheostomies) block the end of the tracheostomy
- Obturators (inserted inside the tracheostomy when first inserting a tube into the patient, Figure 1.9)
- Speaking valves, which should not be used with an inflated cuffed tube (Figure 1.10)
- Blocked humidification devices such as Swedish noses.

Tracheostomies

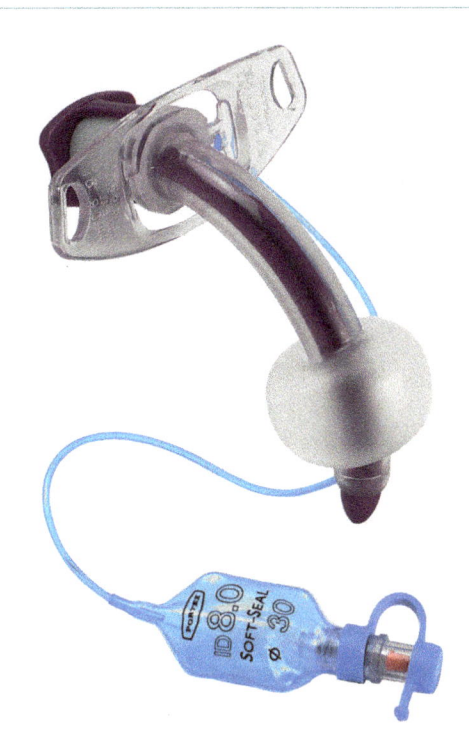

Figure 1.9 A tracheostomy tube with obturator in situ.

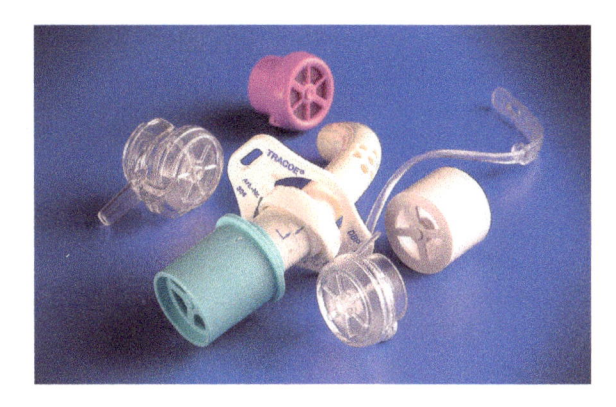

Figure 1.10 A selection of speaking valves. These should never be fitted to cuffed tubes.

If the tracheostomy tube is a double-cannula design, remove the inner cannula, but remember with some types of tubes the connector required for bag-mask ventilation is mounted on the inner cannula. Pass a suction catheter through the tube and into the trachea to check patency. It should pass easily through the tube. Don't use a gum-elastic bougie at this stage as it is more rigid than a suction catheter and might create a false passage in cases where the tube is misplaced. If the suction catheter passes through the tube, suction the tube and attempt to ventilate the patient. Take care not to insert it too far as this will produce severed coughing unless the patient has absent airway reflexes. If this fails and the tube has a cuff, deflate it and reassess the patient using the same look, listen and feel technique as before at both the face and the stoma site.

Next steps

If everything attempted thus far has failed to improve the patient's condition, remove the tube. Reassess the patient again and hopefully they will be breathing. If the patient is in cardiac arrest, continue with BLS/ALS. Attempt to oxygenate the patient via the oral route, but don't forget to cover the stoma site with swabs or a gloved hand. Use standard airway adjuncts to achieve effective ventilation. Alternatively, a paediatric face-mask (with a catheter mount attached to an adult self-inflating bag, if you find it difficult to access the neck) or laryngeal mask airway (LMA) can be placed over the stoma and the patient ventilated. If there is a large air leak from the mouth and/or nose, occlude them both during PPV.

Don't rush to escalate your airway management if you can achieve effective ventilation with basic methods. However, if you still cannot effectively ventilate the patient then you will need to attempt tracheal intubation. This may be possible via the oral route, although you should expect it to be difficult. Use an uncut tube as it will need to be inserted further than normal in order to bypass the stoma.

In patients with an established tracheostomy or who have a known upper airway problem that is going to make intubation difficult, it

Chapter 1 Airway and Breathing

can actually be more straightforward to simply insert another, smaller diameter tracheostomy or endotracheal tube into the stoma. Always use capnography as well as bilateral chest rise to confirm correct placement.[21,22]

Management of the laryngectomy patient

Unlike patients with a tracheostomy, laryngectomy patients do not have any connection between the upper airway and their lungs. Do not attempt to ventilate via the mouth/nose. Laryngectomy patients do not normally have tracheostomy tubes either, but may have a tracheo-oesophageal puncture (TEP) valve fitted to allow for speech. This may be visible inside the stoma, but should not be removed. They usually are fitted with a one-way valve to prevent aspiration.

Since patients have, in effect, no upper airway, it cannot be obstructed by an inappropriate head position and due to the reduction in anatomical dead space, chest compressions typically generate sufficient tidal volume to negate the need for PPV if this proves difficult to administer. Instead, just provide a supply of high-flow oxygen to the stoma site.

Tracheostomies are ten times more commonly performed than laryngectomies, so in the event that there is any uncertainty about whether the stoma is a laryngectomy or tracheostomy site, it is better to apply oxygen to both face and stoma. Take the following steps to manage a laryngectomy emergency:[19,20]

Help and equipment

As for tracheostomy.

Airway and breathing

Check and open the upper airway as normal. Look, listen and feel for breathing at the stoma site for no more than 10 seconds.

If the patient is breathing, apply high-flow oxygen to the stoma site. If the patient is not breathing, making agonal gasps or there are no signs of life, start chest compressions and follow the BLS/ALS algorithms while continuing to troubleshoot the laryngectomy stoma, since this may be the cause of the cardiac arrest.

Laryngectomy stoma patency

Most patients will not have a tube in place, but you should remove any string-vest bibs and stoma covers (sometimes called a 'button') if in place. If a tracheostomy tube is in place and is of a double-cannula design, remove the inner cannula, but remember with some types of tubes the connector required for bag-mask ventilation is mounted on the inner cannula.

Pass a suction catheter through the stoma and into the trachea to check patency. It should pass easily into the trachea. If it does, the stoma is patent, so suction the trachea and attempt to ventilate the patient if they are not breathing. If this fails and there is a cuffed tracheostomy tube in place, deflate it and reassess the patient, preferably with capnography.

Next steps

If everything attempted thus far has failed to improve the patient's condition, remove any tracheostomy tubes, if present. Reassess the patient again and hopefully they will be breathing. If the patient is in cardiac arrest continue with BLS/ALS.

Attempt to ventilate the patient using a paediatric face-mask or LMA placed over the stoma. Don't rush to escalate your airway management if you can achieve effective ventilation with basic methods. If this fails, attempt to intubate the stoma with either a smaller diameter tracheostomy or endotracheal tube. Always use capnography as well as bilateral chest rise to confirm correct placement.

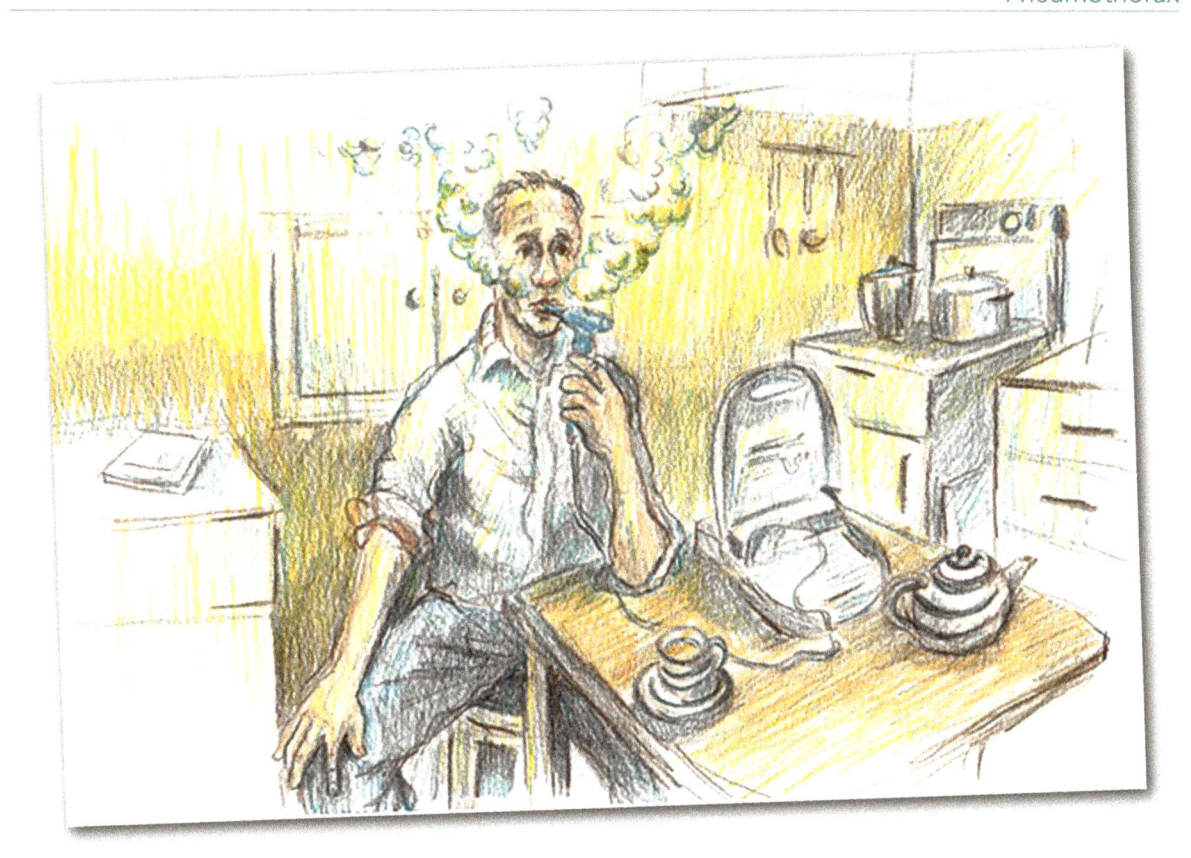

Pneumothorax

You are on standby watching the leaves and litter blow down the street. An involuntary shiver, caused by the thought of all those chronic medical illnesses being exacerbated by the cold weather, leads to your colleague asking if you want the heating turned up. However, your physical and mental well-being will have to wait as the MDT passes you details of a 59-year-old man with chronic obstructive pulmonary disease (COPD).

As you turn onto the patient's street, you see an rapid response vehicle (RRV) parked outside the patient's house, which is good as you won't have to take any equipment in with you. After knocking on the door and entering, you follow the sound of a nebuliser to the kitchen, where the RRV paramedic and patient are located. The patient is propping himself upright, with an elbow on the kitchen table so that he can hold a nebuliser with a mouthpiece, which makes a change from the masks that you usually use. To save having to limit nebulisation to 6 minutes, the RRV paramedic is using the patient's own compressor to drive the nebuliser, but seems to have missed the pulse oximetry reading, which is currently 84%.

Since the RRV paramedic has only just arrived on scene, he tells you that he has not found

Chapter 1 Airway and Breathing

out much, apart from the patient appears to be suffering from an exacerbation of COPD, with increasing shortness of breath for a couple of days and a productive cough with green sputum. You ask the RRV paramedic about low oxygen saturations and he shrugs and says, "The patient's hands are cold." On enquiring about findings on auscultation, he admits that he has not listened to the patient's chest. "You can hear him wheezing from here," he shrugs, again. This is quite true: the patient does have an impressive, and audible, wheeze even from across the room. The RRV paramedic explains that he is hoping that the combination of salbutamol and ipratropium he has poured into the nebuliser chamber will improve the patient's condition, so that he can refer the patient to their own GP. He suggests that you aren't required and can leave.

> What are you going to do: **Leave scene** (read on) or **Listen to the patient's chest** (skip the next paragraph)?

Leave scene

Marvellous. Not only have you avoided taking equipment into the patient's house, but you don't even have to tax your back with a lift. You say your goodbyes and wander back to the ambulance. However, as you sit down in the cab, you can't help feeling concerned about the treatment plan "I bet that paramedic didn't even listen to the patient's chest," your colleague mutters, "and those oxygen saturations. Cold hands, my @$!#." The situation is indeed worrying; your colleague never swears. You open the door of the ambulance, having decided to go back in and listen to the patient's chest and find out more about the history of this exacerbation.

Listen to the patient's chest

Under the guise of testing out your new stethoscope, you have a listen to the patient's chest. The right side of his chest sounds horrible, a blend of low-pitched wheezing and coarse crackles. The left side of his chest, however, has no wheeze, or crackles, or air entry. You recheck all over the left side of his chest and cannot find any air entry on that side. Given this alarming finding, you begin to doubt yourself. Surely, there must be air entry? Just to be sure, you percuss the chest and although the percussion note is hyper-resonant on the right (he is barrel-chested), it is even higher on the left. Just to be sure, you have a listen again. The RRV paramedic seems oblivious to your concern and is busy looking for the GP's number, but your colleague knows the look on your face when something is not right. "What's up?" she enquires. "He's got no air entry on the left side of his chest," you reply.

You quiz the patient about the history of his illness again. In broken sentences, he gives you the same story as the RRV paramedic. However, when you specifically ask about any sudden change, he does admit that this morning while standing outside smoking a cigarette, he suddenly became acutely short of breath. Your colleague leaves, without prompting, to fetch the chair and you attach the patient's nebuliser to oxygen.

As your colleague re-appears with the chair, the RRV paramedic twigs that you are not following his management plan. Unfortunately, he has just managed to get through to the GP surgery and so is a bit flustered with having to do two things at once. You help him out by mouthing "Pneumothorax," which, judging by the way his face flushes, makes him realise his mistake. He splutters "Sorry, wrong number," to the GP receptionist and mops up the patient's medication and his equipment as you coax the patient onto the carry chair. Once in the ambulance, you hook the patient to the monitor and review the results:

18

Airway

Patent

Breathing

Dyspnoeic
Respiratory rate: 24 breaths/min
Prolonged expiratory phase
SpO_2: 90% on oxygen-driven nebuliser
Barrel-chested, movement bilateral
No surgical emphysema
High percussion note, left higher than right
Absent air entry on left, widespread wheeze and crackles on right

Circulation

Heart rate: 120 beats/min
Blood pressure: 186/94 mmHg
Peripheries: cool

Disability

GCS score: 15/15
Blood sugar: 6.4 mmol/l

Exposure/Environment

Temperature: 38.3°C

Given that his oxygen saturations are reasonable for a patient with COPD, you elect to keep him on the oxygen-driven nebuliser and repeat the salbutamol. En route you make a pre-alert call, and as a result, one of the emergency department consultants is waiting with a menagerie of student doctors when you arrive. He fixes you with a stare, usually reserved for his students, and asks whether the patient has a pneumothorax or not. This does not really do much for your confidence, but you hold your ground and state that you think it is. He picks up his stethoscope and auscultates the patient's chest. "Here," he says handing you his stethoscope, "you have a listen." Your heart sinks as you wonder what you've missed. Sadly, despite your best efforts, you cannot hear a thing with his stethoscope and you've left yours in the ambulance. "I can't hear a thing with these," you admit. It does not matter; the consultant gives you something that looks a bit like a smile and says, "That's a pneumothorax," before sauntering off to organise an x-ray and chest drain, leaving you slightly bewildered.

Scale of the problem

Pneumothorax, or air in the pleural cavity, is generally classified as being spontaneous, if there is no obvious causal factor, and traumatic, if there is an external cause. These are further subdivided into:[23]

- Spontaneous
  - Primary – Occurring in people with no known underlying lung disease
  - Secondary – Occurring in people with a diagnosis of lung disease, most commonly COPD
  - Catamenial – A pneumothorax occurring in young women around the time of menstruation
- Traumatic
  - Iatrogenic – Caused by medical intervention, such as inserting a large-bore cannula in the patient's chest
  - Non-iatrogenic – Caused by blunt or penetrating chest injury.

Pneumothorax is the primary diagnosis in approximately 12,600 admissions per year in England with spontaneous pneumothorax being the most common, responsible for around 36% of cases (versus 26% due to trauma).[17]

Physiology

In order for air to enter and exit the lungs, there must be a driving pressure gradient, since air flows from areas of high pressure to low pressure. Since it is not normally possible to alter atmospheric pressure, the pressure

Chapter 1 Airway and Breathing

in the alveoli needs to change to facilitate the movement of gases. This is achieved by applying the principle of Boyle's Law, which states that the volume of a gas is inversely proportional to its pressure.[24] Thus, if lung volume increases, alveolar pressure will decrease and vice-versa.

The lungs are surrounded by a pleural membrane (Figure 1.11). The outer layer (parietal pleura) lines the chest wall, and the inner layer (visceral pleura) covers the lungs. Between them is the pleural space, which is lubricated to ensure that the surfaces glide smoothly over one another as well as creating a surface tension that results in the surfaces 'sticking together'.

During normal quiet breathing, the intra-pleural pressure is always lower than atmospheric. Just prior to inspiration, there is no air flow since alveolar and atmospheric pressure are the same, due to the elastic recoil of the lungs (trying to collapse) and the chest (trying to expand) being equally matched. This results in a sub-atmospheric pressure within the intra-pleural space.

As the diaphragm and external intercostal muscles contract, the volume of the thoracic

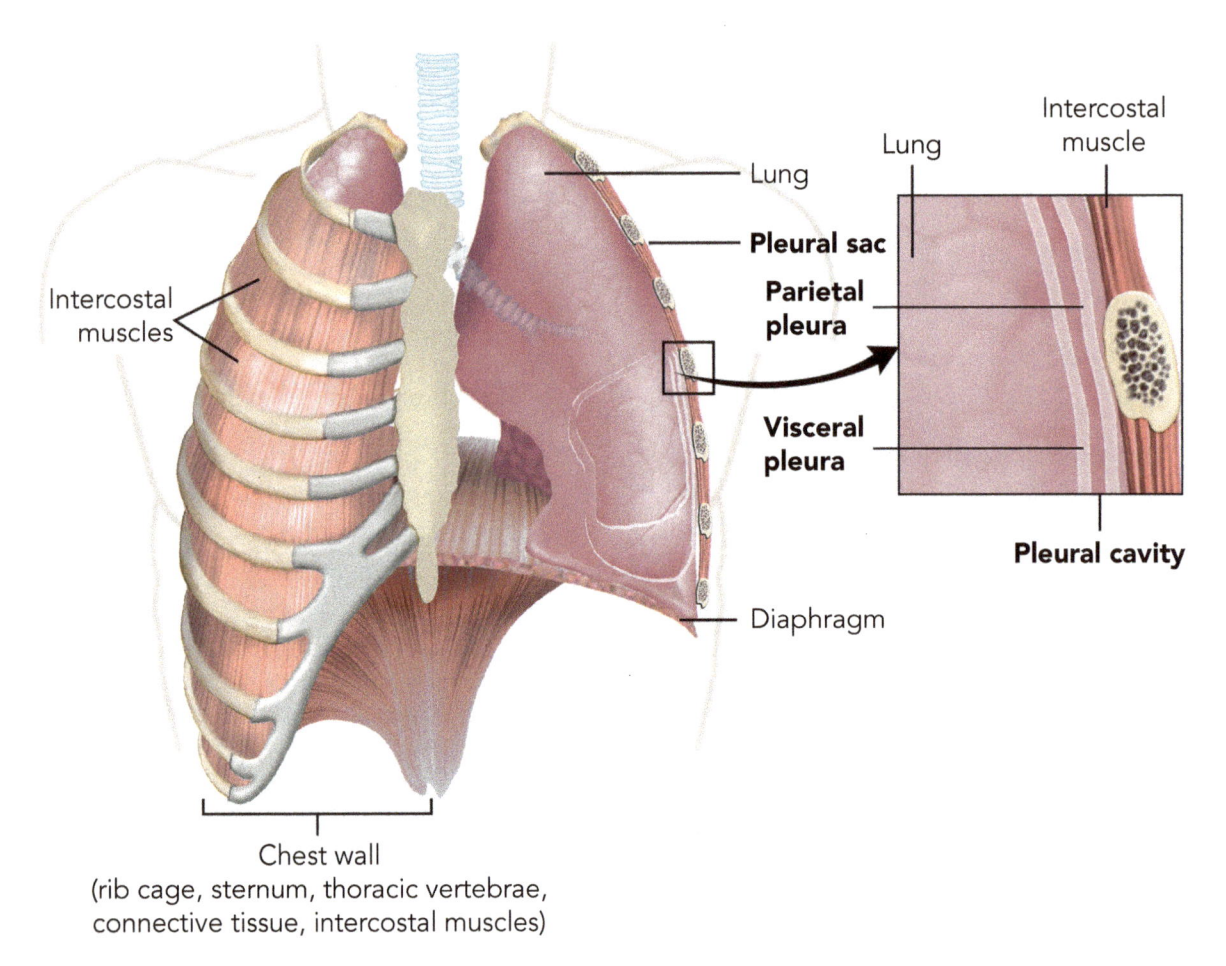

Figure 1.11 The lungs and pleura.
Source: OpenStax College [CC-BY-3.0 (http://creativecommons.org/licenses/by/3.0)], via Wikimedia Commons.

cavity increases. Since the visceral and parietal layers are effectively adhered to each other by surface tension, the lungs expand, increasing in volume. As lung volume increases, the alveolar pressure falls below atmospheric pressure and air moves into the alveoli. This continues while the pressure gradient exists, until an equilibrium of pressures is reached.

In a similar, but opposite, way, exhalation occurs as the elastic recoil of the chest wall causes thoracic volume to reduce, decreasing lung volume at the same time, which in turn increases alveolar pressure above that of atmospheric air, and alveolar gases leave the lungs.

Pathophysiology

In the event that air within the alveoli can escape into the pleural space, or there is an external breach of the thoracic cavity allowing atmospheric air to enter the pleural space, the normal physiology of ventilation is disrupted.

Spontaneous pneumothorax

Since alveolar pressure is greater than pleural pressure, air flows into the pleural space, leading to a progressive lung collapse as a result of its own elastic recoil. Air continues to move into the pleural space until either the pressure equalises, or the lung collapse seals the location of the leak.[25] The exact causes of the air leaks that occur in spontaneous pneumothoraces are not fully understood, but many patients with a primary spontaneous pneumothorax (PSP) have small blisters on the lung surface called blebs and bullae (sometimes referred to as 'emphysema-like changes', with the difference between the two being that blebs are smaller) which can rupture.[23] However, an alternative hypothesis is that cellular changes within the visceral pleura lead to cells being replaced by porous inflammatory cells, leading to the escape of air.[26]

Patients with PSP are more commonly male and taller, which is thought to be related to the fact that the difference in pleural pressure at the apices of the lungs compared to the base is greater in taller people. This may contribute to the development of blebs at the apices, which is the most common location for bleb rupture.[27] Precipitating factors include changes in atmospheric pressure and loud music, but not, surprisingly, exercise.[23]

Secondary spontaneous pneumothoraces (SSP) are usually more serious, since the patient already has underlying lung disease. The most common are conditions that lead to air trapping and destruction of lung tissue such as: COPD, cystic fibrosis, tuberculosis, lung cancer and human immunodeficiency virus-associated pneumonia.[27]

Catamenial pneumothoraces affect women and occur within 72 hours prior to, or after, the onset of menstruation. Although the cause is not fully understood, these women typically have small defects (known as fenestrations), endometrial deposits on their diaphragm and visceral pleura, which may erode the pleura and lead to leakage of air from the abdomen and genital tract.[25]

Traumatic pneumothorax

Iatrogenic pneumothoraces, that is, those caused by medical treatment and/or examination, are even more common than spontaneous pneumothoraces. They are commonly caused by transthoracic needle aspiration, subclavian vessel puncture and thoracentesis.[25]

Non-iatrogenic pneumothoraces are caused by penetrating trauma, such as stab and gunshot wounds or impalements, blunt trauma that leads to rib fractures and increased intrathoracic pressure, and bronchial rupture and barotrauma, where changes in pressure of the air delivered to the lungs leads to expansion. This phenomenon has been reported in air crew and SCUBA divers.[28]

Chapter 1 Airway and Breathing

In an open pneumothorax, air enters the pleural space thanks to a communication between atmospheric air and the pleural space, for example as a result of penetrating trauma. As the chest expands during inspiration, air enters the pleural space. If the wound is large enough, there may be free movement of air into and out of the affected lung during respiration. If the wound is similar in size to the glottic opening to the lower airway, then atmospheric air preferentially enters via the wound, leading to ineffective ventilation of the alveoli. The sound heard as air moves into and out of the wound has led to these types of injury being referred to as 'sucking chest wounds'.

Tension pneumothorax is an uncommon, but life-threatening, condition which can prove rapidly fatal to patients, particularly those who are being ventilated with positive pressure. It most often occurs in:[25]

- Ventilated patients in intensive care
- Trauma
- Cardiac arrest
- Acute exacerbations of asthma and COPD
- Blocked or clamped chest drains
- Non-invasive ventilation.

As with other types of pneumothorax, air enters the pleural space on inspiration, but cannot escape during expiration due to the presence of a one-way valve formed by a pleural defect. This leads to increasing intra-pleural pressure on the affected side of the chest, worsening the lung collapse and causing diaphragmatic depression. In severe cases, and dependent on mediastinal distensibility, this can compress the contralateral lung (Figure 1.12).

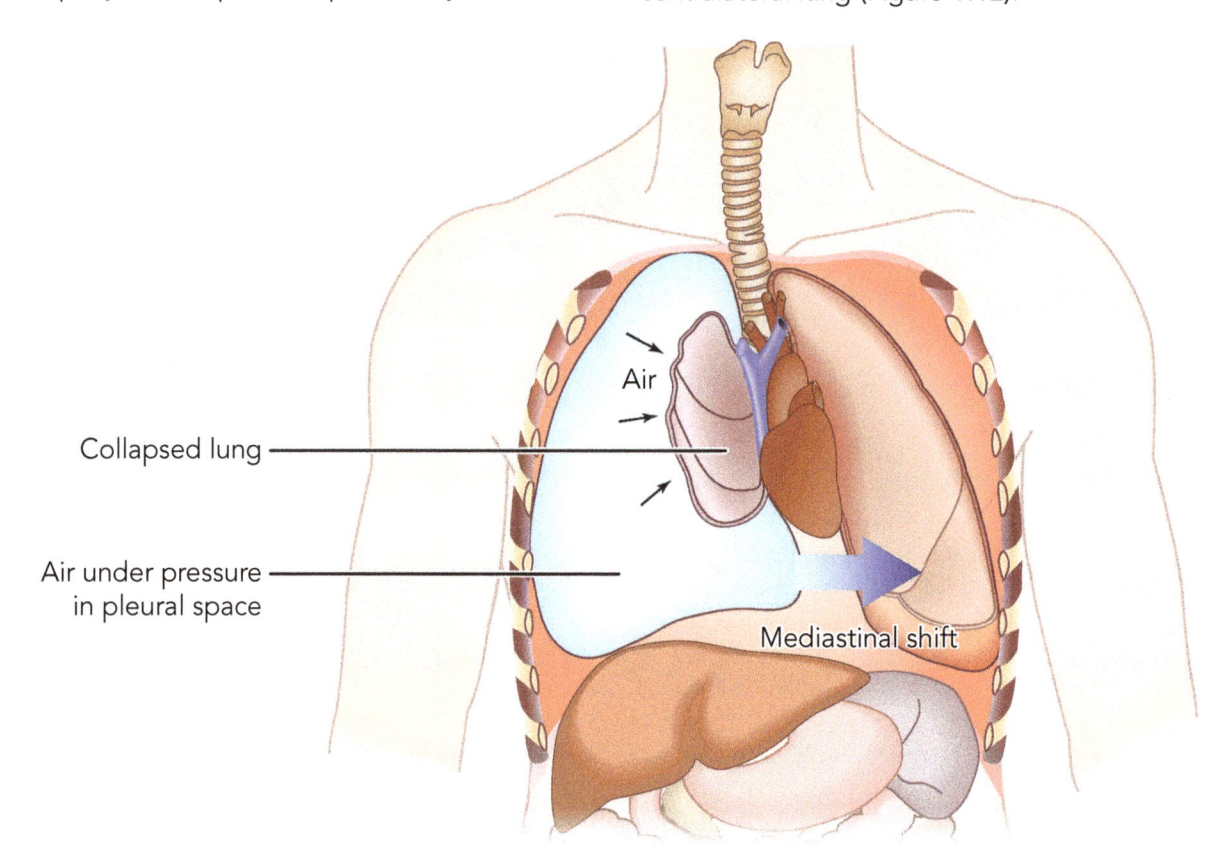

Figure 1.12 A tension pneumothorax including mediastinal shift.

Precisely when an expanding pneumothorax is considered to be under tension is debated, but for clinical purposes it has been suggested that this occurs when the pneumothorax results in significant respiratory or haemodynamic compromise that reverses on decompression alone.[29]

It's worth noting that tension pneumothoraces typically develop far more slowly in spontaneously breathing awake patients, compared to ventilated and sedated patients, who can experience hypotension and a rapid decline in oxygen saturations in just a few minutes, hastened by the administration of PPV.[30]

Assessment

Prior to commencing your assessment, you should start with a suspicion, particularly in patients who have a higher risk of pneumothorax:[31]

- Smoker
- Family history of pneumothorax
- Tall, slender build
- Young males (<40 years)
- Chronic respiratory disease such as COPD/asthma/cystic fibrosis.

Chest pain and dyspnoea are fairly universal findings, with the degree of distress in patients with SSP often completely disproportionate to the actual size of their pneumothorax.[25] If the pneumothorax is large enough, it may be possible to detect reduced chest wall movements, hyper-resonance on percussion and decreased or absent tactile fremitus.[32]

In patients who have a left-sided pneumothorax, have a listen for Hamman's crunch, a distinctive crunching, rasping noise, synchronous with the patient's heartbeat, which is best auscultated over the cardiac apex, although sometimes is loud enough to be heard without a stethoscope.[33]

Most commonly, patients will receive an x-ray to identify the pneumothorax. This typically is a standing erect x-ray taken on inspiration. A pneumothorax is defined as 'large' if the inter-pleural diameter at the level of the hilum is greater than 2 cm. However, if accuracy is important, then a CT-scan is considered to be gold standard. Ultrasound can also be used to diagnose a pneumothorax and has been shown to be more sensitive than x-rays at detecting the presence of a pneumothorax.[34]

Tension pneumothorax

Arguably, the most important type of pneumothorax to recognise is one under tension. However, the clinical course of a tension pneumothorax is not the same for all patients, with the progression of clinical deterioration for an awake, spontaneously breathing patient likely to be considerably longer than those who are being ventilated with PPV.

Signs and symptoms of a tension pneumothorax in awake patients include:[29]

- Reliable and early
  - Pleuritic chest pain
  - Air hunger
  - Respiratory distress
  - Tachypnoea
  - Tachycardia
  - Falling SpO_2
  - Agitation
- Ipsilateral signs
  - Hyper-expansion
  - Hypo-mobility
  - Hyper-resonance
  - Decreased breath sounds
  - Added sounds
- Contralateral signs
  - Hyper-mobility
- Pre-terminal
  - Decreasing respiratory rate
  - Hypotension
  - Decreasing SpO_2
  - Decreasing level of consciousness

- Unreliable signs
  - Tracheal deviation
  - Distended neck veins.

Do not rely on tracheal deviation or distended neck veins as these can be difficult to determine. In one study where tracheal displacement was confirmed by x-ray, there was still only a 50:50 chance of the clinician detecting its presence.[35]

In ventilated patients, the clinical deterioration is likely to be far more alarming. In addition, ventilated patients are more likely to suffer a cardiac arrest, whereas awake patients tend to suffer from respiratory arrest initially. Signs and symptoms of a tension pneumothorax in ventilated patients include:[29]

- Rapid disease progression
- Early reliable signs
  - Immediate decrease in SpO_2
  - Decrease in BP
  - Tachycardia
  - Increased end-tidal carbon dioxide with decreasing amplitude of waveform
- Other signs
  - Increased ventilation pressure
  - Surgical emphysema
- Ipsilateral signs
  - Hyper-resonance
  - Decreased breath sounds
  - Chest hyper-expansion
  - Chest hypo-mobility
  - Added sounds
- Unreliable signs
  - Cyanosis
  - Distended neck veins
  - Tracheal deviation.

Management

Patients with a simple pneumothorax with no signs of cardiovascular compromise, suggesting tension, can be managed conservatively out-of-hospital, but should be closely monitored en route to hospital and preferably positioned upright, or with the healthy lung down.[36] Patients with pneumothorax secondary to a traumatic injury should receive oxygen at the appropriate target range (usually 94–98%, except for patients at risk of carbon dioxide retention, who should be managed at 88–92% or their usual range). If there is an open pneumothorax, then the wound should be covered with a commercial chest seal; the use of three-sided occlusive dressing are no longer recommended.[36] However, these can block, so closely monitor the patient and remove the dressing if the patient shows signs of tension pneumothorax.

Patients with signs of a tension pneumothorax require prompt decompression by needle thoracentesis. An instant egress of air throughout most of the respiratory cycle following cannula insertion into the pleural space is considered diagnostic. For the first attempt, the second intercostal space (ICS), mid-clavicular line should be selected. If this fails, a second attempt should be undertaken, taking a lateral approach (5th ICS, just anterior to the mid-axillary line).

Wherever you elect to insert the needle, remember that they can kink, become displaced, become blocked with skin/blood and are at best a temporary measure. Increasingly, more effective techniques, such as finger thoracostomy, are being performed by appropriately skilled clinicians, including paramedics, out-of-hospital.[37]

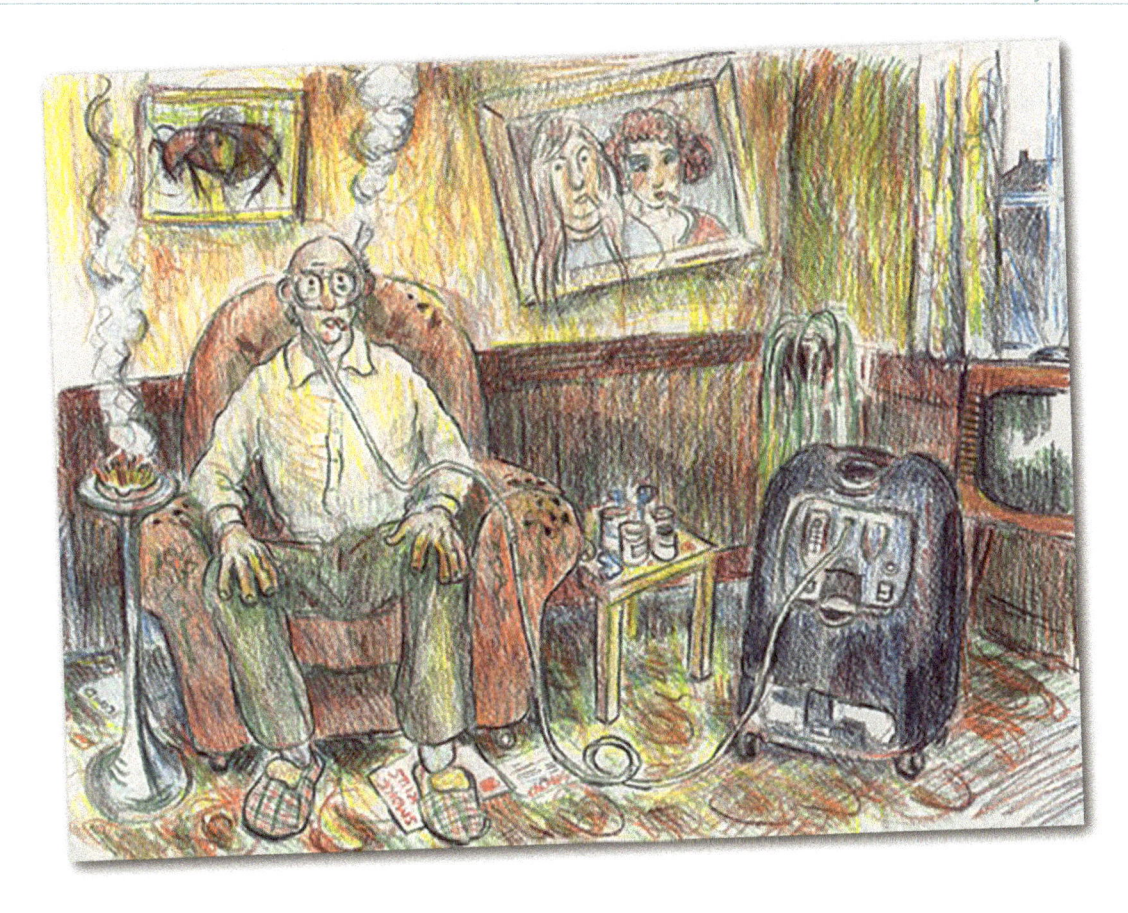

Chronic Obstructive Pulmonary Disease
With Katie Duncan

You are sat on standby enjoying a brief respite from the increased workload caused by winter pressures. It doesn't last long as you are allocated a category 2 call for a 66-year-old man with difficulty breathing. You arrive on scene within 18 minutes; success!

You wrestle your kit out of the vehicle and trudge up three flights of stairs before walking to the end of the landing; a sure sign that the patient is very sick. The haze of cigarette smoke that greets your entrance into the hallway provides a clue as to the cause of the patient's condition. Your colleague mutters something about passive smoking as you both enter the living room.

The patient looks exhausted, but he has managed to find the strength to roll himself a cigarette. It is dangling precariously from the side of his mouth, despite the nasal cannula that is in situ. Fortunately, you can see plenty of burn holes in the metres

Chapter 1   Airway and Breathing

of oxygen tubing that snakes around the living room floor.

The patient wheezily tells you that he's called Eric and that he has chronic obstructive pulmonary disease (COPD) and for the past couple of weeks, a chest infection. His own GP has started him on a course of antibiotics and steroids, but overnight his symptoms have become much worse. His storytelling is interrupted by a wracking cough, which results in him expectorating a large string of green sputum. He captures it in his hanky and offers it to you for closer inspection. While your phlegm-phobic colleague is trying not to gip, you thank him but state that you have seen enough.

The pulse oximeter your colleague attached prior to the coughing fit shows a drop in oxygen saturation (SpO_2) from 86% to 78%. Eric needs treatment and your colleague looks expectantly at you.

> What should you do: **Obtain a peak flow** (read on) or **Give the patient a nebuliser** (skip the next paragraph)?

Obtain a peak flow

You wave off the mask and produce the peak flow meter, as you are certain that it is required to assess the severity of the Eric's breathlessness. He has no idea what his normal peak flow is and despite your coaching fails miserably to produce one for you. On his first attempt he manages to stop the pointer moving with his finger. The second attempt causes another coughing fit and you don't think you ought to put him through the third. Your colleague has filled the nebuliser with 5 mg of salbutamol and connected it to the oxygen supply. You try to explain to her that you need a pre-treatment peak flow reading. "That's for mild and moderate asthma," your colleague retorts and places the mask on the patient.[38]

Give the patient a nebuliser

Eric is in no state to blow into the peak flow meter and you correctly recall that pre-treatment peak flow measurements form part of the assessment for mild and moderate asthma, not COPD. Instead, you use the time it takes for your colleague to prepare the 5 mg salbutamol nebuliser to examine him.

He is sat forward on the chair in a tripod position to better serve his accessory muscles, but his barrel-shaped chest is not helping. You also notice bulging jugular veins as well as clubbed and nicotine-stained fingers. On auscultation you hear a widespread, low-pitched wheeze.

The noise of the oxygen concentrator is drowned out by the sheesh and gurgling sounds coming from the nebuliser. His saturations soon rally and his work of breathing reduces slightly. After six minutes, in accordance with the British Thoracic Society oxygen guidelines,[39] you switch off the nebuliser and reassess the patient's observations:

Airway

Patent

Breathing

Respiratory rate: 32 breaths/min with a long expiratory phase
SpO_2: 90% initially, after several minutes, the SpO_2 drops to 87%.

Circulation

Bounding and irregular radial pulse at a rate of 100 beats per minute
Blood pressure: 150/89 mmHg

Chronic Obstructive Pulmonary Disease

Disability
GCS score: 15/15
Blood sugar: 8.4 mmol/l

Exposure/Environment
Temperature: 37.2°C

> Eric requires oxygen therapy, but at what concentration: **100%** (read on) or **28%** (skip the next paragraph)?

100%

You go for the non-rebreathing mask and up the flow rate to 15 l/min, after all you can't have too much oxygen, right? As you approach Eric to apply the mask, he produces a card and says his breathing doctor gave it to him:

OXYGEN ALERT CARD

Name: *Eric Smith*

I am at risk of type II respiratory failure with a raised CO_2 level. Please use my *28* % Venturi mask to achieve an oxygen saturation of *88* % to *92* % during exacerbations

---

Your colleague hands you a 28% Venturi mask and sets the flow rate to 6 l/min, 50% more than the manufacturer recommends.

28%

You correctly identify the risk of hypercapnic (type II) respiratory failure and start with a low concentration of oxygen, which keeps the oxygen saturation around 90%.

Since Eric's respiratory rate is above 30 breaths per minute, you up the flow rate to 6 l/min, as the patient's minute volume is likely to be higher than the minimum flow rate delivered by the mask at 4 l/min. You repeat the 5 mg of salbutamol and follow this with a nebuliser containing 500 mcg ipratropium bromide, but the post-treatment saturations still drop.

On arrival at hospital, you are directed to one of the resuscitation bays. Another patient with COPD is being attended to by a consultant who spots your uniform, strides over and thrusts a small piece of paper at you. "Look at that, just look at that!" he rasps while gesticulating at what turns out to be a blood gas result. You take a closer look and note the following (normal ranges are in brackets):

pH:	7.3	(7.35–7.45)
PaO_2:	16.0 kPa	(10.0–13.0 kPa)
$PaCO_2$:	8 kPa	(4.7–6.0 kPa)
HCO_3^-:	30 mmol/l	(22–26 mmol/l)

> What does the blood gas show: **Metabolic alkalosis** (read on) or **Respiratory acidosis** (skip the next paragraph)?

Metabolic alkalosis

The words have no sooner left your lips when the consultant launches into a tirade about how ambulance staff know nothing about the physiology of the respiratory system, and you in turn mumble about how you are just an 'ambulance driver' and slink off to book the patient in.

Respiratory acidosis

"That's a severe respiratory acidosis," you tell him brightly, "and with a PaO_2 that high, you'll have to be careful not to remove the oxygen too quickly otherwise he might suffer

Chapter 1 Airway and Breathing

a rebound hypoxaemia." The doctor seems satisfied and returns to his patient.

You return to the ambulance to find that it has already been tidied and a cup of your favourite hot beverage is waiting for you. Since you have been at hospital for only 10 minutes and there are no operations managers to be seen, your colleague asks about COPD and oxygen titration.

Scale of the problem

COPD is characterised by airflow obstruction. The airflow obstruction is usually progressive, not fully reversible and does not change markedly over several months. In the United Kingdom there are over 1.2 million people diagnosed with COPD, but many more are thought to suffer from the condition without knowing.[40,41]

COPD kills approximately 30,000 people a year in the UK, making it the fifth biggest killer. The cost to the NHS is around £800 million a year and COPD is the second leading cause of emergency admission to hospital in the UK.[42]

Risk factors for COPD include cigarette smoking primarily, and second-hand smoke, occupational exposure to dust and chemicals, air pollution and alpha-1 antitrypsin deficiency.[43]

Gases (no, not that sort of gas)

The pressure of a specific gas in a mixture of gases (for example, oxygen in the air) is known as the partial pressure of that gas. Since the partial pressure of oxygen is higher in the alveoli than the capillaries, oxygen moves across into the capillaries. Conversely, carbon dioxide has a higher partial pressure in the capillaries than the alveoli and so moves out of the capillaries and into the alveoli, where it can be expired.

The rate of pulmonary and systemic gas exchange depends on a number of factors such as:

- Partial pressure – gases in air act as if no other gases are present. This is known as Dalton's Law. The greater the difference in partial pressure of the gas in the alveoli and capillaries, the more rapidly it will diffuse across from one compartment to the other.
- Diffusion distance – the further the gas has to travel, the slower gas exchange occurs.
- Solubility – carbon dioxide diffuses much more rapidly than oxygen (about 20 times faster) despite having a lower partial pressure gradient. This is because it is much more soluble than oxygen.
- Surface area – gas exchange is reduced if the surface area decreases.

Oxygen physiology

Oxygen is vital for cell metabolism, but tissues in the body have no mechanism for storing it. Instead, cells rely on a constant supply that can vary depending on cell metabolism.

The arterial oxygen tension (also known as the partial pressure of oxygen, PaO_2) is a measure of the oxygen dissolved in blood plasma. It is not very soluble and as a result, only 1.5% of oxygen is transported in this way.

Most oxygen is carried in the blood (about 98.5%) bound to haemoglobin inside the red blood cells. This makes global oxygen delivery dependent on cardiac output and the oxygen content of the blood. The oxygen content of blood, is in turn, dependent on arterial oxygen saturation (oxygen bound to haemoglobin, SaO_2) and the amount of haemoglobin in the blood.[44]

Normal daily activities consume around 25% of the oxygen delivered to the cells. The remainder is returned to the lungs as a mixed venous saturation and is usually

65% saturated with oxygen. As oxygen consumption increases or supply decreases, the amount of oxygen extracted by the tissue cells increases to maintain aerobic metabolism. This can continue until around 60–70% of oxygen is extracted. If consumption continues to increase or supply decreases, tissue hypoxia will occur.

Oxygen transport

Only dissolved oxygen can diffuse into cells, so the process of binding and dissociating oxygen from haemoglobin is carefully managed, thanks to the design of haemoglobin, which can accept up to four oxygen molecules.

There are a number of factors which control this process, the most critical of which is the partial pressure of arterial oxygen. This relationship between the saturation of haemoglobin (SaO_2) and the partial pressure of arterial oxygen (PaO_2) is shown in the oxyhaemoglobin dissociation curve (blue line on Figure 1.13).

At very low PaO_2, haemoglobin binds few oxygen molecules because the haemoglobin subunits are held together tightly. However, once a single oxygen molecule binds to haemoglobin, it becomes progressively easier for subsequent oxygen molecules to come aboard as the haemoglobin changes shape. This explains why the curve is so steep between a PaO_2 of approximately 2 kPa and 5 kPa.

At the typical PaO_2 found in a healthy lung (13 kPa), the total SaO_2 is around 97%.

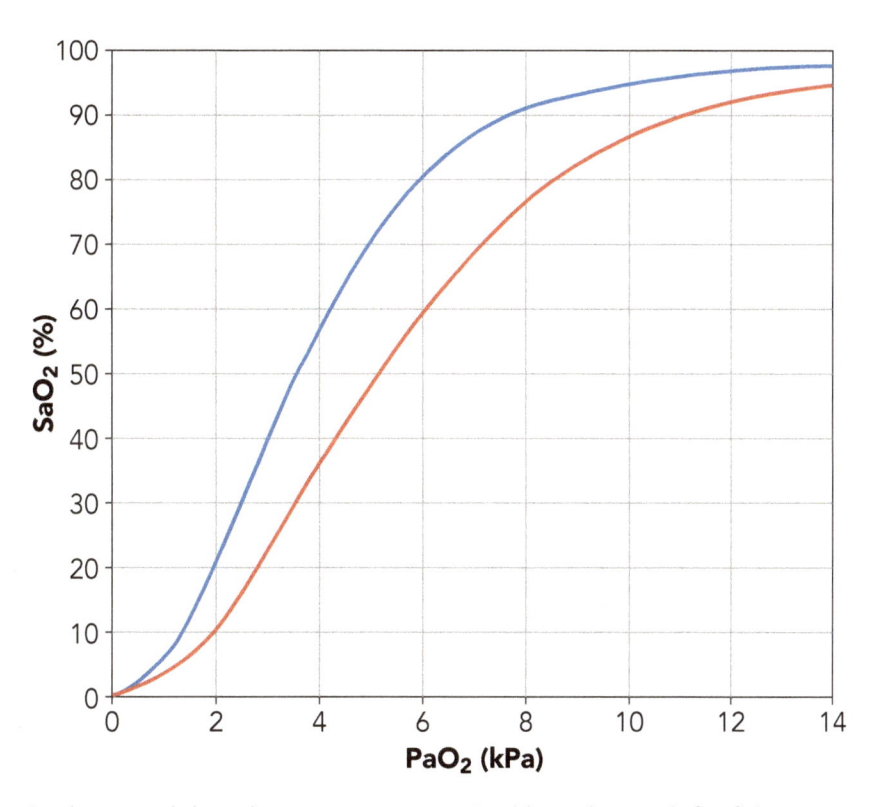

Figure 1.13 Oxyhaemoglobin dissociation curve. Red line shows shift of the curve to the right due to decrease in haemoglobin's affinity for oxygen.

Chapter 1   Airway and Breathing

Other factors affecting haemoglobin's affinity for oxygen include: acidity, the partial pressure of carbon dioxide ($PaCO_2$), temperature and diphosphoglycerate (2,3 DPG, which is usually elevated in COPD patients).

An increase in any of these decreases haemoglobin's affinity for oxygen, resulting in a shift of the oxyhaemoglobin curve to the right (the red line in Figure 1.13), known as the Bohr effect. Thus for any given PaO_2, the saturation of haemoglobin will be lower. In the tissues there is a lower partial pressure of oxygen with increased acidity and high levels of carbon dioxide. With the oxygen only loosely held by the haemoglobin due to the Bohr effect, it is released into the tissues.

Carbon dioxide, hydrogen ion and oxygen transport

Like oxygen, carbon dioxide moves down its concentration gradient. The highest partial pressure is found in the tissues, where it is produced, and the lowest in the lungs, where it is expired. Carbon dioxide is more soluble than oxygen, with 9% dissolved in the blood plasma, 27% combines with haemoglobin to form carbaminohaemoglobin and 64% reacting with water (H_2O) to form bicarbonate (HCO_{3-}) and H^+ (hydrogen ion).

Tissues

Since the partial pressure of carbon dioxide is high in the tissues, it moves into the red blood cells and reacts with water to form carbonic acid (H_2CO_3). Carbonic acid dissociates into H^+ and HCO_{3-} (Figure 1.14). This could present a problem for the cell since the presence of H^+ slows down the conversion of CO_2 and H_2O into H_2CO_3. However, there a number of buffers that 'soak up' the H^+, the most important of which is haemoglobin.

The presence of H^+ encourages haemoglobin to shed oxygen and instead take up H^+. In addition, as the amount of haemoglobin carrying oxygen decreases, the carbon dioxide carrying capacity of the blood increases, a process known as the Haldane effect. This occurs because carbon dioxide binds with haemoglobin to form carbaminohaemoglobin and haemoglobin also buffers H^+ to keep the reaction in Figure 1.14 moving to the right.

$$CO_2 + H_2O \rightarrow H_2CO_3 \rightarrow H^+ + HCO_{3-}$$

Figure 1.14   Reaction at the tissues.

Alveoli

At the lungs, the partial pressures of oxygen and carbon dioxide are high and low, respectively. This causes the reaction to move to the left. The high PaO_2 results in H^+ dissociating from haemoglobin, allowing oxygen to bind to haemoglobin instead. H^+ in turn combines with HCO_{3-} to form H_2CO_3 and then H_2O and CO_2, which can be expired (Figure 1.15).

$$CO_2 + H_2O \leftarrow H_2CO_3 \leftarrow H^+ + HCO_{3-}$$

Figure 1.15   Reaction at the alveoli.

Blood gases

The components of the whole process (PaO_2, $PaCO_2$, H^+, HCO_{3-}) can be measured in the emergency department with an arterial blood gas (ABG). H^+ concentration is usually expressed as an inverse logarithm, pH. This means that as H^+ concentration increases (that is, the solution becomes more acidic), the pH goes DOWN. Conversely, when H^+ concentration decreases, the pH goes UP (more alkalotic).

Normal values for blood gases are shown below:[45]

pH: 7.35–7.45
PaO$_2$: 10.0–13.0 kPa
PaCO$_2$: 4.7–6.0 kPa
HCO$_3$-: 22–26 mmol/l

An acute respiratory acidosis would result in a reduced pH, increased PaCO$_2$ and a normal HCO$_3$-. In acute exacerbations of COPD, it is common to see a compensated respiratory acidosis. Because COPD patients often have chronically elevated levels of PaCO$_2$, the kidneys can produce HCO$_3$- and so maintain a normal pH. A patient with COPD who is between exacerbations, would be expected to have a normal pH, elevated PaCO$_2$ and elevated HCO$_3$-.

An 'acute on chronic' exacerbation of COPD would result in a reduced pH, elevated PaCO$_2$ (probably even higher than normal for the patient) and an elevated HCO$_3$-. Take a look at the ABG results for your next patient with COPD and see if you can work out what is going on.

Pathophysiology of COPD and excessive O$_2$ administration

There is evidence from a single well-conducted randomised controlled trial that pre-hospital titration of oxygen administration to patients with COPD significantly reduces mortality.[46,47] The most significant effect of hyperoxia (excessive oxygen) on the respiratory system is hypercapnic respiratory failure in vulnerable populations (such as patients with severe COPD). This can occur even with a PaO$_2$ within normal or near-normal values. It is thought that there are a number of mechanisms that are responsible:[39]

V/Q mismatch

The pulmonary vasculature maximises PaO$_2$ by ensuring well-ventilated areas of the lung receive the most blood flow. This ventilation (V) to perfusion (Q) matching is mostly achieved by a process called hypoxic pulmonary vasoconstriction (HPV).

Unlike most vessels, pulmonary arterioles actually constrict in response to low alveolar partial pressures of oxygen (PAO$_2$ – note the big A denoting alveoli, as opposed to small a, which denotes arterial). Most vascular beds would dilate in this scenario to maximise blood flow to the area. However, the HPV cannot prevent perfusion to all poorly ventilated areas and some deoxygenated blood will still exit poorly ventilated areas and be mixed with oxygenated blood.

If inspired oxygen is increased, the pulmonary arterioles will dilate, increasing blood flow to poorly ventilated areas. Although the alveolar partial pressure of oxygen will increase, the partial pressure of carbon dioxide in the alveoli remains high, reducing the concentration gradient of carbon dioxide and thus increasing the partial pressure of arterial carbon dioxide. This increase in the partial pressure of carbon dioxide leads to a decrease in pH (that is, the blood becomes *more* acidic).

In a healthy person this would not present a problem as the rate and depth of ventilation could increase. However, this may not be possible in a patient with COPD already operating at the limit of their respiratory function and results in increased carbon dioxide retention.

Ventilatory drive

Hypoxaemia leads to increased ventilation and so it seems reasonable to assume that hyperoxaemia caused by administering high-flow O$_2$ could lead to a decrease in ventilation. This is the basis for hypoxic drive theory.

In fact, if the PaO$_2$ is greater than 8 kPa there is no significant reduction in ventilation

Chapter 1 Airway and Breathing

caused by this mechanism and above 13 kPa, there is no further reduction at all. This mechanism is therefore only important in explaining increases in $PaCO_2$ when PaO_2 increases up to 13 kPa, but not beyond. It is therefore not possible to stop your patient breathing by giving them high-flow oxygen by this mechanism alone.

Haldane effect

Increasing levels of oxygen bound to haemoglobin by upping the inspired oxygen concentration, results in a reduction in haemoglobin available to buffer hydrogen ions and carbon dioxide. This results in increased $PaCO_2$ and a further reduction in pH.

Absorption atelectasis

This is thought to occur due to absorption of oxygen from alveoli with high partial pressures of oxygen beyond obstructed airways and occurs even with inspired oxygen concentrations of 30–50%. As oxygen diffuses out of the alveoli, it is thought that the alveoli collapse.

Hypercapnia in exacerbations of COPD is not universal. Some patients have repeated hypercapnic respiratory failure, whereas others may not. Even in COPD patients with chronic respiratory failure, not all will develop high partial pressures of carbon dioxide and acidosis during acute exacerbations.

Recognition

No doubt you can recall a list of signs and symptoms that are suggestive of COPD, but it is not always clear that the patient in front of you with difficulty breathing has the disease. In the absence of a clear diagnosis of COPD, the British Thoracic Society suggests: If the diagnosis is unknown, patients who are over 50 years of age, who are long-term smokers with a history of chronic breathlessness on minor exertion, such as walking on level ground, and no other known cause of breathlessness should be treated as if having COPD. Patients with COPD may also use terms such as chronic bronchitis and emphysema to describe their condition but may sometimes mistakenly use 'asthma'.[39]

Management

Treating the symptoms of COPD is clearly described in the *JRCALC Clinical Guidelines*.[38] Note that if a patient has an oxygen alert card, the oxygen saturation range will normally be 88–92%, but you may also see 85–88% and 85–90%, based on previous blood gas results.

In-hospital management for exacerbations of COPD that leads to persistent hypercapnic ventilatory failure despite optimal medical therapy is non-invasive ventilation (NIV).[40] There are encouraging results from a number of studies (although none from the UK) that suggest pre-hospital NIV might reduce intubation risk and mortality rates,[48] but a large UK randomised controlled trial is unlikely anytime soon to prove this is the case.[49] However, if you have local critical care/enhanced care teams who can provide NIV, then consideration should be given to contacting them early in cases of acute respiratory failure.

Remember! If you 'overcook' a COPD patient with high-flow oxygen, do not suddenly cease administration as it can lead to a rebound hypoxaemia in patients with hypercapnic respiratory failure. The sudden drop in the alveolar partial pressure of oxygen can cause the partial pressure of arterial oxygen to drop below the pre-treatment level.[39]

References

1. Benger JR, Kirby K, Black S, Brett SJ, Clout M, Lazaroo MJ, et al. Effect of a strategy of a supraglottic airway device vs tracheal intubation during out-of-hospital cardiac arrest on functional outcome: the AIRWAYS-2 randomized clinical trial. *The Journal of the American Medical Association*, 2018 Aug 28;320(8):779–791.
2. Prekker ME, Kwok H, Shin J, Carlbom D, Grabinsky A, Rea TD. The process of prehospital airway management: challenges and solutions during paramedic endotracheal intubation. *Critical Care Medicine*, 2014 Jun;42(6):1372–1378.
3. Gabrielli A, Wenzel V, Layon AJ, von Goedecke A, Verne NG, Idris AH. Lower esophageal sphincter pressure measurement during cardiac arrest in humans: potential implications for ventilation of the unprotected airway. *Anesthesiology*, 2005 Oct 1;103(4):897–899.
4. Robinson M, Davidson A. Aspiration under anaesthesia: risk assessment and decision-making. *Continuing Eduction in Anaesthesia, Critical Care & Pain*, 2014 Aug 1;14(4):171–175.
5. Hennessy M, Goldenberg D. Surgical anatomy and physiology of swallowing. *Operative Techniques in Otolaryngology – Head and Neck Surgery*, 2016 Jun;27(2):60–66.
6. Newell C, Grier S, Soar J. Airway and ventilation management during cardiopulmonary resuscitation and after successful resuscitation. *Critical Care*, 2018 Aug 15;22(1):190.
7. Soar J, Böttiger BW, Carli P, Couper K, Deakin CD, Djärv T, et al. European Resuscitation Council Guidelines 2021: adult advanced life support. *Resuscitation*, 2021 Apr;161:115–151.
8. Truhlář A, Deakin CD, Soar J, Khalifa GEA, Alfonzo A, Bierens JJLM, et al. European Resuscitation Council Guidelines for Resuscitation 2015. Section 4. Cardiac arrest in special circumstances. *Resuscitation*, 2015 Oct;95:148–201.
9. Pilbery R, Young T, Hodge A. The effect of a specialist paramedic primary care rotation on appropriate non-conveyance decisions: a controlled interrupted time series analysis. *medRxiv*, 2020 Aug 7;2020.08.06.20169334.
10. Gautier N, Danklou J, Brichant JF, Lopez AM, Vandepitte C, Kuroda MM, et al. The effect of force applied to the left paratracheal oesophagus on air entry into the gastric antrum during positive-pressure ventilation using a facemask. *Anaesthesia*, 2019;74(1):22–28.
11. Sorour K, Donovan L. Intentional esophageal intubation to improve visualization during emergent endotracheal intubation in the context of massive vomiting: a case report. *Journal of Clinical Anesthesia*, 2015 Mar 1;27(2):168–169.
12. Pilbery R, Teare MD. Soiled airway tracheal intubation and the effectiveness of decontamination by paramedics (SATIATED): a randomised controlled manikin study. *British Paramedic Journal*, 2019 Jun 1;4(1):14–21.
13. McClelland G, Pilbery R, Hepburn S. Soiled airway tracheal intubation and the effectiveness of decontamination by United Kingdom paramedics (SATIATED2): a randomised controlled manikin study. *Australasian Journal of Paramedicine* [Internet]. 2020 Jul 17;17. Available from: https://ajp.paramedics.org/index.php/ajp/article/view/783
14. Root CW, Mitchell OJL, Brown R, Evers CB, Boyle J, Griffin C, et al. Suction Assisted Laryngoscopy and Airway Decontamination (SALAD): a technique for improved emergency airway management. *Resuscitation Plus*, 2020 Mar 1;1–2:100005.
15. DuCanto J, Serrano KD, Thompson RJ. Novel airway training tool that simulates vomiting: Suction-Assisted Laryngoscopy Assisted Decontamination (SALAD) system. *The Western Journal of Emergency Medicine*, 2017 Jan;18(1):117–120.
16. National Tracheostomy Safety Project (Great Britain). *Comprehensive tracheostomy care: the National Tracheostomy Safety Project manual*. McGrath BA, editor. Chichester, West Sussex: John Wiley & Sons Inc; 2014.
17. NHS Digital. Hospital Admitted Patient Care Activity 2019–20 [Internet]. NHS Digital, 2020. Available from: https://digital.nhs.uk/data-and-information/publications/statistical/hospital-admitted-patient-care-activity/2019-20

Chapter 1 Airway and Breathing

18. Cheung NH, Napolitano LM. Tracheostomy: epidemiology, indications, timing, technique, and outcomes. *Respiratory Care*, 2014 Jun 1;59(6):895–919.
19. Lewith H, Athanassoglou V. Update on management of tracheostomy. *BJA Education*, 2019 Nov;19(11):370–376.
20. McGrath BA, Bates L, Atkinson D, Moore JA. Multidisciplinary guidelines for the management of tracheostomy and laryngectomy airway emergencies: Tracheostomy management guidelines. *Anaesthesia*, 2012 Sep;67(9):1025–1041.
21. Whitaker DK. Time for capnography – everywhere. *Anaesthesia*, 2011 Jul 1;66(7):544–549.
22. Kodali BS. Capnography outside the operating rooms. *Anesthesiology*, 2013;118(1):192–201.
23. Noppen M. Spontaneous pneumothorax: epidemiology, pathophysiology and cause. *European Respiratory Review*, 2010 Sep 1;19(117):217–219.
24. Tortora GJ, Derrickson BH. *Principles of anatomy and physiology*. Hoboken: John Wiley Inc; 2017.
25. MacDuff A, Arnold A, Harvey J. Management of spontaneous pneumothorax: British Thoracic Society pleural disease guideline 2010. *Thorax*, 2010 Aug 1;65(Suppl 2):ii18–31.
26. Haynes D, Baumann MH. Pleural controversy: aetiology of pneumothorax. *Respirology*, 2011 May 1;16(4):604–610.
27. Porth C. *Essentials of pathophysiology: concepts of altered states*, 4th edition. Philadelphia: Lippincott Williams and Wilkins; 2014.
28. Society BPGL and BT. British Thoracic Society guidelines on respiratory aspects of fitness for diving. *Thorax*, 2003 Jan 1;58(1):3–13.
29. Leigh-Smith S, Harris T. Tension pneumothorax – time for a re-think? *Emerg Med J*. 2005 Jan 1;22(1):8–16.
30. Roberts DJ, Leigh-Smith S, Faris PD, Blackmore C, Ball CG, Robertson HL, et al. Clinical presentation of patients with tension pneumothorax: a systematic review. Annals of Surgery, 2015 Jun;261(6):1068–1078.
31. Yarmus L, Akulian J. Pneumothorax – symptoms, diagnosis and treatment | *BMJ Best Practice* [Internet]. 2019. Available from: https://bestpractice.bmj.com/topics/en-gb/504/
32. Kirmani BH, Page RD. Pneumothorax and insertion of a chest drain. *Surgery (Oxford) Journal*, 2014 May;32(5):272–275.
33. Jaiganesh T, Wright K, Sadana A. Mobile diagnosis: Hamman's crunch in a primary spontaneous pneumothorax. *Emergency Medicine Journal*, 2010 Jan 6;27(6):482–483.
34. Husain LF, Hagopian L, Wayman D, Baker WE, Carmody KA. Sonographic diagnosis of pneumothorax. *Journal of Emergencies, Trauma, and Shock*, 2012;5(1):76–81.
35. Spiteri MA, Cook DG, Clarke SW. Reliability of eliciting physical signs in examination of the chest. *The Lancet*, 1988 Apr 16;1(8590):873–875.
36. Leech C, Porter K, Steyn R, Laird C, Virgo I, Bowman R, et al. The pre-hospital management of life-threatening chest injuries: a consensus statement from the Faculty of Pre-Hospital Care, Royal College of Surgeons of Edinburgh. *Trauma*, 2017 Jan 1;19(1):54–62.
37. Hannon L, Clair TS, Smith K, Fitzgerald M, Mitra B, Olaussen A, et al. Finger thoracostomy in patients with chest trauma performed by paramedics on a helicopter emergency medical service. *Emergency Medicine Australasia*, 2020;32(4):650–656.
38. Joint Royal Colleges Ambulance Liaison Committee, Association of Ambulance Chief Executives. JRCALC Clinical Guidelines. Cited from JRCALC Plus (Version 1.2.13) [Mobile application software]. Bridgwater: Class Publishing Ltd; 2021.
39. O'Driscoll BR, Howard LS, Earis J, Mak V. BTS guideline for oxygen use in adults in healthcare and emergency settings. *Thorax*, 2017 Jun 1;72(Suppl 1):ii1–90.
40. National Institute for Health and Care Excellence. Chronic obstructive pulmonary disease in over 16s: diagnosis and management [Internet]. NICE; 2019. Available from: https://www.nice.org.uk/guidance/ng115
41. British Lung Foundation. The battle for breath – the impact of lung disease in the UK [Internet]. British Lung Foundation. 2016. Available from: https://www.blf.org.uk/policy/the-battle-for-breath-2016

References

42. Royal College of Physicians. COPD Who cares matters Clinical Audit 2014 [Internet]. London: RCP; 2015. Available from: https://www.rcplondon.ac.uk/projects/outputs/copd-who-cares-matters-clinical-audit-2014
43. Currie GP, editor. ABC of COPD, 3rd edition. Hoboken: Wiley-Blackwell; 2017.
44. Marieb E, Hoehn K. *Human anatomy & physiology*, 11th edition. San Francisco: Pearson; 2019.
45. Nolan J, Resuscitation Council (UK). Advanced life support, 7th edition. London: Resuscitation Council (UK); 2016.
46. Austin MA, Wills KE, Blizzard L, Walters EH, Wood-Baker R. Effect of high flow oxygen on mortality in chronic obstructive pulmonary disease patients in prehospital setting: randomised controlled trial. *The British Medical Journal*, 2010 Oct;341(oct18 2):c5462–c5462.
47. Kopsaftis Z, Carson-Chahhoud KV, Austin MA, Wood-Baker R. Oxygen therapy in the pre-hospital setting for acute exacerbations of chronic obstructive pulmonary disease. *Cochrane Database of Systematic Reviews* [Internet]. 2020;(1). Available from: https://www.cochranelibrary.com/cdsr/doi/10.1002/14651858.CD005534.pub3/full
48. Pandor A, Thokala P, Goodacre S, Poku E, Stevens JW, Ren S, et al. Pre-hospital non-invasive ventilation for acute respiratory failure: a systematic review and cost-effectiveness evaluation. *Health Technology Assessment*, 2015 Jun;19(42):1–102.
49. Fuller G, Keating S, Goodacre S, Herbert E, Perkins G, Rosser A, et al. Is a definitive trial of prehospital continuous positive airway pressure versus standard oxygen therapy for acute respiratory failure indicated? The ACUTE pilot randomised controlled trial. *BMJ Open*, 2020 Jul 1;10(7):e035915.

2   Circulation

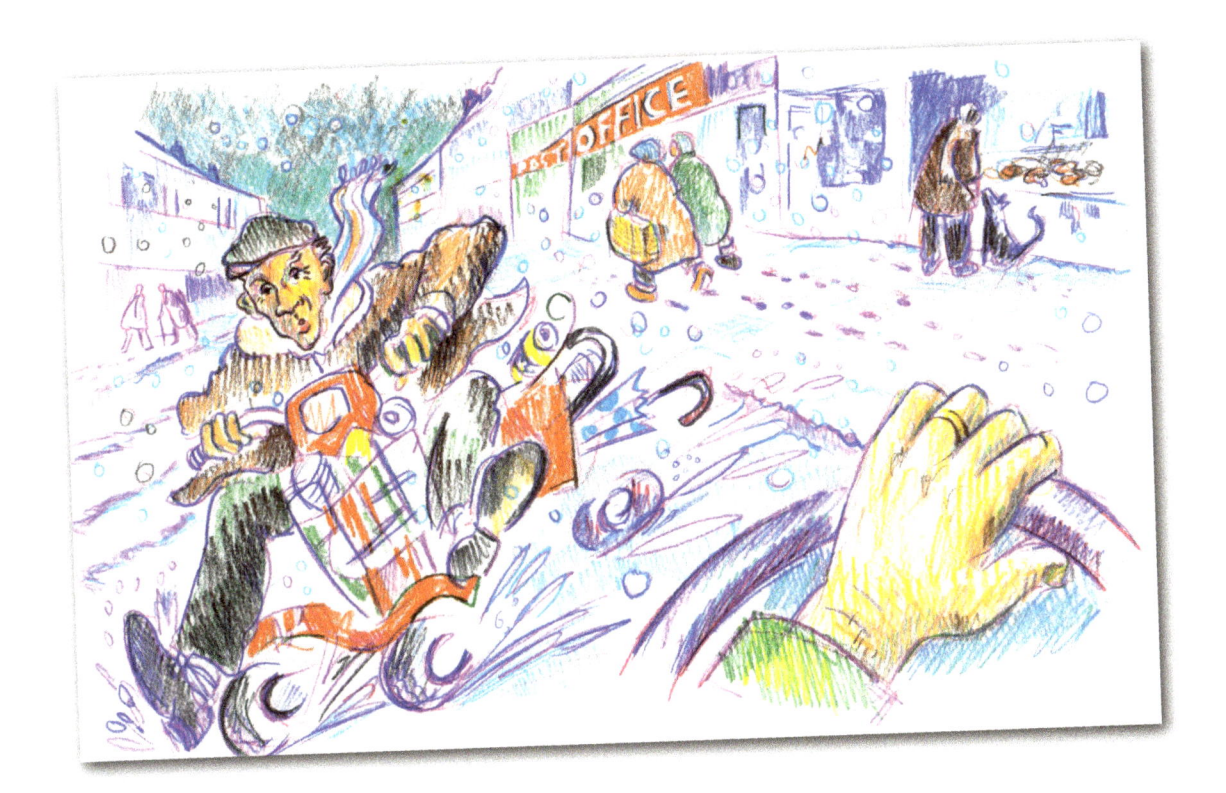

Chest Pain

With Katie Duncan

You are sat on standby on week 10 of the worst winter for years. Not only have you struggled through the snow to work, but now, 20 minutes into your shift, you are sent to the edge of your patch to cover the elderly person's weekly commute to the Post Office.

Not many brave souls have ventured out, although an elderly man on a mobility scooter provides a surreal moment as he slides slowly sideways past your bonnet. Only your immense professionalism prevents you from roaring with laughter. Instead, you produce what you hope is a concerned look on your face and leave the comfortable womb of the vehicle to check that he is alright and discuss the merits of snow chains for mobility scooters.

Your MDT and radio simultaneously light up and flash as you are called to a 70-year-old

Chapter 2 Circulation

male with chest pain. The address is not far away, but means venturing off the relative safety of the gritted main roads and onto a nearby estate. Despite the atrocious conditions, you manage to get very close to the house: the front garden.

Inside you are greeted by the sound of retching and your patient glances up from the toilet bowl looking rather grey and sweaty. His pain, he tells you, is retrosternal and radiates to his jaw and both arms. The rest of his history sounds like a textbook presentation of an acute coronary syndrome.

After checking for drug allergies, your colleague gets busy administering an aspirin and asks if the patient has taken any erectile dysfunction medications in the past 24 hours. You know they are contemplating giving glyceryl trinitrate (GTN) so you take a look at the patient's repeat prescription to see what other drugs they are taking:

- Aspirin
- Atenolol
- Simvastatin
- Levothyroxine
- Allopurinol
- Bendroflumethiazide.

You check the patient's blood pressure (BP) and it comes back as 90/50 mmHg.

> Should you: **Administer GTN** (read on) or **Do an ECG first** (skip the next paragraph)?

Administer GTN

You administer GTN since normally you wouldn't even bother checking a BP; the presence of a radial pulse is enough, isn't it? It works a treat ... his BP plummets, he goes into PEA and eventually asystole. You scratch your head wondering what just happened and wishing you had done an ECG first.

Do an ECG first

You wire the patient up to the 12-lead ECG (Figure 2.1) while your colleague gets IV access. Your patient looks up at you, contemplates asking you if he is going to die and then thinks better of it ... instead he asks, "What does it show?"

You tell him:

A: "It looks fine, better than mine."
B: "It shows an anterior MI, you're having a heart attack, but don't worry, you're in safe hands."
C: "It shows a lateral MI, it's probably just indigestion, but let's treat you as if it's a heart attack ... just in case."
D: "It shows an inferior MI, it looks like you're having a heart attack."

A, B or C

Your colleague looks at you in disbelief. "That is clearly an inferior MI and with the ST elevation in III, greater than II, don't you think you ought to consider right ventricular involvement?"

D

Everyone agrees that it is an inferior MI. Interestingly, the ST elevation in lead III is greater than that of lead II, which could suggest a right ventricular infarct.

You need to get the patient to the nearest cardiac catheter lab. The thing is, there is a LOT of snow outside and he has just stopped vomiting, although he still feels nauseous.

> What should you do: **Carry him** (read on) or **Let him walk** (skip the next paragraph)?

Carry him

You elect to carry him and crunch your way through the snow, on what turns out to be

Chest Pain

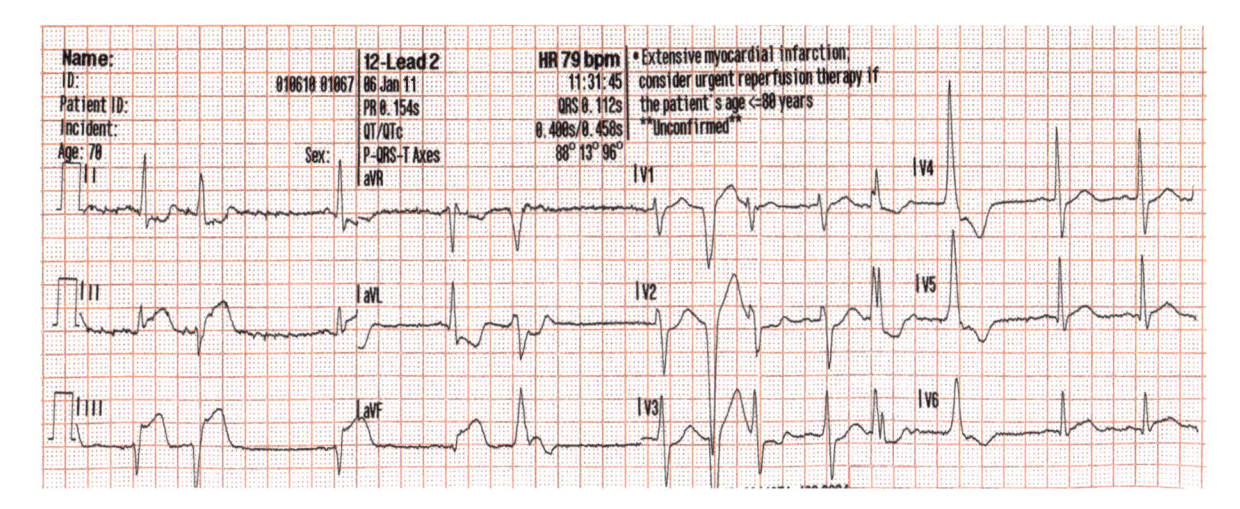

Figure 2.1 The patient's ECG.

a rare collection of snow-covered gnomes. Without warning, the patient projectile vomits all over you (if only you had taken the head end, eh?), causing you to slip. In slow motion, the chair flips over and the patient lands head first in the snow. The sudden exposure of his head to the freezing snow causes a reflex slowing of his heart rate ... to zero. Despite a valiant attempt at resuscitation in the snow, your patient does not survive and you get frostbite. Letting him walk seems like a good option now, why not try it (read on)?

Let him walk

After completing a thorough risk assessment taking into account the need for traversing a snow-covered gnome garden, you elect to walk the patient to the ambulance. It is cold, but amazingly, you remembered to turn on the heater on the way to the call and the back of the ambulance is nice and warm.

After assisting the patient onto the ambulance trolley, you set about getting a set of observations. Once this has been completed your colleague takes a look at the monitor. "His BP is dropping." Sure enough, his BP is now 80/40 mmHg.

The scale of the problem

Approximately 100,000 people per year in the UK are admitted to hospital due to a heart attack; that's 280 admissions daily or 1 every 5 minutes.[1] Between 40–50% of those will have an inferior wall myocardial infarction (MI). This is generally good news for the patient(!) as the mortality rate is around 2–9%, which is more favourable than patients suffering from an anterior MI. However, patients with inferior wall MI and associated right ventricular involvement generally have a worse prognosis due to their pre-load sensitivity, and can develop severe hypotension, especially after administration of vasodilators such as GTN.[2,3]

This group of patients who have right ventricular involvement are important to recognise, as the standard treatment ambulance staff provide for MIs generally, may be detrimental to these patients.

Anatomy

Figure 2.2 and Table 2.1 summarise this section, so feel free to use them to make things clearer!

Chapter 2 Circulation

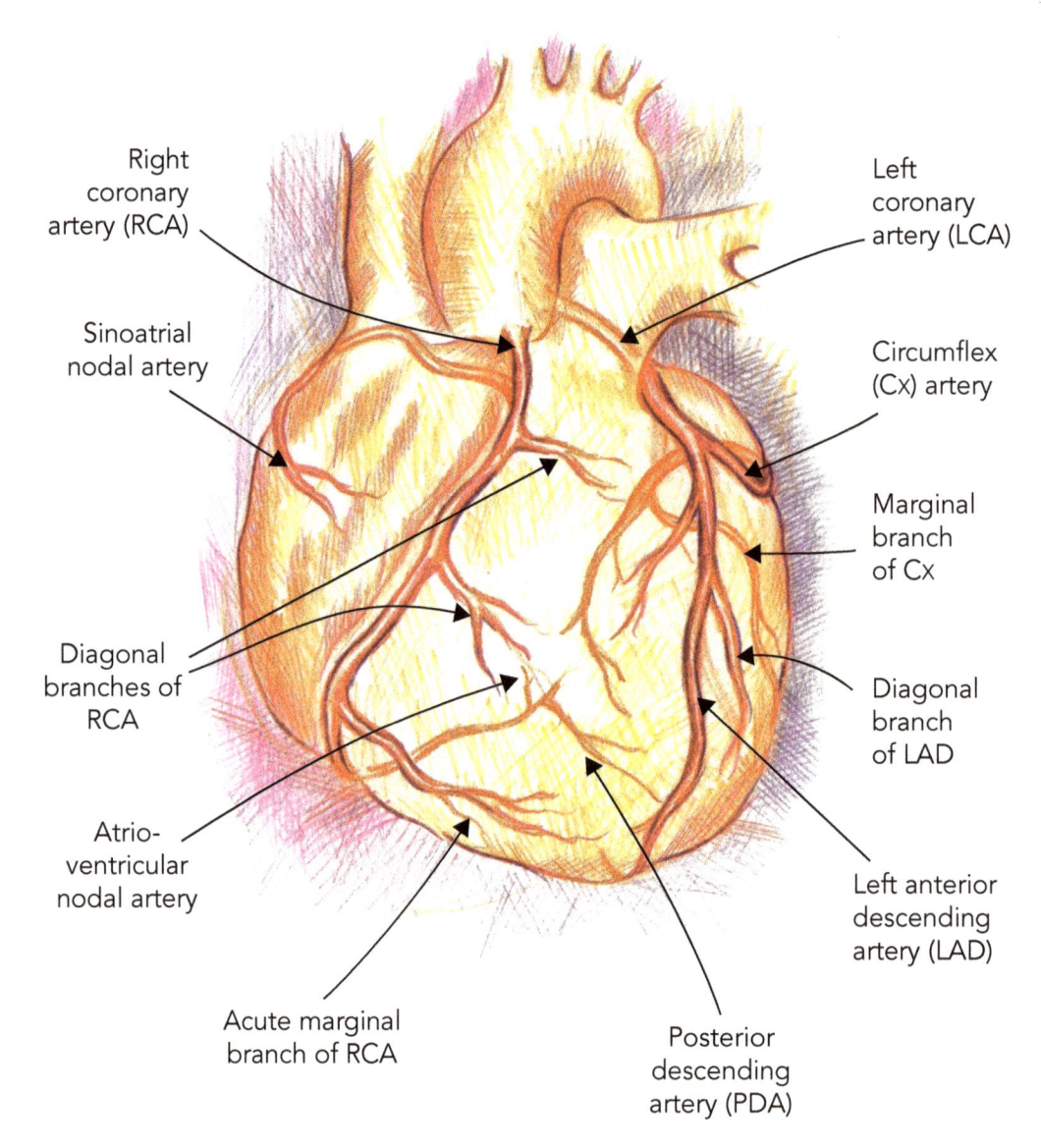

Figure 2.2 Coronary artery anatomy.

The right and left coronary arteries originate at the base of the ascending aorta, from the aortic sinuses.

Right coronary artery

The right coronary artery (RCA) runs down the right side of the heart in the coronary sulcus (depression) between the right atrium and ventricle. In 50–60% of people, the first branch off the RCA is the conus artery (not shown), which supplies the right ventricular outflow tract (in 20–30% this artery runs off the aorta).[4] The second branch in around half the population is the sinoatrial nodal artery (in the rest, this artery runs off the circumflex

40

Table 2.1 Summary of coronary arteries, branches and regions of myocardium served.

Coronary artery	Branches	Region of myocardium served
Right	Sinoatrial nodal branch	Sinoatrial node Bachmann bundles Free wall of right and left atria
Right	Conus	Right ventricular outflow tract
Right	Diagonals	Anterior wall of right ventricle
Right	Acute marginal	Lateral wall of right ventricle
Right	AV nodal branch	AV node
Right	Posterior descending (PDA) artery	Inferior wall of left ventricle Postero-inferior third of intraventricular septum
Left	LAD Diagonals	Anterior wall of the left ventricle, most of the interventricular septum, the Bundle of His and the bundle branches
Left	Circumflex Obtuse marginals	Lateral wall of left ventricle and atrium, posterior and high lateral portions of the left ventricle

artery, CX). The next branches are called diagonals and they supply the anterior wall of the right ventricle. Just before the RCA heads posteriorly, the large acute marginal branch heads off to supply the lateral wall of the right ventricle. Once the RCA reaches the inferior margin of the heart it turns posteriorly, continuing in the sulcus and branching to supply the atrioventricular (AV) node (90% of the time). Most people (around 80%) are right dominant; the RCA gives rise to the posterior descending artery (PDA). In around 8%, this artery arises from the left Cx artery (termed left dominance), with the remainder being served by both arteries.[5] The PDA serves the inferior wall of the left ventricle as well as the inferior part of the septum.

Left coronary artery

The left coronary artery (LCA) passes behind the pulmonary trunk and splits almost immediately into two branches, the anterior interventricular branch (often referred to as the left anterior descending artery, LAD) and the circumflex artery (Cx). The LAD descends obliquely towards the apex of the heart in the anterior interventricular sulcus, supplying the anterior part of the septum and anterior wall of the left ventricle via one or two diagonal branches.[6]

The Cx branch lies in the left coronary sulcus and supplies the lateral wall of the left ventricle via obtuse marginal branches. It carries on towards the base of the heart, usually ending before it reaches the posterior interventricular sulcus.

Pathophysiology

The heart is actually two pumps in one, although they are connected in a closed system by the pulmonary and systemic circulations. The right side of the heart only has to overcome the low pressure of the pulmonary circulation, so it is much less muscular and consumes less oxygen. This, coupled with a good collateral blood supply, makes the right ventricle resistant to irreversible ischaemic injury.[7,8] The left side of the heart has to overcome the peripheral vascular resistance of the systemic circulation and so is more muscular and as a result has greater oxygen demands. Despite these

Chapter 2   Circulation

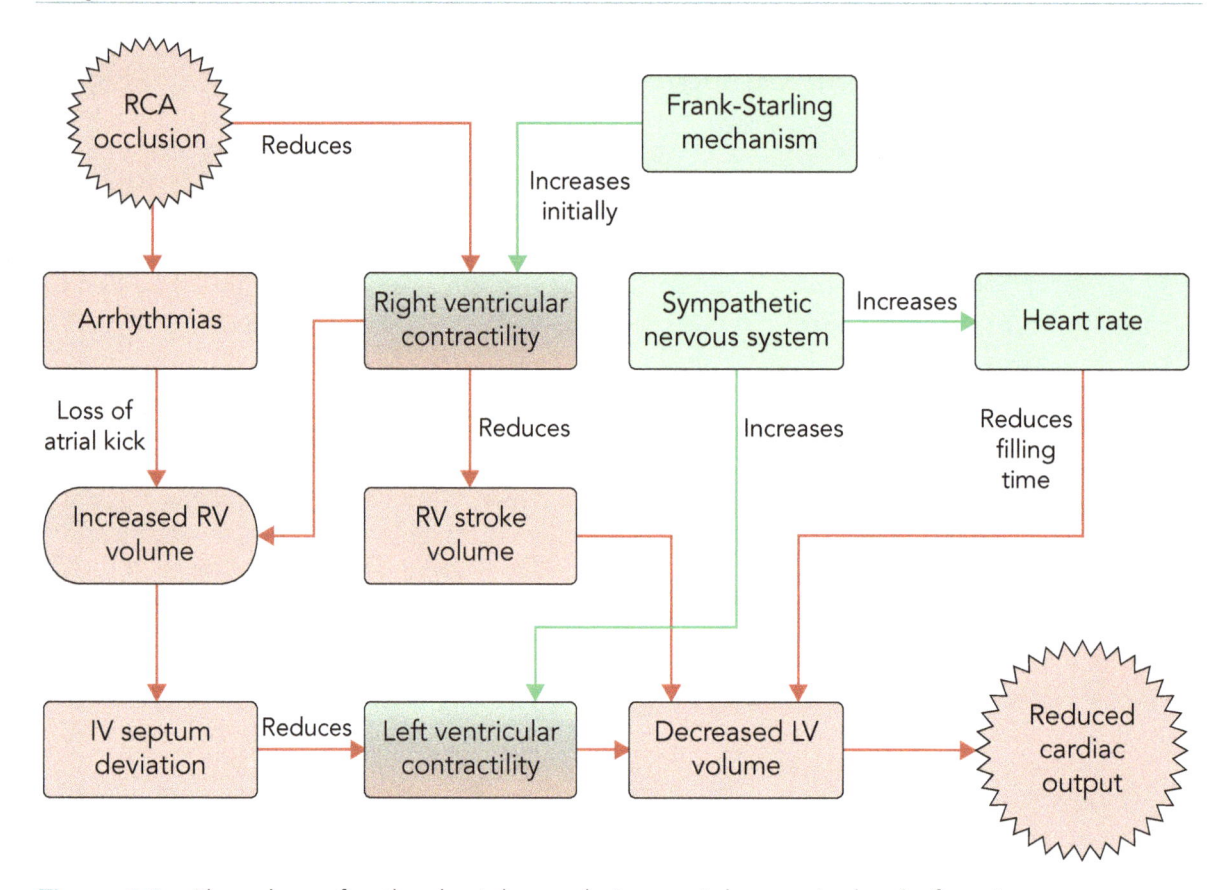

Figure 2.3   Flow chart of pathophysiology relating to right ventricular dysfunction.

differences, cardiac output is essentially the same from both sides.

When the RCA is occluded proximal to the diagonal branches serving the right ventricle, this balance can be disrupted. Right ventricular dysfunction results in less blood being ejected into the pulmonary circulation and returned to the left ventricle, which can ultimately lead to a decreased cardiac output (Figure 2.3).

There are a number of compensatory mechanisms to maintain adequate cardiac output. When the atria contract, a modest amount of blood is ejected into the ventricles prior to ventricular systole. However, it is common in proximal RCA occlusions for the sinoatrial and atrioventricular nodes to become affected, resulting in arrhythmias (such as atrial fibrillation and flutter) and blocks, reducing the efficiency of the 'atrial kick'. Increased end diastolic volume in the ventricles stretches the muscle fibres and creates a reflex increase in contractility, according to the Frank-Starling law of the heart.[7] However, excessive right ventricular volume will overcome this mechanism, causing blood to back up into the right atrium and venae cavae.

Usually when right ventricular contractility is reduced, right ventricular systolic pressure can be maintained by left ventricular septal contractions as the intraventricular septum is displaced into the right ventricle. In right ventricular dysfunction where the ventricle is abnormally dilated, the increased intrapericardial pressure coupled with increased right ventricular end diastolic pressure shifts the intraventricular septum towards the left ventricle. This has the effect of reducing left ventricular volume and alters the geometry of the ventricle, reducing contractility. In addition, the reduced volume of blood returned from the pulmonary circulation reduces stroke volume even further. The sympathetic nervous system tries to offset the reduction in stroke volume by increasing the heart rate (recall that cardiac output = heart rate × stroke volume). However, this has the effect of reducing filling time available to the ventricles and ultimately reduces cardiac output further.

Recognition

Faced with a history suggestive of an acute MI, you will record a set of observations and a 12-lead ECG as a matter of course. On a standard 12-lead ECG, the following are indicative of right ventricular involvement:[3,9]

- Presence of an inferior MI (ST elevation in leads II, III and aVF)
- ST elevation in III greater than II
- ST elevation in V1

The *JRCALC Clinical Guidelines* also advocate using V_3R and V_4R as additional leads to identify a right ventricular infarction. These leads are positioned in the same location as V_3 and V_4 but on the right side of the chest.[10]

The clinical examination can also provide several clues suggesting right ventricular involvement, in particular jugular venous distension (JVD) with clear lung fields. JVD is often seen in acute left ventricular failure or congestive cardiac failure, but you will recall that these patients typically have a bubbling chest or at least some basal crackles. JVD with a clear chest suggests three diagnoses: pulmonary embolism, pericardial tamponade and right ventricular infarction. The history and examination should provide an indication as to which of the three it is.

Management

One of the critical factors in right ventricular infarction (RVI) is the maintenance of preload, since this and the atrial kick are key in keeping flow to the left side of the heart. Large volumes of fluid are unnecessary and indeed may be detrimental, but fluid boluses coupled with frequent reassessment are appropriate in shocked patients. If the patient responds to fluid boluses, the administration of nitrates should be avoided due to their venodilatory effects.[3] Morphine is not contraindicated, but should be used with caution since the histamine release it causes can have venodilatory effects.

If the patient is normotensive or even hypertensive, then careful administration of nitrates could be considered, but monitor your patient closely. The best treatment for RVI is reperfusion via primary percutaneous coronary intervention (PPCI) and evidence suggests that the right ventricle usually makes a full recovery.[11]

> What are you going to do: Lie the **patient flat and elevate his legs** (read on) or **Administer a fluid bolus** (skip the next paragraph)?

Lie the patient flat and elevate his legs

Great, the patient's BP rallies to 85/40 mmHg ... for about 7 minutes. You need to do something else; why not administer a fluid bolus?

Chapter 2 Circulation

Administer a fluid bolus

You administer a 250 ml bolus, which has little effect, but another 250 ml boosts his BP up to 105/55 mmHg and a further bolus raises his BP to 118/65 mmHg.

Despite the Entonox, the patient is still in pain, so while en route to the nearest cath lab, you administer morphine and for once give it at a rate of 1 mg/min. After 6 mg, the patient's pain score is down to 3/10 and although his BP has dropped back to 105/55 mmHg, it seems to be holding.

Due to the snow, all elective procedures have been cancelled and thanks to your pre-alert, the staff are ready to pounce. The patient is stripped off, consents and is having a wire inserted up his radial artery before you have even made up the ambulance trolley, giving you a chance to have a nosy at the angiograms. They show, as you suspected, an occluded right coronary artery.

The patient has been saved and since this is a fictitious case study you receive gushing thanks, both verbal and written from the patient and his family, resulting in your mugshot appearing in the Service 'good news' circular and being the butt of station jokes for the next week.

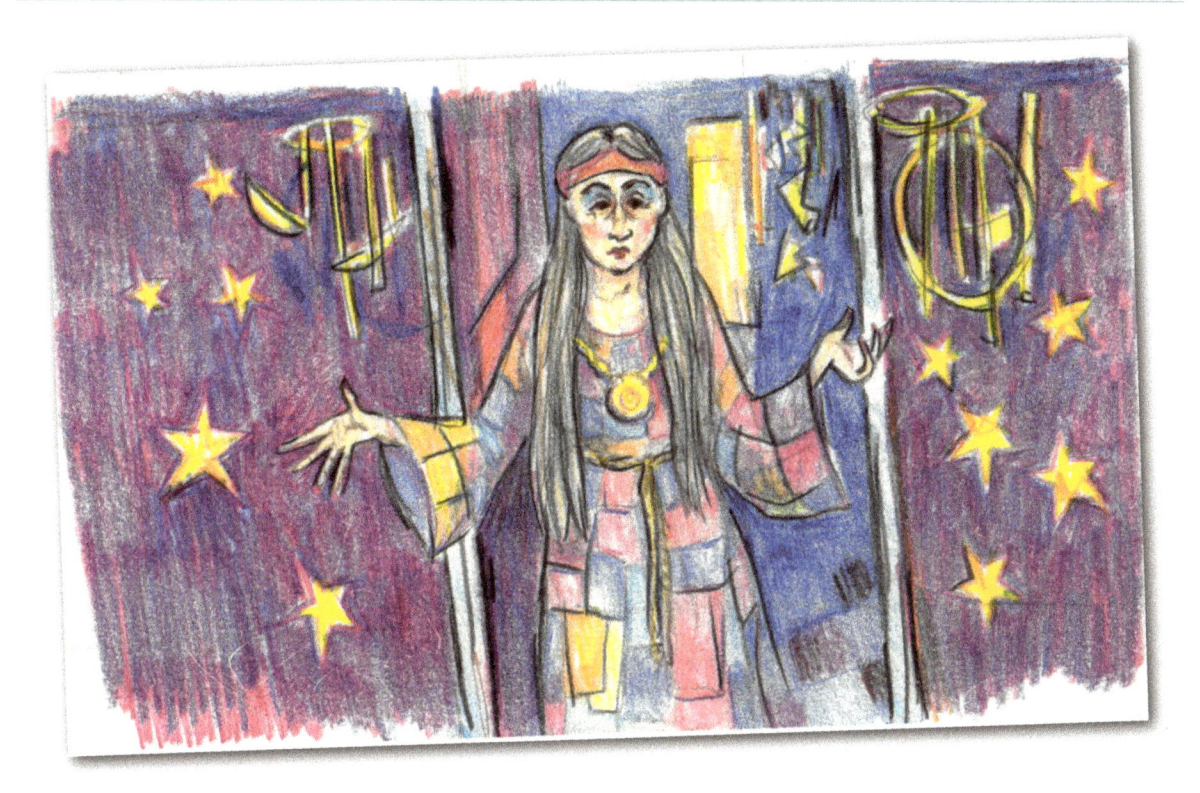

Pacemakers and ICDs

You are on standby enjoying the spring sunshine and watching a local tai-chi group gracefully, and slowly, moving in unison through a range of moves. It's quite hypnotic and your eyelids are starting to get heavy when the MDT bleeps into life with your next patient. Your colleague peers over at the screen and tuts. The screen reads: 71-year-old female, feeling stressed, hearing a beeping sound from inside her body. "Just when I thought I'd seen it all," sighs your colleague. The address is not far and, despite the low categorisation of the call and your colleague's steady driving, it takes only 10 minutes to arrive on scene.

"This must be the place," says your colleague as you pull up alongside a house that has been painted vivid purple. "The stars are a nice touch, though," she continues. You walk up the gravelled pathway to the front door, which looks like it has a crystal hanging from the door knocker. The door creaks open, unveiling the patient, resplendent in a full-length patchwork dress. "Come in," she says slowly and in an unusually low-pitched voice. You enter the hall and dodge the wind chimes, which seems odd inside the house, although your colleague mouths "Good feng shui?" at you. On entering the living room, you introduce

Chapter 2   Circulation

yourself and ask how you can help. "I can hear a beep from within," your patient, Sybil, tells you. "It starts and stops, starts and stops." Your colleague turns her back to you both, apparently to examine a tapestry on one of the walls, but the gentle jiggling up and down of her shoulders betrays the real reason.

You give yourself a virtual slap and focus. You run through a range of questions, and although Sybil is a frustrating historian thanks to her 'mystical' method of delivery, you ascertain that the beeping started this morning, when she put on her new magnetic necklace. "It's made from neodymium and helps my blood to flow," she breathes. You're not quite sure that her blood needs assistance from magnets to flow, but whatever. The beep is a constant tone that "doesn't last very long" and has been heard on several occasions, particularly after she has spent time poring over her very large jigsaw puzzle.

> What are you going to do: **Obtain a set of observations** (read on) or **Ask Sybil to carry on with her jigsaw** (skip the next paragraph)?

Obtain a set of observations

You ask your colleague, who seems to have regained some of her composure, to record a set of observations to buy you some time to work out your next move. She comes back with the following:

Airway
Patent

Breathing
Respiratory rate: 12 breaths/min
SpO_2: 96% on air

Circulation
Good radial pulse at a rate of 60 beats/min
Blood pressure: 130/80 mmHg

Disability
GCS score: 15/15
Blood sugar: 6.8 mmol/l

Exposure/Environment
Temperature: 36.8°C

These seem reassuringly normal, but don't help you work out what is going on. You decide to ask Sybil to repeat the actions that led to the beeping.

Ask Sybil to carry on with her jigsaw

You need a set of observations, but your initial impression is that Sybil is likely to be primary survey negative, so you ask her to resume completing her jigsaw. She goes through a well-rehearsed, if over the top, ritual involving removing her necklace and placing it around a jewellery stand. Next she picks up her half-moon spectacles from a shelf before retrieving a box containing pieces. She hovers over the jigsaw for several minutes and … nothing happens. Your colleague finds a home for a couple of pieces in the jigsaw, but this is not helping you get to the bottom of things.

You ask Sybil if she wouldn't mind stopping completing the jigsaw and ask her about her past medical history. However, your questions go unanswered until she has returned the half-moon glasses to their place and retrieved her necklace and placed it around her neck. Right on cue, you hear a beeping from her chest. You lean in to better determine the exact location and decide it seems to be coming from the left side of her upper chest.

Pacemakers and ICDs

> What are you going to do now: **Ask to see her chest** (read on) or **Something else** (skip the next page)?

Ask to see her chest

You ask Sybil if you can take a closer look at her chest and she pauses. "I've not been asked that question for a long time," she muses. You quickly add that it is just to determine where the beeping is coming from, but it doesn't stop your blushing, as well as the dread that is associated with the "just wait until I tell everyone in the mess room" look on your colleague's face. Sybil seems keen to remove her top, but you intervene, asking her just to lower the neckline on the left-hand side. You spot a scar just under her collarbone, with a small bulge under the skin. "Do you have a pacemaker, Sybil?" you enquire. "Yes, I do," she replies.

Something else

You don't fancy asking to see Sybil's chest, so you get your colleague to do it instead.

A 12-lead ECG seems like an appropriate test since the beep appears to be chest-related. It's a bit of a faff, but despite Sybil, your colleague manages to obtain a 12-lead ECG (Figure 2.4).

Putting everything together, you realise that Sybil has a pacemaker, and every time she wears her magnetic necklace, it is triggering it. The question is, what type of pacemaker and what does the beeping mean? Fortunately, Sybil is able to produce a card that the cardiologist who fitted the device gave her. It has some contact details which, although incorrect, do at least point to the correct hospital. Luckily, since it is midweek and in office hours, you are able to get hold of a junior doctor who works for the consultant and explain the situation. The doctor explains that this is probably an indication that the battery is nearing the end of its life, since the device has been in place for over 9 years. They arrange an outpatient appointment for Sybil that day.

Scale of the problem

Modern cardiac electrophysiology can be traced back to the late 18th century thanks to scientists such as Luigi Galvani and his

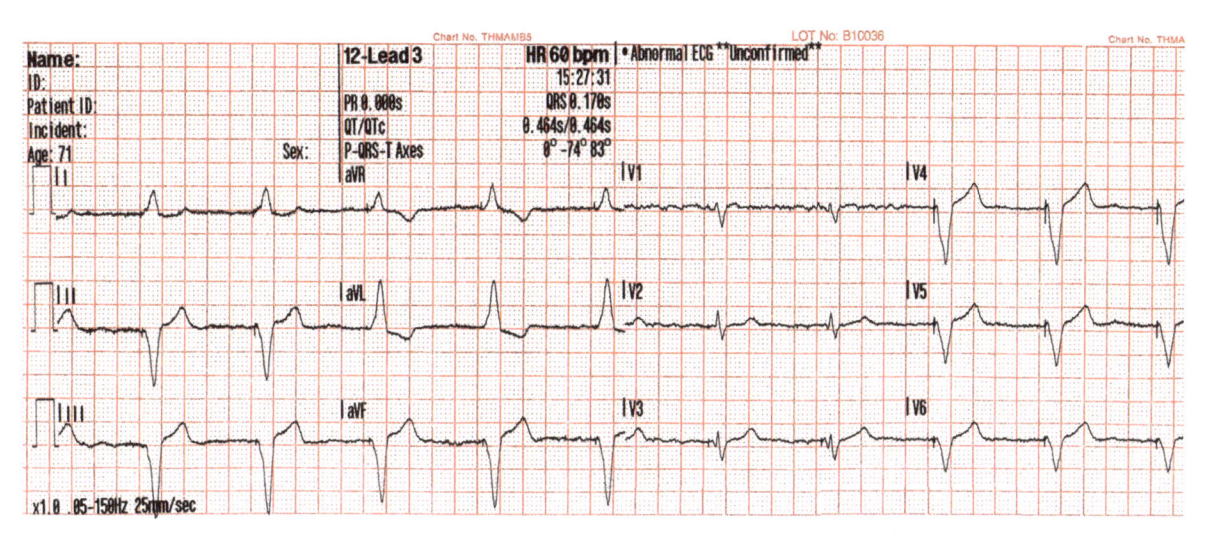

Figure 2.4 Sybil's ECG.

47

Chapter 2 Circulation

experiments on frogs (Figure 2.5), and Xavier Bichat, who would eagerly await victims of the guillotine during the French Revolution so that he could conduct tests on their hearts.[12] Implantable pacemakers arrived in the 1960s and developed over the next 50 years to include non-invasive programming, dual-chamber, rate-responsive and bi-ventricular pacemakers, and steroid-eluting leads among others.

While there was much excitement about the in-hospital management of arrhythmias, it was not until two cardiologists, Michel Mirowski and Morton Mower, produced the first internal cardio-defibrillator (ICD) in 1969 that the problem of sudden cardiac death in the community could be addressed. The first implantation in humans did not take place until 1980, however. Like pacemakers, these devices have also undergone rapid development, becoming smaller and capable of pacing and synchronised cardioversion as well as defibrillation.[13]

In the 21st century, approximately 33,000 pacemakers, 6,000 ICDs and 8,600 cardiac resynchronisation pacemakers are implanted each year in the UK.[14]

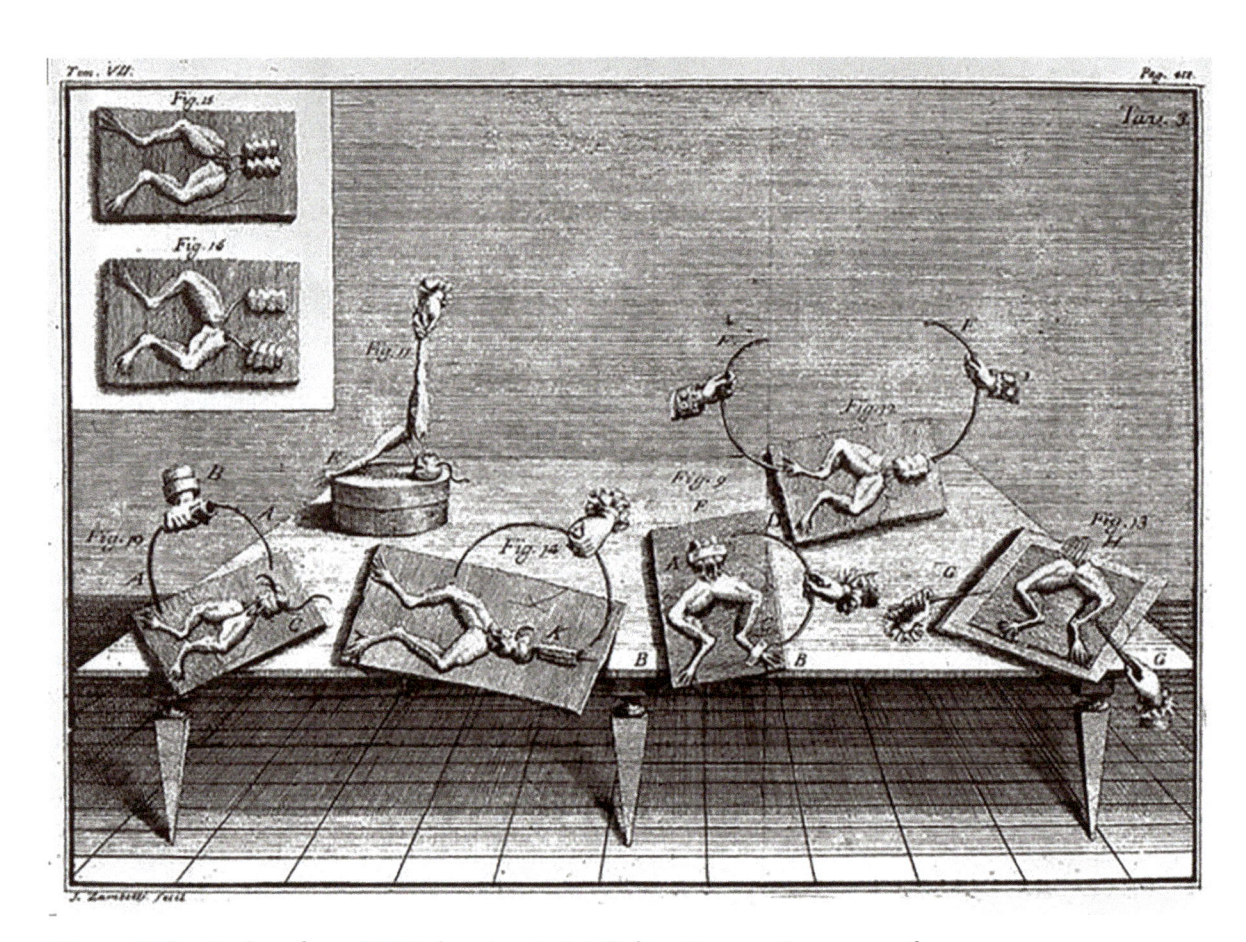

Figure 2.5 A plate from 1791 showing Luigi Galvani's experiments on frogs.
Source: Wellcome Collection [CC BY 4.0 (https://creativecommons.org/licenses/by/4.0/)].

Anatomy of a pacemaker

Pacemakers consist of a battery and programmable circuitry, encased in a titanium box (often referred to as the 'can') that is welded to make it air- and water-tight (Figure 2.6). There are also connectors for the pacing leads, which are typically made of plastic and are fixed to the outside of the can. Since the 1970s, lithium iodide batteries have been used, as they have an average life span of around 10 years, depending on the frequency and amplitude of pacing events.[15]

The circuitry incorporates the various functions of the pacemaker, including sensing and pacing algorithms, a timing clock and data collection systems. Some also have telemetry built in so that non-invasive access to the data is possible. Most pacemakers have a reed switch, which responds to magnets placed over the pacemaker and either provides feedback on the status of the device or amends/disables certain functions.

Pacing leads

Pacing leads are flexible insulated wires with a connector pin at one end (to attach to the pacemaker) and an electrode tip at the other. Leads have two types of fixator at the electrode end, which fix the lead either passively or actively. The most common is the passive type, which consists of tines (a bit like fish hooks) that act as an anchor, fixing the lead to the myocardial trabeculae. Over time, there is fibrosis of the myocardium around the tip, further securing the attachment. The other type, active, consists of a retractable screw that can be inserted into the myocardium. This is typically used in right ventricular placement high up on the septum.[15]

Leads are usually unipolar or bipolar. Unipolar leads have a single wire core and electrode tip, with the can acting as the other electrode. This causes a large pacing spike on the ECG as the current tracts through the body. Bipolar pacing leads on

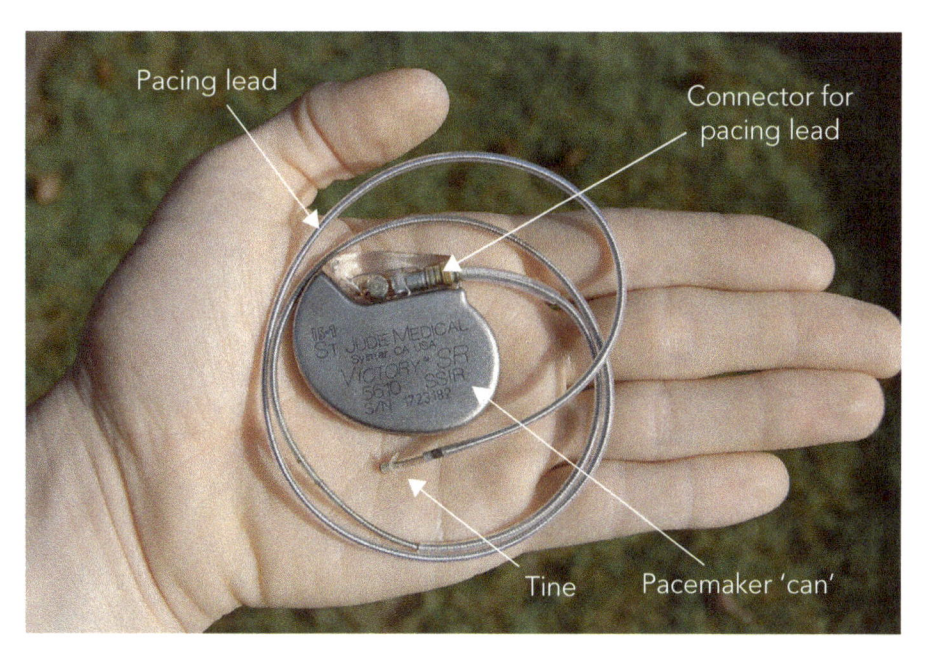

Figure 2.6 A pacemaker.
Source: Steven Fruitsmaak [CC BY 3.0 (https://creativecommons.org/licenses/by/3.0)], via Wikimedia Commons.

Chapter 2 Circulation

the other hand consist of two inner wires within the lead. This means that the pacing and sensing circuits have to travel across only a few millimetres of myocardium, resulting in a much smaller pacing spike.[16]

More recently, leadless pacemakers have been developed. However, they can only detect a single chamber (the right ventricle) and there have been a number of serious complications. As such they are not recommended for use outside of clinical research studies.[17,18]

Pacemaker codes

It's difficult to read anything about pacemakers without coming across cryptic codes such as VVI or DDDR. The code was created by the North American Society of Pacing and Electrophysiology Mode Code Committee and The British Pacing and Electrophysiology Group (NASPE/BPEG), and is known as the NASPE/BPEG generic (NBG) code (Table 2.2). A combination of at least three letters from the code create the pacemaker 'mode'. The first three letters highlight the bradycardia functions of the pacemaker, the fourth identifies whether the pacemaker is programmable and the presence of rate modulation, and the fifth, whether the device has any anti-tachyarrhythmia functions.[19]

First letter

This identifies the location of the actual pacing, which can be none, atrium only, ventricles only or atrium and ventricles (dual).

Second letter

The second letter denotes where the device 'senses' the intrinsic electrical activity of the heart. Remember, it cannot 'see' the surface ECG that you will record with electrodes on the skin. The sensitivity of pacemakers is important, because the voltage at which sensing occurs determines when the pacemaker response will be triggered. Sensing at very low voltages will lead to over-pacing (inappropriate additional pacemaker responses) and vice versa. As with pacing location, this can take the values of none, atrium or ventricle only and dual sensing.

Third letter

The third letter denotes the response to sensed events. This can be either no response, triggered, inhibited or dual (both triggered and inhibited, depending on the chamber). As the name implies, if set to trigger when sensing occurs, the pacemaker will immediately deliver an output in the same chamber (or after an appropriate atrioventricular delay, to the ventricle when set to dual mode).

Table 2.2 The NBG code.

Letter position	1	2	3	4	5
Function	Chamber(s) paced	Chamber(s) sensed	Response to sensing	Rate modulation	Multi-site pacing
Options	O: none A: atrium only V: ventricle only D: dual (atrium and ventricle)	O: none A: atrium only V: ventricle only D: dual	O: none T: triggered I: inhibited D: dual (both triggered and inhibited)	O: none R: rate modulation	O: none A: atrium only V: ventricle only D: dual

Source: Bernstein et al., 2002.

If set to inhibit, the escape interval, that is the maximum allowed time from either a spontaneous or a paced ventricular wave, is reset and no pacing output is delivered.

Fourth letter

This letter serves to identify whether the pacemaker can adapt the pacing rate (rate modulation). These features typically consist either of a blended sensor, with an accelerometer that can tell if you are moving and a minute ventilation monitor to determine increased exertion, or of a closed-loop stimulation system, which detects cardiac contractility.[19]

Fifth letter

This denotes whether there is multiple pacing occurring within the same chamber (typically the left ventricle). The options are none, atrium only, ventricle only or dual (both chambers).

Two common modes are VVI and DDD. Using the NBG code, you'll be able to determine that in the case of VVI, the pacemaker only paces and senses in the ventricle and the response to a sensed event is to inhibit ventricular pacing. A DDD pacemaker, on the other hand, will sense and pace the atrium and the ventricle, and will respond to a sensed event in either chamber by inhibiting pacing, but will deliver a pacing stimulus to the ventricle when an atrial event is sensed, which is not associated with an appropriate ventricular response by the heart after a maximum pre-programmed interval.[15]

Pacemaker implantation

Pacemakers (and ICDs) are typically placed on the left side of the chest. This is because it is easier for right-handed cardiologists to perform the procedure and makes it easier to place the pacing leads (particularly leads in the right atrium). In order to house the pacemaker, a pocket is formed, most commonly in the pectoral region; other sites include the axilla (especially in children) and abdomen (for epicardial and femoral pacemaker systems).

Placement in the pectoral region can be either subcutaneous or sub- or intra-muscular. A subcutaneous placement is usually sufficient for most people unless they have very little adipose tissue, in which case sub-muscular pockets offer better protection for the pacemaker. The pacing leads are typically inserted through the cephalic, subclavian or axillary veins, although less common routes include the internal jugular and femoral veins.[20]

Indications for a pacemaker

Pacemakers treat bradyarrhythmias. As a result they are indicated for:[21]

- Sinus node disease when symptoms are directly caused by bradycardia, sinus arrest or sinus-atrial block
- Acquired AV block, either Mobitz Type II or complete heart block
- Recurrent, unpredictable reflex syncope due to sinus arrest or AV block, or both
- Asymptomatic sinus pauses of over 6 seconds
- Bundle branch block (BBB) unexplained syncope and abnormal electrophysiological study
- Alternating BBB (also known as bilateral BBB, where ECGs show RBBB and then LBBB on successive ECGs, or vice versa).

Cardiac resynchronisation therapy

A special type of pacemaker can be used for the severest categories of heart failure. These are patients with New York Heart Association functional classification types III or IV:[22]

- Type III: Marked limitation of physical activity. Comfortable at rest, but minor exercise, for example, a 20 metre walk, results in severe symptoms.
- Type IV: Symptoms even at rest. Patients are mostly bedbound.

Congestive heart failure is typically associated with cardiomyopathy (following a myocardial infarction, for example) and conduction abnormalities, such as left bundle branch block (LBBB). These can result in asynchrony of ventricular contraction, reducing the pumping efficiency of the heart (usually measured as left ventricular ejection fraction, LVEF).[23]

Cardiac resynchronisation therapy (CRT) devices are essentially pacemakers, but differ from those used to treat bradycardias because they pace the left ventricle, either alone, or in conjunction with the right ventricle. A common configuration is right atrial sensing, with a fixed 100–120 ms atrioventricular delay before simultaneous pacing of the left and right ventricles.[21]

There are two types of CRT device:

- CRT-P: Devices that only pace
- CRT-D: Devices that also have a built-in implantable cardioverter-defibrillator.

Implantable cardioverter defibrillators

ICDs have been used in patients for over 30 years, with the majority implanted as for a regular pacemaker, with transvenous leads in the right side of the heart and with the addition of an intracavitary right heart coil(s). In patients who have recurrent problems with vascular access, or if the ICD has been removed because of infection, or for patients who are young and likely to require ICDs long-term, subcutaneous ICDs can be fitted. Unlike their transvenous cousins, the ICD and leads are all outside of the heart. However, they are limited by their inability to pace (except for 30-second bursts of transcutaneous pacing following a shock) and/or provide CRT.

They are generally recommended for the following patients:[24]

- Recorded ventricular fibrillation (VF) or haemodynamically unstable ventricular tachycardia (VT) in the absence of reversible causes

- Recurrent sustained VT following MI who are already receiving optimal medical therapy.

When things go wrong

There are a number of complications that can occur in patients with pacemakers and ICDs (collectively referred to as cardiovascular implanted electronic devices, CIEDs). These can be loosely organised into:[25,26]

- Implant-related complications
- Pacemaker malfunction
- The shocking ICD.

Implant-related complications

There are a number of implant-related complications, including:[26]

- *Pocket haematoma*: Bleeding is a common early complication, but is generally treated conservatively, unless the haematoma is large and/or very painful.
- *Pocket infection*: Up to 8% of patients can get an infection. You should consider the CIED as a potential source of infection in patients who have a pyrexia of unknown origin.
- *Lead infection*: Infections that affect the CIED long after implantation has been performed are more likely to involve the leads. These can be serious pathologies, including sepsis, endocarditis and pulmonary embolism (PE).
- *Pericardial effusion*: This is uncommon and occurs soon after implantation.
- *Pneumothorax*: This occurs in around 1% of implantations and is a consequence of the close proximity of the subclavian vessels and the apex of the lung. Unless the pneumothorax is of a significant size, it is generally managed conservatively.
- *Superior vena cava syndrome*: Deep vein thrombosis (DVT) can occur following CIED implantation. Patients will typically present with fever and upper extremity and/or facial swelling.

Pacemaker malfunction

Pacemaker malfunctions are generally due to one of three failures:

- *Failure to pace*: This can be observed on the ECG by the absence of a pacing spike and pacemaker-induced QRS complex. Instead, the underlying rhythm of the patient is presented. Note that many pacemakers are on demand, that is, they only pace when required. If the patient has a natural heart rate above 60 beats/min, for example, then it is quite likely that the pacemaker will not fire.
- *Failure to capture*: This can also be seen on the ECG, as a pacing spike, but no ventricular activity in response. This is typically caused by lead displacement or fracture, a dying battery or electrolyte abnormalities which result in a raised depolarisation threshold.
- *Failure to sense*: In order to pace properly, the pacemaker has to be able to detect, or sense, the underlying rhythm of the patient. This is a fine balance. Oversensing, where the pacemaker typically interprets the underlying heart rate as higher than it actually is, results in the pacemaker not providing an impulse to depolarise the ventricles when it should do. The opposite, undersensing, leads to inappropriate ventricular contraction.

Pacemaker-mediated tachycardia

In dual-chamber pacemakers, a re-entrant loop tachycardia can develop if a premature ventricular complex or paced ventricular depolarisation is conducted in a retrograde fashion to the atria, where it is sensed by the atrial lead as a P wave, leading to another ventricular impulse.

Twiddler's syndrome

In patients with a large pocket or loose subcutaneous tissue, fiddling with your CIED can become a bit of a habit. The problem with this is that with persistent fiddling (or twiddling) the pacemaker leads become twisted and coiled, leading to fracture and/or dislodgement. This requires surgical correction.[27]

The shocking ICD

There are two basic scenarios when an ICD will shock the patient:

- *Appropriate*: The patient is in ventricular fibrillation or requires termination of a ventricular tachyarrhythmia.
- *Inappropriate*: The patient is not experiencing either of the above. The most common causes of inappropriate shocks are supraventricular tachycardia and atrial fibrillation. However, new onset of LBBB can lead to inappropriate shocks as can device-related problems, such as lead fracture and insulation damage.

Management

The management of patients with ICDs is explained in published ambulance guidelines,[10] so for brevity is not repeated here. However, a key component of management is the use of a magnet. Magnets trigger the reed switches on CIEDs, typically causing the following behaviours:

- *Pacemakers*: Revert to asynchronous mode (that is, ignore the patient's underlying heart rate) at a fixed rate around 60 beats/min
- *ICDs*: Disables the shocking function. Pacing mode usually remains functional.

In the case of ICDs, remember that if you disable the defibrillator, you will be responsible for providing any subsequent shocks should the patient develop VF or pulseless VT. Defibrillator pads should be placed at least 8 cm from the ICD, which can be achieved by placing the pads in the anterior–posterior position in cases of right-sided or axilla implantations.[28]

Chapter 2   Circulation

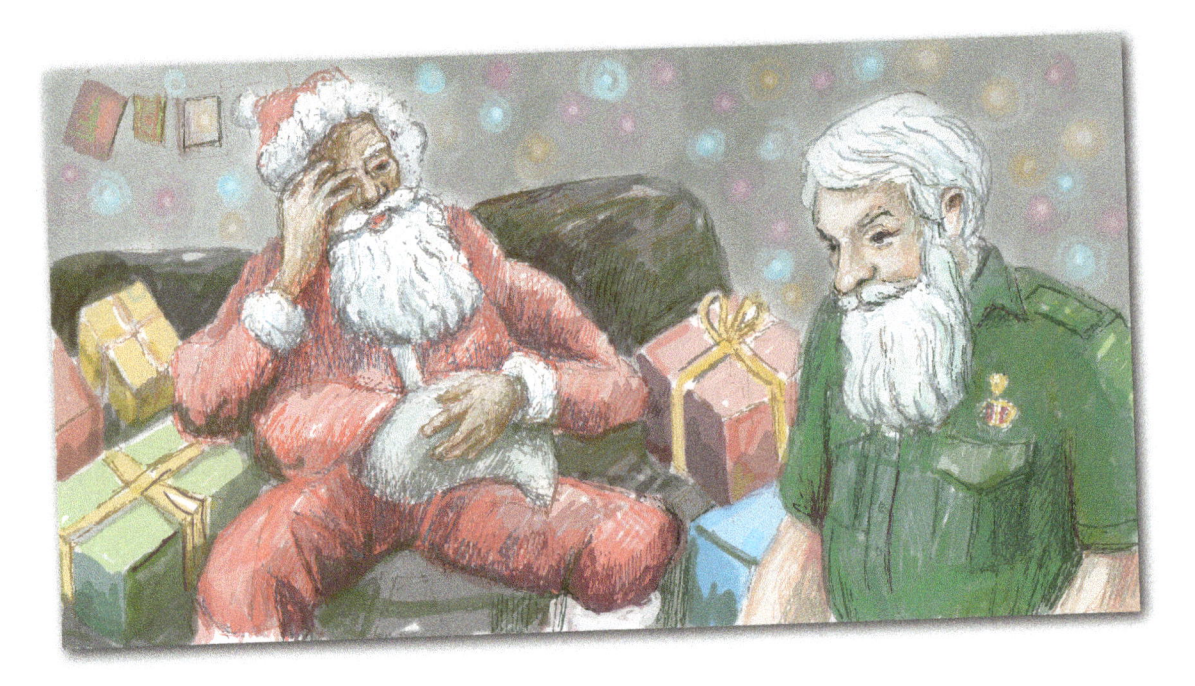

Sickle Cell Disease

You are on standby on the night before Christmas. Well, the afternoon before Christmas. Next to you in the cab is Pete, one of the longest serving ambulance technicians in the service. For the majority of the year, he is nicknamed 'Big Daddy' on account of his rotund abdomen and in homage to an 80s wrestler by the same name. This is lost on most of the younger members of staff and every time the issue of the origin of his name is raised, an internet search is required before an understanding is reached. However, in the run-up to Christmas (a longish, three-month run-up), Pete starts to grow his beard ready for his annual role as Father Christmas at his village community centre. His abdomen needs no further encouragement, but as he points out, it's the authenticity of his 'natural' stuffing and beard that makes him perfect for the job.

Indeed, he now has a monopoly following a disastrous year where the centre, wanting to get through as many children in as short a period of time as possible, elected to have four Father Christmases handing out presents simultaneously. This worked well until a curious child pulled back the curtain acting as a divider, revealing all of them. Much damage limitation followed with parents pointing out that no, they were not the real Father Christmas, just helpers, and yes, that one did look rather like the father of one of their friends. "Now it's just me," says Pete proudly, for around the tenth time during the shift.

Hopes of an on-time finish are dashed by the MDT, which passes details of a 35-year-old

Sickle Cell Disease

male with all-over body pain. Pete tuts and sets off for the address, which is a block of flats 14 minutes away.

As you arrive on scene, you elect to take all of the response kit up with you, as the flat number indicates it is near the top. However, in contrast to most tower blocks you attend, this one is rather more upmarket and you risk leaning on the sides of the lift as it ascends.

The doors open on the 24th floor and you swiftly locate the address. You ring the doorbell and are greeted by the patient's partner, a green Christmas elf (judging by her costume), who flashes Pete a big smile before inviting you both in. You find your patient in the living room, sitting on the sofa and squirming with pain. The hi-fi in the corner appears to be playing Christmas classics and 'Jingle Bells' has just started. Your patient is quite a sight. He is dressed as Father Christmas, but it is clear that his beard and 'stuffing' are not natural.

Pete glowers at the Santa imposter, muttering "You're not Father Christmas … you're, you're … ," "Black?" volunteers the patient. "No," replies Pete, "young." "I made a promise to my father that I'd take over his role, when he was admitted to hospital," explains the young Father Christmas, who is called Daniel. "But it looks like I'm going to be letting down the local children too." This clearly strikes a chord with Pete, whose demeanour instantly softens. "Well, we'd better see if we can get you back on your feet, then." You take this as your cue to introduce yourself and find out the reason for the emergency call.

Daniel explains that he has sickle-cell anaemia. He usually manages to control his symptoms himself, but with the upheaval caused by his father's admission to hospital and then preparing for Christmas, he has not been taking his medication and his pain has gotten out of control. You ask him where his pain is located and he tells you that he has pain in his abdomen, all of his joints, shoulders, upper arms, hips, thighs, knees and toes, knees and toes (there's a song in there somewhere).

As he reaches for his management plan, he temporarily gives in to the pain and it takes a few minutes for him to regain his composure. You cast your eyes over the plan, which describes his pre-hospital management as: Entonox, morphine, transport to hospital and keep well oxygenated.

> What are you going to do: **Follow the plan** (skip the next paragraph) or **Administer IV paracetamol** (read on)?

Administer IV paracetamol

You're not prepared to dole out strong analgesia to just anyone. Besides, IV paracetamol is just as good as morphine, right? You state your plan and set about trying to find a vein. However, Daniel points out that he has taken his co-codamol less than three hours ago. With that course of action ruled out, you decide to follow Daniel's action plan.

Follow the plan

Daniel is clearly the expert here on his condition and his plan has been put together by a haematology consultant you've never heard of, but you recognise the hospital. You've got Entonox to hand and he gratefully inhales the analgesic gas while you record a set of observations and plan your exit.

> What are you going to do: Encourage Daniel to **Walk** back to the ambulance (read on) or send Pete for the **Carry chair** (skip the next paragraph)?

Chapter 2 Circulation

Walk

As a rule, Pete generally only carries patients who are older than him: a shrinking pool of individuals as he approaches retirement. You suggest to Daniel that he should walk with you to the ambulance. He tries to stand, but the pain in his joints is too severe and he crumples into the coffee table and rolls about on the floor in agony. Pete sighs and heads out the door.

Carry chair

Despite Pete's usual rule of not carrying patients younger than him, when you suggest that Daniel might struggle to walk, he shrugs his shoulders and heads out the door to fetch the carry chair from the ambulance.

By the time he returns, Daniel's pain has reduced to a 7/10 from a high of 10/10. You elect to administer 5 mg of morphine subcutaneously and let Daniel continue with the Entonox while you fasten him into the chair and wheel him to the lift. By the time you arrive at the emergency department, and with another 5 mg of morphine administered, Daniel's pain is coming under control with a pain score of 5/10 and he looks more relaxed. You see Pete chatting with Daniel's partner and as you meet up at the ambulance having handed over, he is looking very pleased with himself. "What?" you enquire. "Santa's little helper has got him a second gig dishing out presents to children," he replies.

The scale of the problem

Sickle cell disease (SCD, or more accurately, homozygous sickle-cell anaemia) is the most commonly inherited red blood cell (RBC) disorder and is characterised by haemolysis and vaso-occlusion. It is typically found in people of African, Mediterranean and Asian descent and is associated with a range of symptoms and complications (Figure 2.7) including:[29]

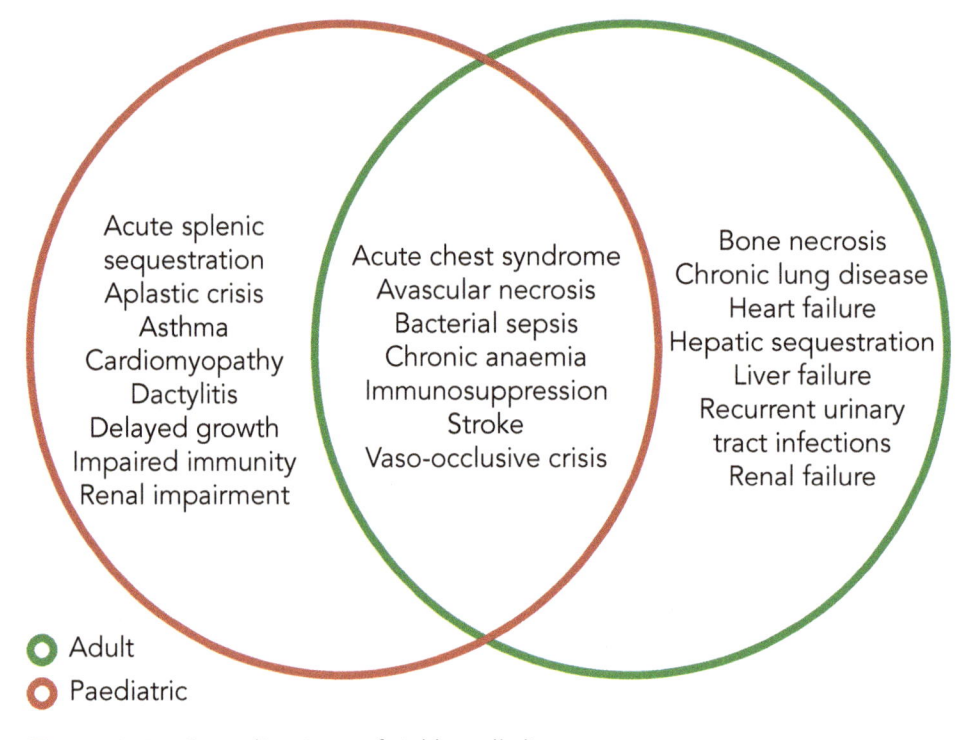

Paediatric only:
- Acute splenic sequestration
- Aplastic crisis
- Asthma
- Cardiomyopathy
- Dactylitis
- Delayed growth
- Impaired immunity
- Renal impairment

Both (Adult and Paediatric):
- Acute chest syndrome
- Avascular necrosis
- Bacterial sepsis
- Chronic anaemia
- Immunosuppression
- Stroke
- Vaso-occlusive crisis

Adult only:
- Bone necrosis
- Chronic lung disease
- Heart failure
- Hepatic sequestration
- Liver failure
- Recurrent urinary tract infections
- Renal failure

○ Adult
○ Paediatric

Figure 2.7 Complications of sickle cell disease.

- Acute and chronic pain
- Vaso-occlusive crises
- Multi-organ injury
- Decreased lifespan and quality of life.

There are in the region of 14,000 people with SCD in the UK, although this may be an underestimate due to immigration and new births.[30]

A quick primer in genetics

All human cells, except reproductive cells (gametes), contain 23 pairs of chromosomes: thread-like structures that contain DNA. One chromosome comes from the father and the other from the mother. They form pairs (homologues) that contain genes (portions of DNA that 'code' for a particular trait). If there are multiple forms of a gene that code for the same trait and that are found in the same position within a homologous chromosome, they are known as alleles.[7]

The possible combinations of these alleles, that result when a sperm fuses with an ovum at the moment of conception to create a zygote, are known as genotypes. In some cases, one allele will dominate over another as it is more likely to be passed on to the parents' children. Unsurprisingly, this is known as a dominant allele, whereas the less dominant allele is known as the recessive allele.

If the same alleles are found on homologous chromosomes, then they are said to be homozygous. If there are different alleles on a homologous chromosome, then they are heterozygous.

Anatomy and physiology

There are in the region of 5.4 million RBCs (erythrocytes) in the adult male, and 4.8 million RBCs in the adult female, per micro-litre of blood. They are biconcave discs with a strong and flexible membrane that tolerates being squeezed, as occurs when they travel around the micro-circulation (for example, capillaries). They are simple structures, with no nucleus or other organelles, such as mitochondria. As a result, they cannot reproduce or 'repair' themselves, and use anaerobic metabolism to create adenosine triphosphate (ATP, the energy source for the cell), which means that none of the oxygen carried by the cell is metabolised by itself.[7]

Haemoglobin

The lack of organelles in the RBC makes room for haemoglobin (Hb). In fact, each RBC contains approximately 280 million Hb (Figure 2.8). These are the oxygen-carrying proteins that contain a pigment (heme) that is responsible for giving RBCs their characteristic red colour. Normal adult haemoglobin (HbA, which replaces fetal haemoglobin, HbF, in infancy) contains four globin chains (alpha-1, alpha-2, beta-1, beta-2), each with a non-protein heme bound to it. At the centre of each heme is an iron ion (Fe^{2+}) which can bind reversibly with one oxygen molecule.[31]

The typical lifespan of a RBC is 120 days, due to the wear and tear caused by squeezing

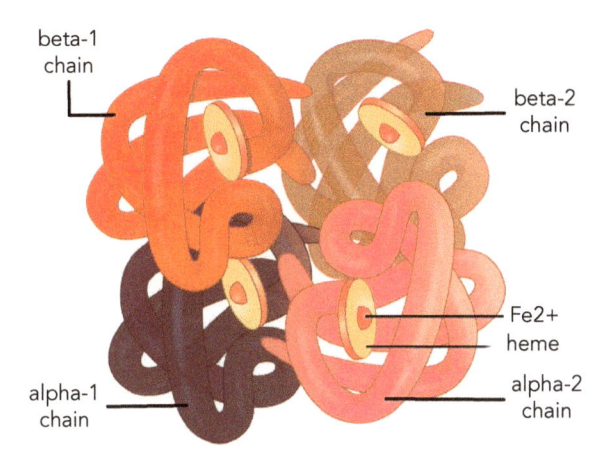

Figure 2.8 A haemoglobin molecule.
Source: OpenStax College [CC BY 3.0 (http://creativecommons.org/licenses/by/3.0)], via Wikimedia Commons.

Chapter 2 Circulation

through capillaries. Over time, the plasma membrane becomes increasingly fragile, making it prone to rupture. Should this occur, fixed phagocytic macrophages located in the liver and spleen remove them from the circulation and destroy them.[7]

Pathophysiology

SCD arises because of a genetic mutation of the beta-2 subunit of Hb, which leads to the formation of abnormal, sickle haemoglobin (HbS). Children with the homozygous dominant genotype form normal Hb; those with the heterozygous genotype are said to have the sickle-cell trait (HbAS). They are generally free from symptoms and have some protection from the most common type of malaria. However, since a proportion of their haemoglobin is HbS, they can become symptomatic when hypoxic, for example, due to severe respiratory illness, anaesthesia or travel in unpressurised aircraft.[32] Finally, there are those children who inherit the homozygous recessive genotype. They have homozygous sickle-cell anaemia (HbSS).

In addition, there are other, rarer, forms of SCD that arise when HbS combines with other forms of abnormal haemoglobin such as type C, E or beta-thalassaemia, for example. The most severe of these is HbSS and beta-thalassaemia major.

HbS differs from normal haemoglobin because the two beta chains bind together to form a polymer nucleus, which enlarges to fill the RBC. This process adversely affects the flexibility of the cell. When oxygen availability is reduced or demand is high, such as in hypoxia, stress or acidosis, HbS becomes dehydrated and changes shape forming stiff, rod-like structures which bend the RBC into its characteristic sickle (crescent) shape (Figure 2.9).[7]

These RBCs are fragile, with a reduced lifespan (typically 10–20 days), and due to their shape they can occlude the micro-circulation, which leads to ischaemia and infarction, and chronic haemolytic anaemia (a lack of RBCs due to abnormal RBC destruction).[33]

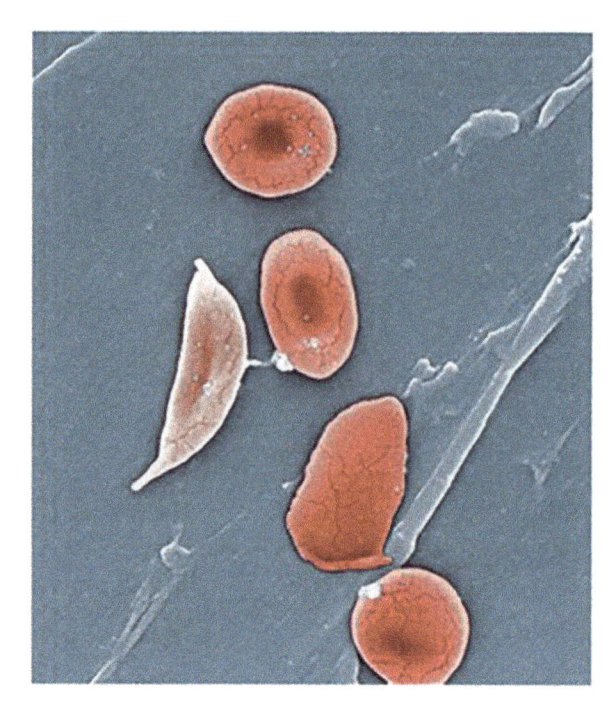

Figure 2.9 Sickle haemoglobin (left).
Source: OpenStax College [CC BY 3.0 (http://creativecommons.org/licenses/by/3.0)], via Wikimedia Commons.

Vascular occlusion occurs due to interaction between HbS and white blood cells (WBC). In addition, inflammatory processes increase adhesion between the vascular endothelium, HbS and WBC in the post-capillary venules. In the pre-capillary arterioles, the deformed, 'sickled' HbS causes obstruction. The dynamic interaction between the vascular endothelium and HbS causes a cycle of vascular occlusion followed by reperfusion that leads to tissue injury as a result of oxidative stress, and vascular enzyme and inflammatory cytokine release (Figure 2.10).[29,34]

Sickle Cell Disease

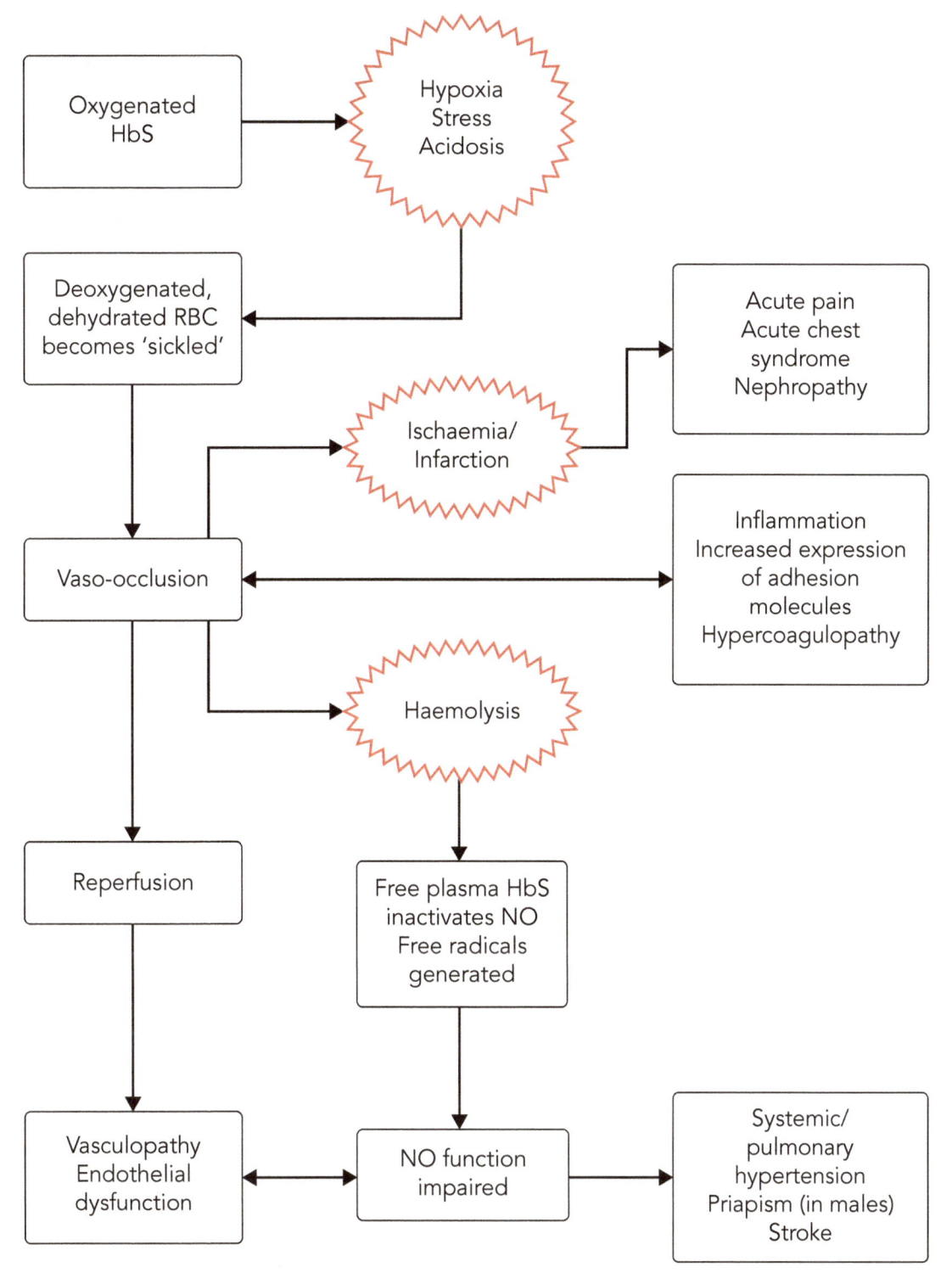

Figure 2.10 Pathophysiology of sickle cell disease.

Chapter 2 Circulation

Another important disease process in SCD is haemolytic anaemia, which is thought to be a contributory factor to vessel disease. The anaemia manifests as hypertension (systemic and pulmonary) as well as causing damage to vascular endothelium and smooth muscle.

Haemolysis also causes the release of HbS into the blood plasma, where it causes the generation of reactive oxygen species ('free radicals'). Some of these interfere with nitric oxide (NO) signalling. This is important because NO plays a key role in regulating base-level vascular tone and inhibits platelet activation and clotting, and reduces expression of endothelial adhesion molecules. Over time, the blood can become hypercoagulable.

Signs and symptoms

SCD is a multi-organ disease, leading to a range of symptoms and complications (generally covered by the umbrella term 'sickle cell crisis'), which vary in severity but generally worsen with age. Pain is the most common presenting symptom.

Vaso-occlusive crisis

This is the most common cause of admission in patients with SCD.[35] It is typically due to microvascular occlusion and is triggered by cold, dehydration, infection or hypoxia. In children less than 3 years of age, there may be painful swelling of the hands and feet (dactylitis). If the mesenteric circulation is affected, ischaemia can cause abdominal pain, while bone marrow involvement leads to back, pelvic, rib and long bone pain. Vaso-occlusion of the penis can lead to priapism (an unwanted, painful erection). If the central nervous system is affected, the patient can present with stroke or convulsions.[29]

Acute chest syndrome

The second most common reason for admission in SCD, this can be caused by infection, fat embolism caused by bone marrow necrosis or pulmonary infarction. This causes a range of signs and symptoms, including:[32]

- Shortness of breath
- Tachypnoea
- Hypoxia
- Cough
- Fever.

Splenic sequestration

This is mainly a complication in children since by adulthood, the spleen has atrophied. Splenic sequestration causes acute enlargement of the spleen with pooling of RBCs, severe anaemia and hypovolaemic shock. Sequestration can also occur in the liver.

Bacterial sepsis

Decreasing splenic function leads to increased susceptibility to infections. Newborn screening, prophylactic antibiotics and vaccines for *Haemophilus influenzae* and *Streptococcus pneumoniae* have helped to reduce child mortality, but they remain at increased risk of sepsis.

Aplastic crisis

This is caused by the parvovirus B19 which, in patients with sickle cell disease, can lead to a dramatic and sudden reduction in RBC production.[33]

Assessment

Patients with SCD who display any of the following signs or symptoms require urgent referral to hospital:[36]

- Severe pain not controlled by simple analgesia or low-dose opioids
- Dehydration caused by severe vomiting or diarrhoea
- Severe sepsis: temperature >38.5°C or >38°C if under 2 years old, temperature <36°C, or hypotension

- Symptoms or signs of acute chest syndrome including tachypnoea, oxygen saturation more than 5% below steady state, signs of lung consolidation
- New neurological symptoms or signs
- Symptoms or signs of acute fall in haemoglobin
- Acute enlargement of spleen or liver over 24 hours, particularly in young children
- Marked increase in jaundice
- Haematuria
- Sudden and severe priapism lasting more than two hours or worsening of recurrent episodes.

Follow the standard patient assessment approach, and if you see time-critical signs, promptly transport the patient to hospital and make a pre-alert call. If the patient has a treatment plan, follow it where possible.[10]

Management

Hydroxycarbamide (hydroxyurea) is the only drug that has been proven to reduce the incidence of painful crisis and acute chest syndrome.[37] However, it is not useful in the acute phase. Blood transfusions are important for reducing the risk of stroke in patients with SCD, but recurrent transfusions can lead to iron deposition in the organs, causing damage.

All patients with a sickle cell crisis should receive supplemental oxygen and it is better to over-oxygenate while preparing pulse oximetry measurement than to withhold oxygen. Aim for an SpO_2 of 94–98% and administer high concentrations to children. Patients who are wheezing due to bronchoconstriction may benefit from salbutamol.[35]

Perform a 12-lead ECG in patients with chest pain and always offer analgesia. Patients with severe pain ideally require opiate analgesia, but Entonox can be effective, although it should not be used for prolonged periods due to the risk of peripheral neuropathy.[38]

The UK clinical practice guidelines advocate giving morphine via the subcutaneous route where possible, with dosages guided by the patient's plan (if they have one). Where possible discourage patients from walking to the ambulance as this can exacerbate the effects of tissue hypoxia.[10]

If you have the option in your locality, transfer the patient to a specialist centre.

Chapter 2 Circulation

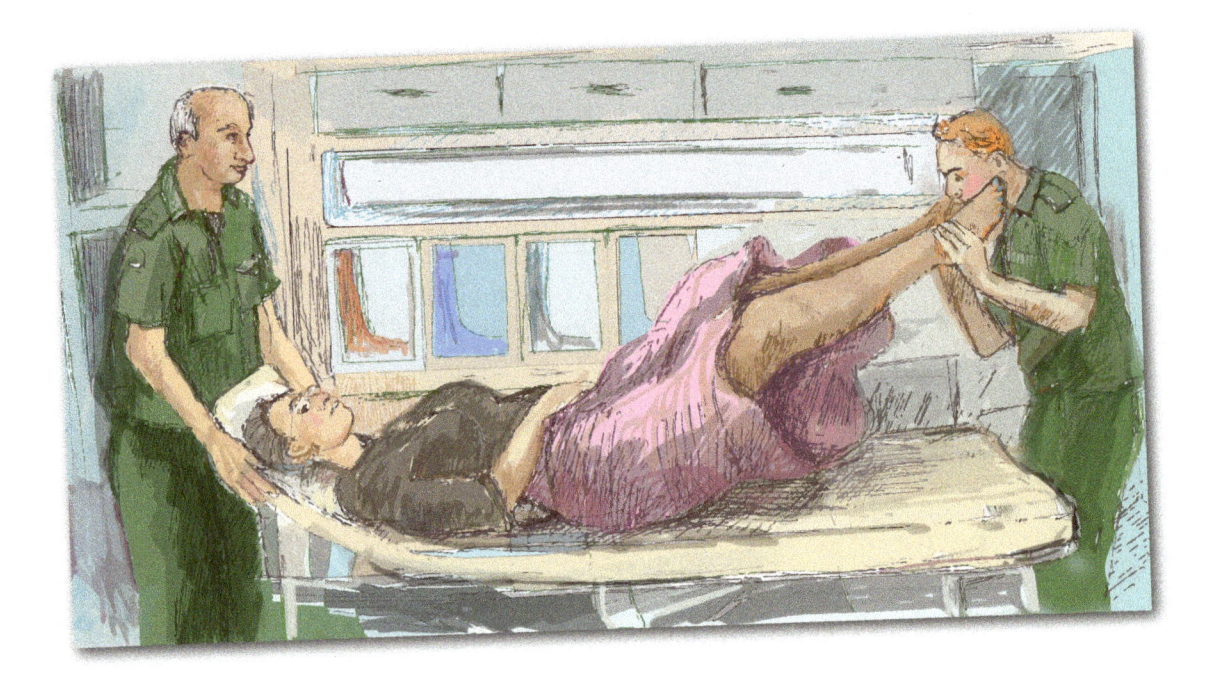

Tachyarrhythmias

You are on standby catching your breath after another relentless morning of emergency calls. The paramedic student who is riding along with you is busy trying to complete an essay that is due to be submitted in four days. By the looks of things, he hasn't actually got very far. Your colleague offers helpful words of advice about how you shouldn't leave things to the last minute, but you take pity on the furrow-browed student (called Niall) and offer to review one of the articles he is frantically trying to read. He explains that he is writing a case study related to a patient who had supraventricular tachycardia (SVT), who failed to revert with Valsalva manoeuvres and required adenosine in the emergency department (ED). Unfortunately, he has lost the notes he made about that case study and so is trying his hand at 'creative writing', which is not going well.

Although the title of the paper you've picked up is a bit of a mouthful (Postural modification to the standard Valsalva manoeuvre for emergency treatment of supraventricular tachycardias (REVERT): a randomised controlled trial),[39] the results look impressive. There's even a video showing how to perform the technique. You hand the article back to the student and suggest he reads this. His eyes widen but then his shoulders drop. "What's the chance we are going to see a patient with SVT today, though?" As if on cue, the MDT passes details of your next call: a 65-year-old woman with chest pain and palpitations … and a rapid heart rate.

You set off for the address, which is not far away, and before long you turn into the patient's street, where an anxious family member is frantically waving to attract your

Tachyarrhythmias

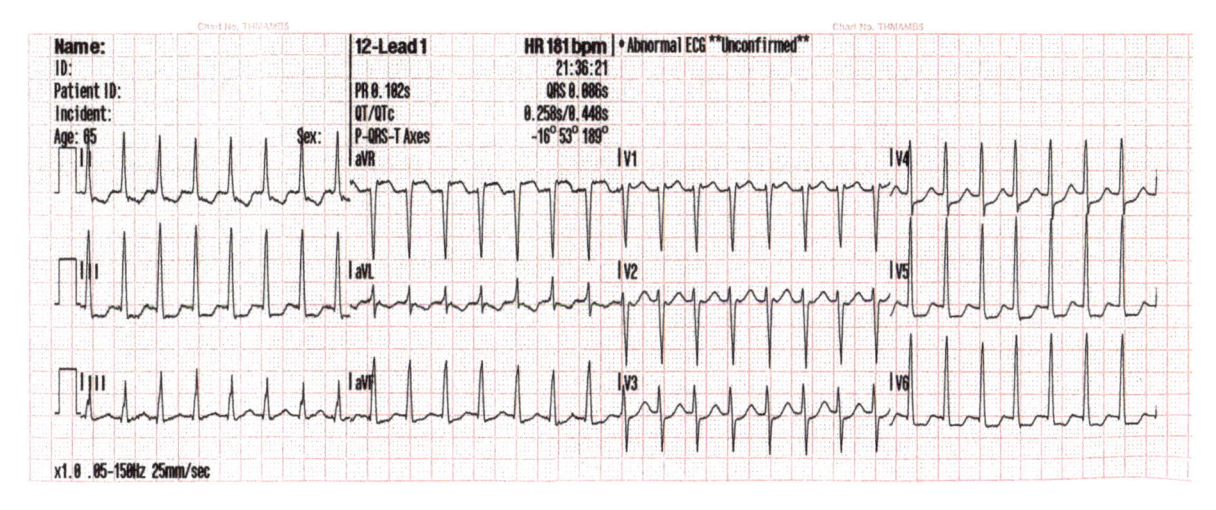

Figure 2.11 Brenda's initial ECG.

attention. You let Niall take the lead and he does a great job of introducing himself and encouraging the worried relative to lead the way to the patient, while you and your colleague follow up with the rest of the response kit.

In the living room, you find Brenda, the patient. She is looking a little pale and you notice that she is clutching her GTN spray. Niall is busy obtaining a set of baseline observations. He places his hand on Brenda's radial artery and looks up at you. "It must be over 150 beats per minute," he exclaims. Brenda explains that she has paroxysmal SVT and despite cutting out all of her 'pleasures' (smoking, alcohol and caffeine) as advised by her doctor, episodes of SVT are becoming more frequent. She is on a waiting list for an ablation but has not received a date for the procedure. While your colleague obtains a manual blood pressure, Niall gets busy connecting up the 12-lead ECG and recording a trace. While the machine acquires the ECG, Niall summarises the primary survey, noting that only the heart rate is abnormal. The monitor spits out the 12-lead ECG (Figure 2.11).

> What does it show: **Broad complex tachycardia** (read on) or a **Narrow complex tachycardia** (skip the next paragraph?

Broad complex tachycardia

You are just about to pronounce your diagnosis when Niall pipes up that it looks like a narrow complex tachycardia and, given the widespread ST-segment depression and Brenda's chest pain, cardiac ischaemia due to the high heart rate is likely. You knew that, didn't you?

Narrow complex tachycardia

You spot straight away that it's a narrow complex tachycardia, which is confirmed by the QRS duration being calculated as <0.12 seconds. Niall offers to interpret the ECG and comes to the correct conclusion, also noting that the widespread ST-segment

Chapter 2 Circulation

depression and chest pain are likely to be due to a heart rate-induced cardiac ischaemia. What a credit to your mentorship skills Niall is (apart from poor time-management with essay submissions, of course).

Brenda explains that she has tried all her usual vagal manoeuvres and they have failed to work. Previous episodes have only been terminated with adenosine, except for one, which was resolved with IV cannulation during a previous ambulance call-out. Given the history, Niall suggests that a trip to the local ED is necessary and asks your colleague if they would mind fetching the carry chair while he administers oxygen. The transfer from living room to ambulance trolley goes without a hitch. Brenda's signs and symptoms are unchanged.

> What are you going to do now: **Set off for hospital** (read on) or **Something else** (skip the next paragraph)?

Set off for hospital

There's nothing you can do for Brenda out-of-hospital: it sounds like she is going to need adenosine again. You turn to Niall to see what he suggests and you can see him staring at the attendant's seat. You follow his eye-line and spot the journal article about the modified Valsalva manoeuvre. He looks at you expectantly and after a pause, you shrug your shoulders. One attempt can't hurt, can it?

Something else

You spot Niall staring at the research article on the modified Valsalva manoeuvre and decide that it won't hurt to have one attempt before you set off. Niall gets busy dismantling the manual sphygmomanometer and trying to connect the manometer to a piece of oxygen tubing. It doesn't fit, but you point out that the 40 mmHg of pressure the patient is supposed to generate while blowing down the oxygen tubing is about the same pressure required to move the plunger on a 10 ml syringe. He explains the procedure to Brenda who, although she is sceptical, is happy to consent to having one attempt. Niall instructs her to blow into the syringe for 15 seconds with enough pressure to move the plunger. As soon as 15 seconds are up, you swiftly lay the patient flat while Niall elevates Brenda's legs. Everything goes according to plan, apart from Niall inadvertently splaying Brenda's legs as he elevates them, forcing him to look quickly away and causing his cheeks to turn scarlet.

Your colleague acquires a 12-lead ECG (Figure 2.12), but you can already see the result on the monitor: Brenda has reverted back to a normal sinus rhythm.

> What are you going to do now: **Set off for hospital** (read on) or **Something else** (skip the next two paragraphs)?

Set off for hospital

Over the next 5 minutes, Brenda's symptoms (including her chest pain) completely resolve and serial 12-lead ECGs continue to show a normal sinus rhythm and the ST-segments return to the baseline. Still, you need to transport Brenda, just in case, right? You explain that she needs a check-up at the local ED, which she is not too thrilled about.

Twenty minutes later, you arrive at a packed ED and given that Brenda's observations are back to normal, the consultant triaging shrugs his shoulders and sends Brenda into the waiting room. You can't help thinking that you could have done something else.

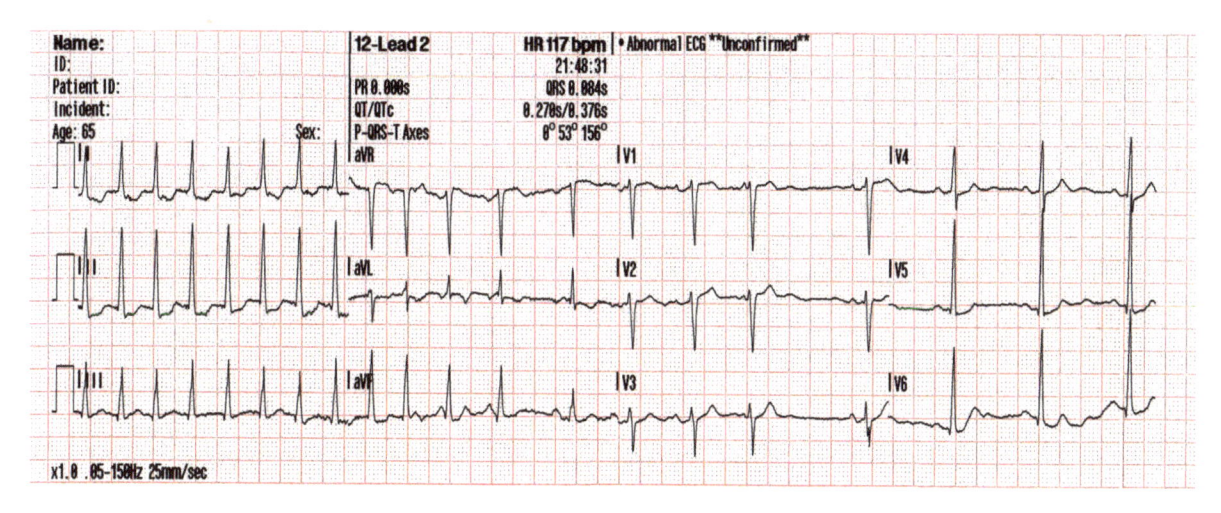

Figure 2.12 Brenda's 12-lead ECG after performing the modified Valsalva manoeuvre. Note the change back to normal sinus rhythm in leads V4–V6.

Something else

Repeated observations and enquiry into how Brenda is feeling reveal that she appears to be back to 'normal'. She even manages to stand up for three minutes, while you check for postural hypotension. You ask Brenda what she wants to do and she states that she really does not want to go to the ED on a Monday afternoon.

You enquire further about her cardiology referral and she mentions a letter she received relating to her last outpatient's appointment. An idea pops into your head. You escort Brenda back into the house, which she manages unaided. She digs out the letter and you ring the cardiology consultant's secretary and explain the situation. As luck would have it, the consultant's afternoon clinics have not started yet and she puts you through to her.

You nervously introduce yourself and explain what has happened. She is particularly impressed at you using the modified Valsalva manoeuvre and agrees that Brenda will not benefit from attending the ED. Instead, she makes her an outpatient's appointment for later in the week and agrees that Brenda has been waiting too long for her ablation and that she will "sort something out."

You relay your discussion with the consultant and Brenda is thrilled that a) she won't have to go to the ED now and b) that she is going to get her ablation organised. Niall has been busy completing the patient report form, ensuring appropriate safety netting is in place and providing written and verbal advice about when Brenda or her family should call back.

Scale of the problem

As the name implies, a tachyarrhythmia is an arrhythmia with a rate of 100 beats/min or greater. Importantly, this does not include sinus tachycardia. There are a number of different classifications of tachyarrhythmias, but in this instance, we are going to keep things simple and only consider whether the tachyarrhythmia has broad or narrow complexes and is regular or irregular.

Atrial fibrillation (AF) is the most common arrhythmia, with an estimated prevalence of 0.4–1%. This increases with age to around 9% of patients aged 80 years and above having AF.

Chapter 2 Circulation

Atrial flutter is far less common (incidence of 88 cases per 100,000 person-years), and is more common in males, older people and patients with chronic obstructive pulmonary disease and heart failure. It's over twice as common as the paroxysmal supraventricular tachycardias (PSVT), such as AV-nodal re-entry tachycardia (AVNRT), AV re-entry tachycardia (AVRT) and atrial tachycardia. PSVTs are more common in women and those over 65 years of age. The majority of PSVTs are due to AVNRTs.[40]

The incidence of ventricular tachyarrhythmias may be as high as 4%. They are more common in patients with coronary artery disease, post-myocardial infarction and cardiomyopathies.[41]

Re-entry tachycardias

The term re-entry refers to the return of an electrical impulse back to an area of the heart that had previously depolarised during the same complex. Ordinarily, cell-to-cell depolarisation, although slower than impulses travelling down the established conduction pathway, is fast enough that any electrical impulses returning to a previously depolarised area would find the cells still in their refractory period and unable to depolarise again.

The key to re-entry is the presence of an area of tissue where conduction is slowed, perhaps due to myocardial tissue damage, ischaemia, electrolyte abnormalities or increased wall tension because of high filling pressures.[40] In these cases, if the impulse returns to a previously depolarised area, the cells may be in their relative refractory period or completely repolarised and ready to depolarise again. This sets off another round of depolarisation, and the re-entry circuit (sometimes called a circus movement) is established.[42]

Re-entry circuits can be small (termed micro re-entry circuits), limited to a specific area of the heart, for instance the atrioventricular (AV) node, or large (macro), involving large areas of tissue in the atria or ventricles.

Atrial flutter

Atrial flutter is a macro re-entry circuit that can arise in the right atrium and causes depolarisation of both atria. The electrical impulse can travel around the atrium clockwise or anti-clockwise, which will affect the morphology (shape) of the wave on the electrocardiogram (ECG). There is no return to the isoelectric line in atrial flutter as it self-perpetuates. Instead, the ECG shows a constant stream of F (flutter) waves, which are referred to as sawtooth in appearance (Figure 2.13).

Atrial flutter generates approximately 300 F waves per minute. However, the AV node does not normally conduct every impulse, leading to a conduction ratio of 2:1 (that is, one ventricular impulse for every two atrial impulses) or 4:1, for example.[42]

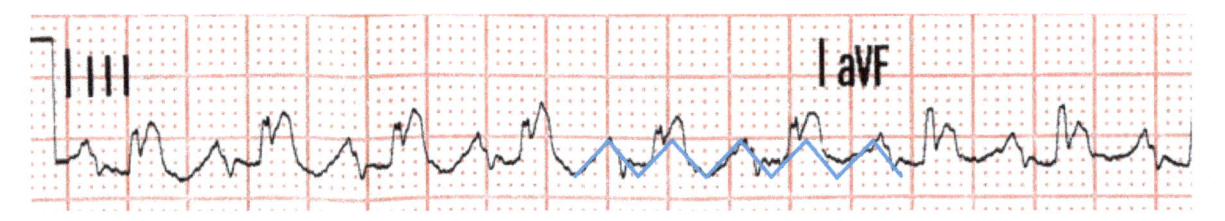

Figure 2.13 Atrial flutter. Note that conduction is 2:1, with half of the flutter waves obscured by the T-wave, which is abnormally elevated by the positive voltage of the flutter wave. Flutter waves are shown in blue.

Atrial fibrillation

This is probably the tachyarrhythmia you are most familiar with. It's an irregularly, irregular rhythm characterised by the absence of P waves. Instead, the chaotic atrial activity can be seen in the form of fibrillatory 'f' waves. As with their ventricular cousin, these can vary in coarseness, but are generally best seen in lead V1. AF comes in three flavours: paroxysmal, persistent and permanent. The first two can be corrected by cardioversion or drugs if treatment is commenced early.[43]

The AV node

The AV node is located within the triangle of Koch, an area of the right atrium bordered by the coronary sinus ostium, tendon of Todaro (I promise I'm not making these names up!) and septal leaflet of the tricuspid valve. It consists of two distinct areas: the compact node and lower nodal bundle, which is continuous with the Bundle of His. Surrounding the compact node is the transitional zone, so-called because the cells there share the morphology and function of both atrial and compact node cells.[44]

There are two extensions of the AV node, one extending proximally from the lower nodal bundle towards the coronary sinus (known as the inferior nodal or rightward extension) and the other extending from the compact node towards the coronary sinus (known as the leftward extension). Collectively, the AV node, extensions and surrounding atrial tissue are referred to as the AV junction, as there is considerable overlap in cell morphology and function.

Electrophysiology of the AV junction

The AV junction has two primary functions:[45]

- Protecting the ventricles from atrial tachyarrhythmias
- Serving as a backup pacemaker.

Just as anatomically there are two extensions of the AV node, there are also two conduction pathways within the AV junction. These are roughly in the same location as the lower nodal bundle extension and compact node extension. As the wave of atrial depolarisation spreads to the AV junction, both of these pathways are excited. However, the pathway closest to the compact node extension conducts impulses faster than the other. Thus, they are referred to as fast and slow pathways, respectively. In keeping with most excitable tissue in the body, the faster pathway has a longer refractory period than the slow pathway.

Normally, by the time the electrical impulse from the slow pathway arrives at the AV node, the cells are in their refractory period, having already been depolarised by the fast pathway. This means that neither antegrade (normal or forward direction) depolarisation towards the Bundle of His nor retrograde (reverse of backward direction) depolarisation up the fast pathway is possible.

AV-nodal re-entry tachycardia

If a premature atrial complex (PAC) is generated and arrives when the slow pathway is no longer in its refractory period, but the fast pathway is, then the electrical impulse propagates down the slow pathway (seen on the ECG as a prolonged PR interval). The AV node will depolarise as normal, but the impulse will also travel up (that is, retrograde) the fast pathway.

Once the impulse exits the fast pathway, the atria and AV junction will be depolarised (producing a P wave known as an 'echo beat'). However, by this time, the slow pathway, with its shortened refractory period, will be ready to depolarise again, and transmits the electrical impulse originating from the fast pathway antegrade towards the AV node via the slow pathway, and so the cycle, or re-entry

Chapter 2 Circulation

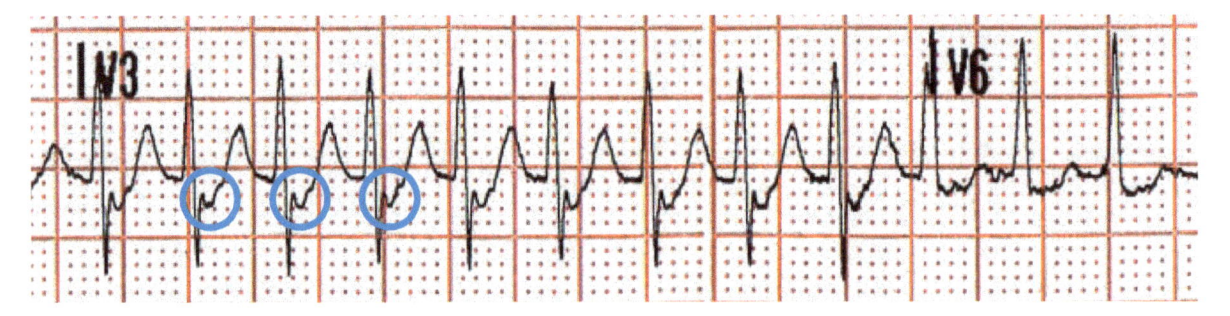

Figure 2.14 An example of a slow-fast AVNRT. The rate is around 220 beats/min and the retrograde P waves are shown by the blue circles.

circuit, begins again, leading to an AV-nodal re-entry tachycardia (AVNRT). This type of AVNRT is the most common and is referred to as a slow-fast AVNRT (due to the re-entry travelling down the slow pathway and then back up the fast, Figure 2.14).[46]

AV re-entry tachycardia

Ordinarily, the atria and ventricles are electrically insulated from one another, with the only access being the AV node. However, if the patient has an accessory pathway that connects the atria and ventricles, then a macro re-entry circuit can be created. The most common accessory pathway is the Bundle of Kent, producing a characteristic ECG complex famously described by Drs Wolff, Parkinson and White. However, there are others, such as Mahaim fibres, but they are not covered here.[47]

Unlike the AV node, the accessory pathway does not delay conduction between the atria and ventricles and so propagates electrical impulses as soon as they are received. Typically, impulses arrive at the AV node and accessory pathway at the same time. The AV node holds its impulse, while the accessory pathway initiates cell-to-cell depolarisation of the ventricle. This causes a wide and bizarre pattern on the ECG since it is much slower than normal conduction via the Bundle of His, bundle branches and Purkinje fibres. However, once the AV node releases its impulse, normal conduction can resume and the remainder of the ECG complex looks normal. However, the initial ventricular depolarisation is visible as a slurred upstroke on the QRS complex known as a delta wave, which results in a shortened PR interval and wide QRS (Figure 2.15).[42]

In the event that a PAC occurs during the accessory pathway refractory period, but is able to conduct through the AV node, the impulse follows the usual conduction pathway and depolarises the ventricle. However, by the time the impulse arrives

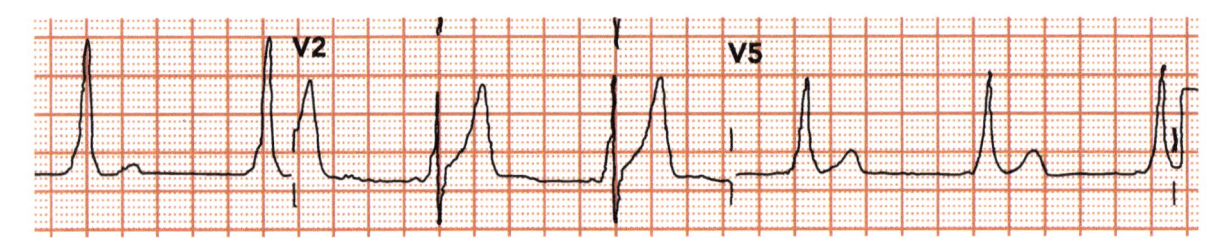

Figure 2.15 Wolff–Parkinson–White ECG complexes.

at the accessory pathway, it is no longer refractory and is able to transmit the impulse in a retrograde fashion to the atria, causing atrial depolarisation and another impulse to be sent to the AV node. This results in a tachycardia referred to as orthodromic AVRT, and is the most common form. The key advantage of this form of AVRT is that the AV node still has control over the propagation of atrial impulses. This means that drugs which delay AV-nodal conduction can terminate the arrhythmia.

The less common variant (<10% of cases) is antidromic AVRT. As the name suggests, impulses travel in the opposite direction, travelling in a retrograde fashion through the AV node, where conduction is not delayed. As a result, ventricular and atrial rates become harmonised. So, if the patient is in atrial flutter for example, then the ventricular rate will attempt to match the atrial rate of 300 beats/min, which can increase the risk of VF.[40]

Drugs that slow AV conduction do not work on accessory pathways and in the case of antidromic AVRT can actually make the problem worse.

Ventricular tachycardia

Ventricular tachycardias (VT) are most commonly seen in patients with cardiac disease, although some cases are idiopathic. If VT lasts for less than 30 seconds it is termed 'non-sustained'.[41] Can you guess what it is called if it lasts for more than 30 seconds?

Sustained VT most commonly occurs as a result of an interventricular re-entry circuit. These typically arise in patients who have a previous history of myocardial infarction or cardiomyopathy. The damaged myocardium and/or scarring leave areas of non-conductive tissue. However, if there is collateral circulation, small 'bridges' of living and conductive myocardium can exist and link to other undamaged tissue. If this 'bridge' depolarises at a slower speed than tissue it links to, a re-entry circuit can be created.

Other, less common causes of VT include those that directly affect the cardiac action potential by causing abnormal depolarisation (afterdepolarisation). If they interrupt phases 2 or 3 of the action potential, they are termed early afterdepolarisation (EAD), and late if they occur during phase 4. EADs are responsible for torsade de pointes, a rotating polymorphic tachycardia.

Assessment and management

Although there are numerous tachyarrhythmias and a precise diagnosis can be challenging, you only need to consider three questions:

1. Is the patient stable?
2. Is the QRS narrow or broad?
3. Is the QRS complex regular?

Adverse signs

When deciding if your patient is stable, look for the following adverse signs:[28]

- Shock – Signs of increased sympathetic activity, for example, pallor, sweating, cool peripheries, hypotension (usually taken to be systolic BP <90 mmHg) and altered level of consciousness
- Syncope – Loss of consciousness
- Myocardial ischaemia – Cardiac chest pain and/or indicative 12-lead ECG, for example, widespread ST-segment depression
- Severe heart failure – Acute pulmonary oedema, raised jugular venous pressure and hepatic engorgement.

Note: unstable tachyarrhythmias are uncommon if the heart rate is less than 150 beats/min.

Cardioversion

Current resuscitation guidelines recommend that patients with adverse signs should be cardioverted. This is problematic for most ambulance staff as conscious sedation is not routinely available. However, cardioversion is painful, so unless your patient is unconscious, you will not be able to undertake this procedure.

Cardioversion is defibrillation with one important difference: the timing of the shock. Delivering a shock during the up-slope or peak of the T-wave is a reliable way of inducing VF. In fact, this is used to test ICDs.[48] Although you know how to treat VF, sending your patient into cardiac arrest in order to revert their arrhythmia is frowned upon.

The procedure for cardioversion varies by device, but the general principles are the same:

1. For broad complex tachycardias (likely to be the only tachyarrhythmia you are permitted to cardiovert), place defibrillator pads on the patient as you would for defibrillation.
2. Remove oxygen.
3. Press the sync button and check that each R wave has a marker signifying that the monitor has detected the complex.
4. Select the correct energy setting. You'll need to follow local guidance on this.
5. Press and hold the shock button until the defibrillator discharges. There is likely to be a small delay as the shock will be timed with the next R waves.
6. After each shock, reassess the patient, their pulse and the ECG. Check to see whether the sync function is disabled after the shock. If it is, make sure you turn it back on before your next shock.
7. After the third shock, administer amiodarone, 300 mg IV over 10–20 minutes. Note that amiodarone is only indicated for cardiac arrest in the clinical practice guidelines,[10] so you'll need a patient group direction (PGD) for this.

Amiodarone is a membrane stabilising drug, increasing action potential duration and the refractory period of both atrial and ventricular myocytes. It can cause hypotension, although this is more often due to the solvents used in the preparation, which cause histamine release, rather than the amiodarone itself. This side effect is related to the speed of administration, which is why it is given over a longer time in stable arrhythmias.[49]

Narrow complex tachycardia

If your patient has no adverse signs, they are stable (for now), then you have time to examine the rhythm in more detail. If the QRS complex is <0.12 seconds, it's a narrow complex tachycardia (NCT).

Remember, the most common NCT is sinus tachycardia. This rhythm does not need cardioverting or anti-arrhythmic drugs. Instead, you should identify the underlying causes and treat those.

If the rhythm is regular and you have excluded sinus tachycardia, the most likely cause is AVNRT. There are two treatments for this: vagal manoeuvres (such as the Valsalva manoeuvre) and adenosine. It is unlikely that you will be administering adenosine, so we'll focus on vagal manoeuvres.

Valsalva manoeuvres

Evidence from REVERT suggests that lying patients flat, elevating their legs and asking them to blow into a 10 ml syringe with sufficient force to move the plunger, as in the case study, can dramatically increase the chance of the procedure working. Two attempts are recommended, but this should be avoided in some cases:[39]

- Aortic stenosis
- Recent MI

- Glaucoma
- Retinopathy
- Third trimester of pregnancy.

Broad complex tachycardia

The 2021 resuscitation guidelines introduced vagal manoeuvres for broad complex tachycardias in addition to SVT. However, if these are ineffective, then amiodarone, 300 mg IV over 10–60 minutes can be administered.[28] Follow your PGD. Irregular broad complex tachycardias (BCTs) are most likely to be caused by atrial fibrillation with a bundle branch block. The mainstay of treatment is rate control drugs, which is beyond the scope of most ambulance crews.

Chapter 2 Circulation

References

1. British Heart Foundation. UK Factsheet [Internet]. 2020. Available from: https://www.bhf.org.uk/-/media/files/research/heart-statistics/bhf-cvd-statistics-uk-factsheet.pdf
2. Burns E, Buttner R. Inferior STEMI [Internet]. Life in the Fast Lane (LITFL). 2021. Available from: https://litfl.com/inferior-stemi-ecg-library/
3. Ibanez B, James S, Agewall S, Antunes MJ, Bucciarelli-Ducci C, Bueno H, et al. 2017 ESC Guidelines for the management of acute myocardial infarction in patients presenting with ST-segment elevationThe Task Force for the management of acute myocardial infarction in patients presenting with ST-segment elevation of the European Society of Cardiology (ESC). *European Heart Journal*, 2018 Jan 7;39(2):119–177.
4. Smithuis R, Willems T. Coronary anatomy and anomalies [Internet]. The Radiology Assistant. 2008. Available from: https://radiologyassistant.nl/cardiovascular/anatomy/coronary-anatomy-and-anomalies
5. Goldberg A, Southern DA, Galbraith PD, Traboulsi M, Knudtson ML, Ghali WA. Coronary dominance and prognosis of patients with acute coronary syndrome. *American Heart Journal*, 2007 Dec;154(6):1116–1122.
6. Drake RL, Vogl W, Mitchell AWM, Gray H. *Gray's anatomy for students*, 3rd edition. Philadelphia, PA: Churchill Livingstone/Elsevier; 2015.
7. Marieb E, Hoehn K. Human Anatomy & Physiology, 11th edition. Pearson; 2019.
8. Haddad F, Hunt SA, Rosenthal DN, Murphy DJ. Right ventricular function in cardiovascular disease, Part I: anatomy, physiology, aging, and functional assessment of the right ventricle. *Circulation*, 2008 Mar 18;117(11):1436–1448.
9. Saw J, Davies C, Fung A, Spinelli JJ, Jue J. Value of ST elevation in lead III greater than lead II in inferior wall acute myocardial infarction for predicting in-hospital mortality and diagnosing right ventricular infarction. *American Journal of Cardiology*, 2001 Feb 15;87(4):448–450.
10. Joint Royal Colleges Ambulance Liaison Committee, Association of Ambulance Chief Executives. JRCALC Clinical Guidelines. Cited from JRCALC Plus (Version 1.2.13) [Mobile application software]. Bridgwater: Class Publishing Ltd; 2021.
11. Goldstein JA. Pathophysiology and management of right heart ischemia. *Journal of the American College of Cardiology*, 2002 Sep 4;40(5):841–853.
12. Ward C, Henderson S, Metcalfe NH. A short history on pacemakers. *International Journal of Cardiology*, 2013 Nov 15;169(4):244–248.
13. Deyell MW, Tung S, Ignaszewski A. The implantable cardioverter-defibrillator: from Mirowski to its current use. British Columbia Medical Journal, 2010;52(5):248–253.
14. National Institute for Cardiovascular Outcomes Research. National Audit of Cardiac Rhythm Management (NACRM) summary report [Internet]. 2020. Available from: https://www.nicor.org.uk/national-cardiac-audit-programme/cardiac-rhythm-management-arrhythmia-audit/
15. Timperley J, Leeson P, Mitchell AR, Betts T, editors. *Pacemakers and ICDs*, 2nd edition. Oxford: OUP Oxford; 2019.
16. Ellenbogen KA, Kaszala K. Cardiac Pacing and ICDs [Internet]. Hoboken/UK John Wiley & Sons, Incorporated; 2014. Available from: http://ebookcentral.proquest.com/lib/shu/detail.action?docID=1650822
17. Verma N, Knight BP. Update in cardiac pacing. Arrhythmia & Electrophysiology Review, 2019 Jul;8(3):228–233.
18. National Institute for Health and Care Excellence. Leadless cardiac pacemaker implantation for bradyarrhythmias [Internet]. 2018. Available from: https://www.nice.org.uk/guidance/ipg626/resources/leadless-cardiac-pacemaker-implantation-for-bradyarrhythmias-pdf-1899873986002117
19. Bernstein AD, Daubert J-C, Fletcher RD, Hayes DL, Lüderitz B, Reynolds DW, et al. The revised NASPE/BPEG generic code for antibradycardia, adaptive-rate, and multisite pacing. Pacing and Clinical Electrophysiology, 2002;25(2):260–264.
20. Rajappan K. Permanent pacemaker implantation technique: part I. *Heart*, 2008 Nov 25;95(3):259–264.

21. Brignole M, Auricchio A, Baron-Esquivias G, Bordachar P, Boriani G, Breithardt O-A, et al. 2013 ESC Guidelines on cardiac pacing and cardiac resynchronization therapy. European Heart Journal, 2013 Aug 1;34(29):2281–2329.
22. The Criteria Committee of the New York Heart Association. *Nomenclature and criteria for diagnosis of diseases of the heart and great vessels*, 9th edition *by Dolgin, Martin (1994) Paperback*. Boston: Little, Brown and Co; 1994.
23. National Institute for Health and Care Excellence. Implantable cardioverter defibrillators and cardiac resynchronisation therapy for arrhythmias and heart failure [Internet]. 2014. Available from: https://nice.org.uk/guidance/ta314
24. Al-Khatib SM, Stevenson WG, Ackerman MJ, Bryant WJ, Callans DJ, Curtis AB, et al. 2017 AHA/ACC/HRS Guideline for management of patients with ventricular arrhythmias and the prevention of sudden cardiac death. Journal of the American College of Cardiology, 2018 Oct;72(14):e91–220.
25. McMullan J, Valento M, Attari M, Venkat A. Care of the pacemaker/implantable cardioverter defibrillator patient in the ED. *American Journal of Emergency Medicine*, 2007 Sep;25(7):812–822.
26. Allison MG, Mallemat HA. Emergency care of patients with pacemakers and defibrillators. Emergency Medicine Clinics of North America, 2015 Aug;33(3):653–667.
27. Salahuddin M, Cader FA, Nasrin S, Chowdhury MZ. The pacemaker-twiddler's syndrome: an infrequent cause of pacemaker failure. *BMC Research Notes*, 2016 Jan 20;9(1):32.
28. Soar J, Böttiger BW, Carli P, Couper K, Deakin CD, Djärv T, et al. European Resuscitation Council Guidelines 2021: Adult advanced life support. *Resuscitation*, 2021 Apr;161:115–151.
29. Piel FB, Steinberg MH, Rees DC. Sickle Cell Disease. Longo DL, editor. New England Journal of Medicine, 2017 Apr 20;376(16):1561–1573.
30. Dormandy E, James J, Inusa B, Rees D. How many people have sickle cell disease in the UK? *Journal of Public Health*, 2018 Sep 1;40(3):e291–295.
31. Mehta A, Hoffbrand V. *Haematology at a glance*, 4th edition. Chichester: Wiley-Blackwell; 2014.
32. Wilkinson IB, Raine T, Wiles K, Goodhart A, Hall C, O'Neill H. *Oxford handbook of clinical medicine*, 10th edition. Oxford: OUP Oxford; 2017.
33. Kanter J, Kruse-Jarres R. Management of sickle cell disease from childhood through adulthood. *Blood Reviews*, 2013 Nov;27(6):279–287.
34. Rees DC, Williams TN, Gladwin MT. Sickle-cell disease. *The Lancet*, 2010;376(9757):2018–2031.
35. Brousse V, Makani J, Rees DC. Management of sickle cell disease in the community. *British Medical Journal*, 2014 Mar 10;348(mar10 11):g1765–g1765.
36. Chakravorty S, Williams TN. Sickle cell disease: a neglected chronic disease of increasing global health importance. *Archives of Disease in Childhood*, 2015 Jan 1;100(1):48–53.
37. Qureshi A, Kaya B, Pancham S, Keenan R, Anderson J, Akanni M, et al. Guidelines for the use of hydroxycarbamide in children and adults with sickle cell disease. *British Journal of Haematology*, 2018;181(4):460–475.
38. Rees DC, Olujohungbe AD, Parker NE, Stephens AD, Telfer P, Wright J. Guidelines for the management of the acute painful crisis in sickle cell disease. *British Journal of Haematology*, 2003;120(5):744–752.
39. Appelboam A, Reuben A, Mann C, Gagg J, Ewings P, Barton A, et al. Postural modification to the standard Valsalva manoeuvre for emergency treatment of supraventricular tachycardias (REVERT): a randomised controlled trial. *The Lancet*, 2015;386(10005):1747–1753.
40. Shadman R, Rho RW. Assessment of tachycardia [Internet]. 2018. Available from: https://bestpractice.bmj.com/topics/en-gb/830
41. Kusumoto F, Butendieck R. Non-sustained ventricular tachycardias [Internet]. 2020. Available from: https://bestpractice.bmj.com/topics/en-gb/831
42. Garcia TB, Garcia DJ. *Arrhythmia recognition: The art of interpretation*, 2nd edition. Burlington, Massachusetts: Jones and Bartlett Publishers, Inc; 2019.

43. Hindricks G, Potpara T, Dagres N, Arbelo E, Bax JJ, Blomström-Lundqvist C, et al. 2020 ESC Guidelines for the diagnosis and management of atrial fibrillation developed in collaboration with the European Association for Cardio-Thoracic Surgery (EACTS). *European Heart Journal*, 2021 Feb 1;42(5):373–498.
44. Kurian T, Ambrosi C, Hucker W, Fedorov VV, Efimov IR. Anatomy and electrophysiology if the human AV node. Pacing and Clinical Electrophysiology, 2010 Jun 1;33(6):754–62.
45. Mani BC, Pavri BB. Dual atrioventricular nodal pathways physiology: A review of relevant anatomy, electrophysiology, and electrocardiographic manifestations. Indian Pacing and Electrophysiology Journal, 2014 Jan 1;14(1):12–25.
46. Iaizzo PA, editor. *Handbook of cardiac anatomy, physiology, and devices*, 3rd edition. Springer; 2015.
47. Bhatia A, Sra J, Akhtar M. Preexcitation syndromes. Current Problems in Cardiology, 2016 Mar;41(3):99–137.
48. Day JD, Doshi RN, Belott P, Birgersdotter-Green U, Behboodikhah M, Ott P, et al. Inductionless or limited shock testing is possible in most patients with implantable cardioverter- defibrillators/cardiac resynchronization therapy defibrillators results of the multicenter ASSURE study (Arrhythmia Single Shock defibrillation threshold testing versus Upper limit of vulnerability: Risk reduction Evaluation with implantable cardioverter-defibrillator implantations). *Circulation*, 2007 Aug 5;115(18):2382–2389.
49. Lindquist DE, Rowe AS, Heidel E, Fleming T, Yates JR. Evaluation of the hemodynamic effects of intravenous amiodarone formulations during the maintenance phase infusion. Annals of Pharmacotherapy, 2015 Dec 1;49(12):1317–1321.

3

Disability

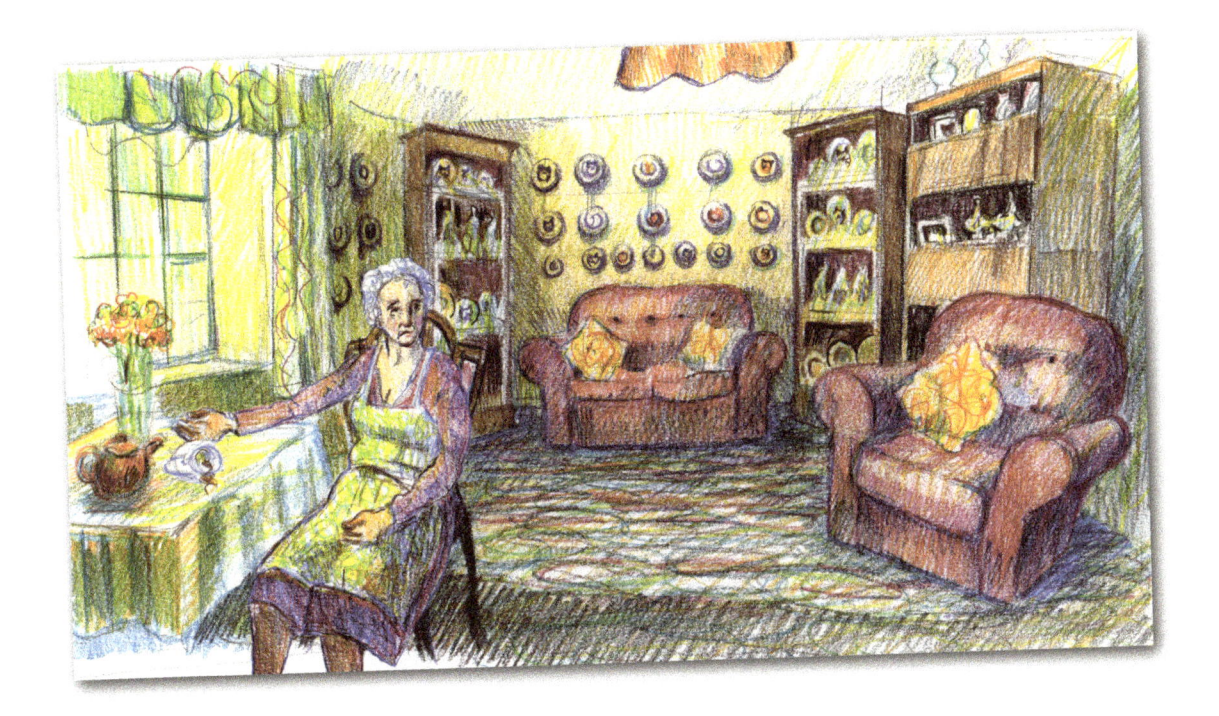

Brain Attack

With Katie Duncan

You are on standby, mulling over the redecoration of your living room. Having been unable to settle on the colour scheme, you decide to take note of the décor of your patients' homes.

You do not have to wait long as you are sent to a 65-year-old female. As you arrive on scene, you find a very smart-looking house with an impeccable frontage. You are looking forward to seeing the interior design of this house … as well as providing top-quality, evidence-based healthcare for the patient, of course.

The patient's husband greets you at the door and leads you into the living room. The door opens and your jaw drops. The walls are covered in a collection of the most nausea-inducing cat plates. It takes you a moment to recover and spot the patient, who is sat next to a table. Her morning cup of tea is beside her and appears to have been knocked over.

"Good morning," you say by way of introduction, "I am from the ambulance service. How can I help you today?"

Chapter 3 Disability

Your patient, Betty, tries to say something, but no words come out. You can clearly see a right-sided facial weakness and her right arm is resting on the table. Her husband tries to fill in the silence with a quip, "Normally, I can't get her to stop talking," he jokes, but as the smile runs away from his face, it's replaced by a look of anxiety. Since the patient cannot speak, you obtain a brief history from her husband, who informs you that just after he brought Betty her tea, she started to slur her speech and, soon after, stopped speaking altogether. This occurred around 20 minutes before you arrived. She has never suffered anything like this before and her medical history is as follows:

- Diabetes mellitus
- Hypertension
- Hypercholesterolaemia
- Previous myocardial infarction.

What are you going to do now: **Administer oxygen** (read on) or **Check the blood glucose** (skip the next paragraph)?

Administer oxygen

As you reach for your oxygen bag and pull out a mask, your colleague waves their phone in front of your face. They have the *JRCALC Clinical Guidelines* app (JRCALC Plus) open on the oxygen administration page. You are reminded that with the exception of COPD (and other risk factors for hypercapnia), oxygen saturations should be maintained in the range 94–98%.[1] Since the patient's oxygen saturations are currently 94%, you revise your decision to administer oxygen and go digging in your response bag for the blood glucose machine instead.

Check the blood glucose

You recall that hypoglycaemia can mimic the signs of a stroke and since the patient is a diabetic, this is a possibility. You check her blood sugar and relish the prospect of 'curing' the patient with a swift bolus of 10% glucose. Alas, her blood sugar is 8.1 mmol/l.

You load the patient onto the ambulance and get Betty comfortable, taking care to avoid trapping her arm which dangles over the side of the ambulance trolley. Your colleague asks if you are ready to go to hospital and suggests the closest emergency department (ED) as the destination, since it is only 10 minutes away. It is generally recognised as the worst in the region and the hospital does not have a CT scanner. There is another hospital with an acute stroke unit, but that is 25 minutes away.

Where should you go: **The nearest ED** (read on) or **The hyper acute stroke unit (HASU)** (skip the next paragraph)?

The nearest ED

The patient is really sick, bypassing a local hospital is always really risky, right? I mean, what if they don't make it to the one further away? You pre-alert the ED and after carefully explaining the patient's signs, symptoms and giving your estimated time of arrival, they are rather off-hand with you and ask if you had considered taking them to the acute stroke unit. Not fancying the reception you are going to get if you carry on, you elect to change destination and head for the HASU.

The hyper acute stroke unit

You know that this patient will not be adequately cared for in the local ED and elect to bypass it in favour of the HASU, where you know the patient can have a CT scan and perhaps be thrombolysed or undergo clot retrieval (thrombectomy), if appropriate.[2] You explain to Betty and her husband the reason for the change of destination.

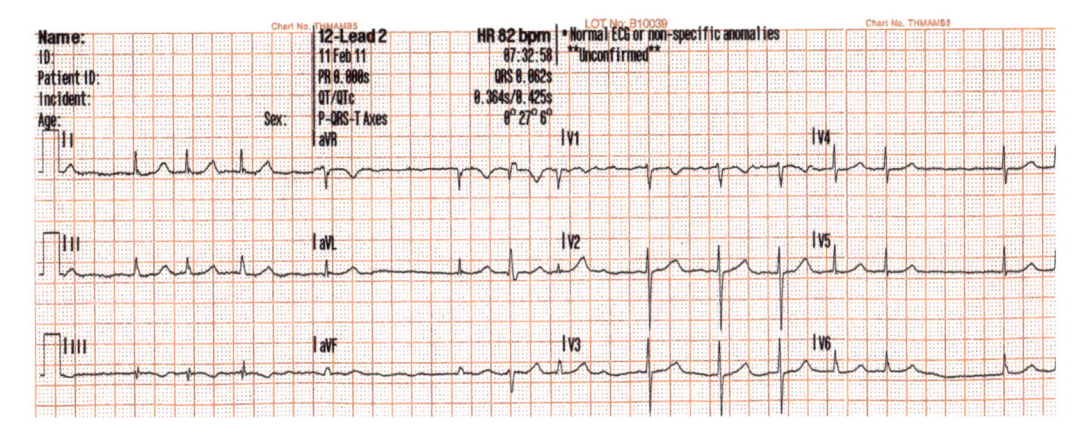

Figure 3.1 Betty's 12-lead ECG.

Due to the increased travel time to hospital, you record a 12-lead ECG en route (Figure 3.1) in addition to the 3-lead ECG monitoring, and have a rustle through the bag that Betty's husband placed her medication in. You find the following:

- Gliclazide
- Aspirin
- Amlodipine
- Bendroflumethiazide
- Atorvastatin
- Insulin (Humulin M3).

On arrival, you are met by the stroke nurse and hand over. You find out later that the CT scan showed an ischaemic stroke and that Betty was thrombolysed. She is now doing really well.

The scale of the problem

Stroke is defined as a clinical syndrome, of presumed vascular origin, typified by rapidly developing signs of focal or global disturbance of cerebral functions lasting more than 24 hours or leading to death.[3] A transient ischaemic attack is essentially the same thing as a stroke, with the exception of the duration of symptoms, which are less than 24 hours and not caused by a haemorrhage.

Stroke is the fourth biggest killer in the UK and over 100,000 strokes occur in the UK every year. Stroke is the second leading cause of death worldwide, causing around 6.2 million deaths each year. Anyone of any age can have a stroke, including babies and children, and there are over 400 childhood strokes occurring every year in the UK.[4] Around £3 billion a year is spent by the NHS in direct care costs for patients who have suffered a stroke.[5]

Anatomy and physiology

The brain cannot store oxygen or glucose and so is dependent on a constant supply of blood, which is provided by two pairs of vessels, the vertebral and internal carotid arteries (Figure 3.2). These arteries are interconnected in the cranial cavity to produce an arterial circle (the Circle of Willis, Figure 3.3), which provides an alternative pathway for blood flow should one of the vessels become occluded.[6]

The internal carotid arteries carry over 70% of the cerebral blood flow and branch into several arteries including the ophthalmic, posterior communicating, and anterior choroidal.

Chapter 3 Disability

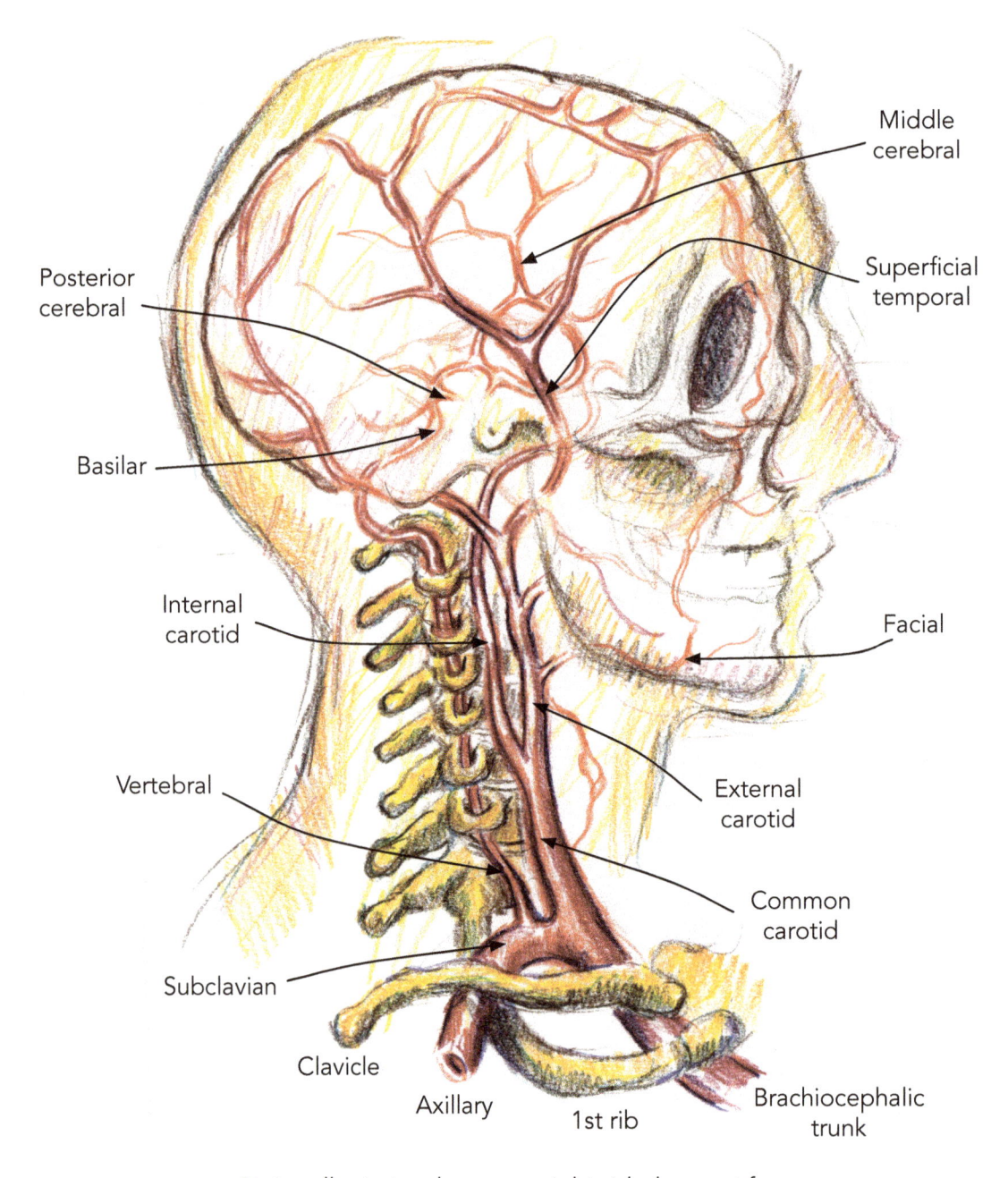

Note: all arteries shown are right sided except for the basilar artery and brachiocephalic trunk

Figure 3.2   Lateral view of arteries supplying the brain.

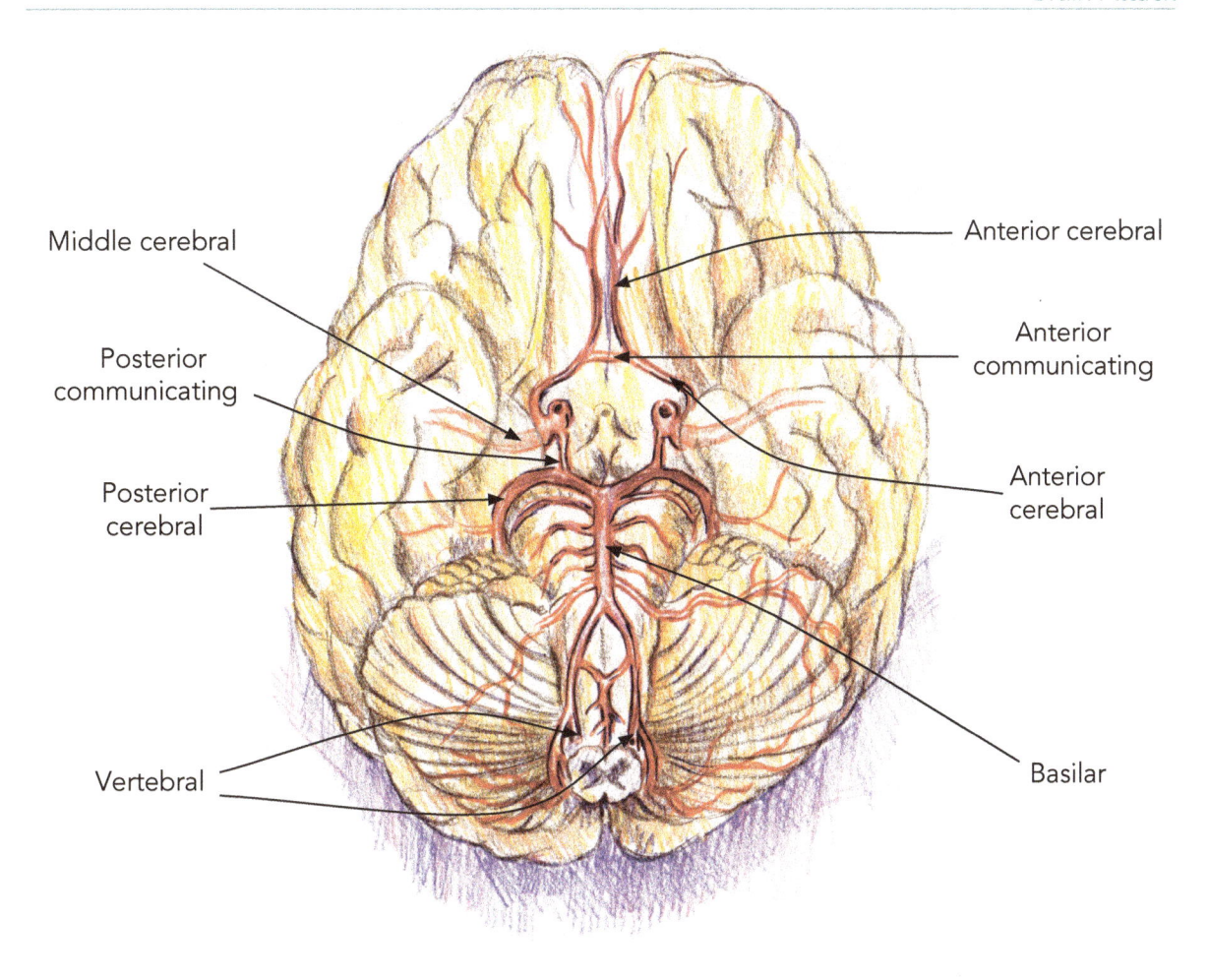

Figure 3.3 Inferior view of the arteries of the brain.

The internal carotid arteries terminate by dividing into the anterior and middle cerebral arteries. The anterior cerebral arteries supply most of the medial and superior surfaces of the brain and frontal lobe. The middle cerebral artery supplies the lateral surface of the brain, including the primary motor and sensory areas of the face and upper limbs, the optic radiations and speech areas of the brain (in the dominant hemisphere).[7]

The two vertebral arteries join together to form the basilar artery. Branches of these arteries supply the brainstem and cerebellum. The basilar artery terminates by splitting into the two posterior cerebral arteries, which supply the occipital and inferior regions of the temporal lobes and the thalamus.[7]

Risk factors

Non-modifiable risk factors for stroke include age, sex, race and family or previous medical history of stroke, transient ischaemic attacks or myocardial infarction. The chance of having

Chapter 3 Disability

a stroke roughly doubles each decade after the age of 55 years and although it is more common in men, over half of all stroke deaths occur in women. People of South Asian, African or African-Caribbean origin are more likely to suffer from a stroke.[8]

Modifiable risk factors include hypertension, smoking, atrial fibrillation, diabetes, diet, physical activity, alcohol consumption, blood cholesterol and obesity.[9,10]

Causes and pathophysiology

Strokes can be classified as either ischaemic or haemorrhagic in origin. Ischaemic strokes are the most common, responsible for around 80–85% of all new strokes, and are the focus for the rest of this issue.[4,9] There are a number of causes of ischaemic stroke (Figure 3.4), although in many cases, the exact cause is never found (and labelled cryptogenic). Possible causes include:[11]

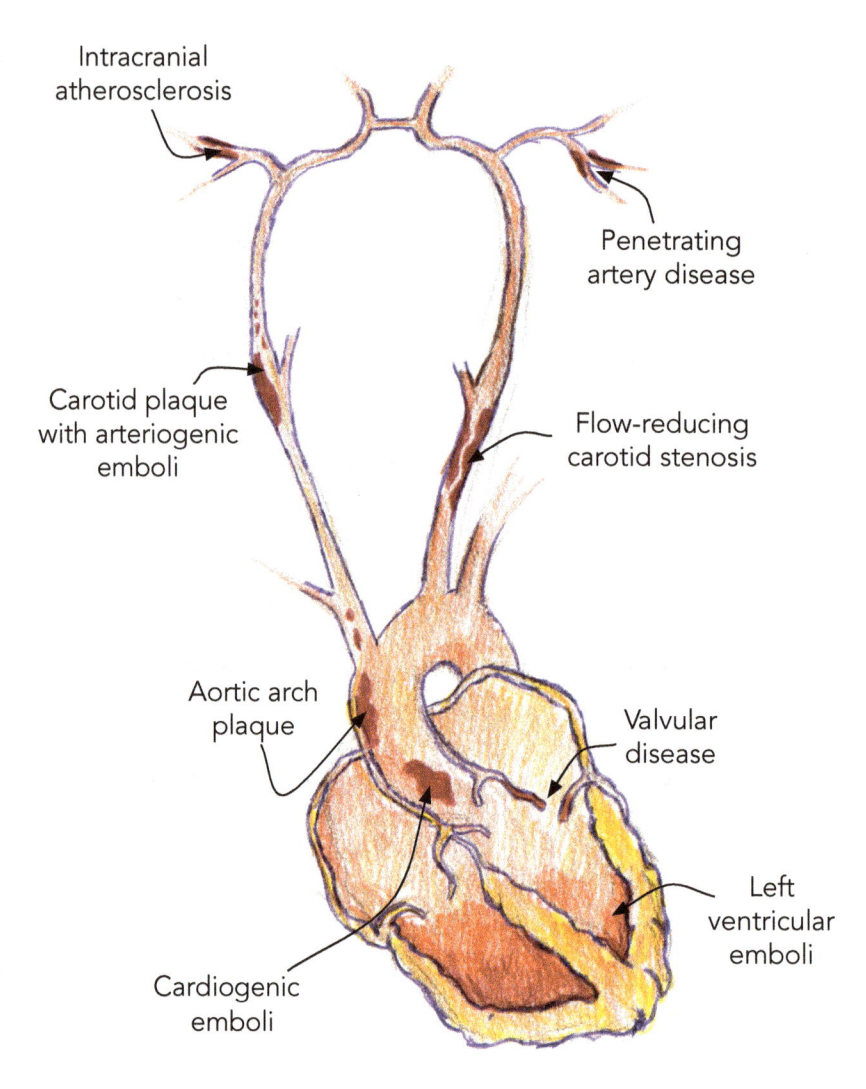

Figure 3.4 Sites of arterial and cardiac abnormalities causing ischaemic stroke.

- Atheromatous changes, mostly in the internal carotid arteries, close to where they split from the common carotid arteries
- Stenosis and occlusion of internal carotid or vertebral arteries, restricting blood flow
- In situ stenosis and occlusion of small, penetrating cerebral arteries, which lack collateral supplies. These are called lacunar infarcts as they leave behind small cavities or lacunae (lakes)
- Emboli including those originating from the heart due to arrhythmias (such as atrial fibrillation), or emboli that are result of structural changes caused by myocardial infarction.

Whatever the cause, once a cerebral artery is occluded, the area of the brain (or brain stem) it serves will infarct if there is no collateral supply. The infarcted tissue (the core) is surrounded by an area of ischaemic, but salvageable tissue known as the ischaemic penumbra. Time is brain and with each passing minute 1.9 million neurons, 14 billion synapses and 12km (7.5 miles) of myelinated fibres are destroyed. This equates to the premature 'ageing' of the brain to the tune of 3.6 years for each hour without reperfusion treatment.[12]

Recognition

All NHS ambulance trusts train their staff to use the Newcastle Face Arm Speech Test (FAST, Table 3.1) for stroke.[13] This is in line with current guidance, which recommends that in any acute onset of neurological symptoms, a validated tool (such as FAST) should be used outside of hospital. In addition, blood glucose should be checked as hypoglycaemia can mimic the signs of a stroke.[14]

The problem with FAST is that it does not recognise symptoms such as unilateral leg weakness or non-traumatic unilateral vision loss; both of which may indicate a stroke, so it is important to use your clinical judgement in cases where a patient is FAST negative. A variety of other scores have been advocated for out-of-hospital use but were either designed to identify patients suitable for thrombolysis and therefore included age and/or disability exclusion criteria (for example, the Los Angeles Prehospital Stroke Scale), or were hospital tools that have not yet been demonstrated to perform better than FAST

Table 3.1 Newcastle Face Arm Speech Test.

Components	Instructions
Facial palsy	Ask patient to smile or show teeth Look for new lack of symmetry This is positive if there is an unequal smile or grimace or obvious facial asymmetry
Arm weakness	Lift the patient's arms to 90° (45° if lying), ask them to hold the position for 5 seconds, then let go Look for one arm drifting or falling rapidly
Speech impairment	During the course of a conversation (if patient can speak) Look for new speech disturbance (you may need to ask someone who knows the patient) Specifically look for slurred speech and word-finding difficulties Ask patient to identify common objects (such as a set of keys, cup, chair, pen) If there is a severe visual disturbance, place an object in the patient's hand and ask them to name it

Adapted from: Harbison et al., 2003.

when used out-of-hospital (for example, National Institutes of Health Stroke Scale and Recognition of Stroke in the Emergency Room).[3,15]

The symptoms of an ischaemic stroke will vary, depending on the artery affected. Table 3.2 summarises the signs and symptoms, although these are dependent on the hemisphere (dominant vs. non-dominant) and collateral supply. Most sensory and motor signs occur on the contralateral side to the stroke due to the decussation (the crossing over) of nerve fibres.[7,11]

Table 3.2 Potential signs and symptoms of stroke by cerebral artery territories.

Artery	Signs and symptoms
Anterior cerebral	Weakness/loss of sensation in contralateral leg
Middle cerebral (most common)	Dysphasia/aphasia (dominant hemisphere) Contralateral hemiplegia of face and arm Homonymous hemianopia Inability to turn eyes towards affected side Left-right confusion
Posterior cerebral	Homonymous hemianopia and other visual defects such as colour blindness
Basilar and vertebral	Ataxia Cranial nerve palsies Decreased level of consciousness

Adapted from: Marieb et al., 2019.

Management

The most important components of pre-hospital management of stroke patients is early recognition and prompt transport to a HASU (where possible).

Establishing a time of onset is vital as it can have a significant bearing on the eligibility of patients for thrombolysis or thrombectomy if their stroke is ischaemic. Thrombolysis with drugs such as alteplase usually needs to be started within 4.5 hours of symptom onset. The window for thrombectomy is longer (usually 5 hours, but up to 24 hours in some very specific circumstances), but can only be performed on more proximal, large vessel occlusions.[3] If you are unable to establish an 'onset time' (such as in instances of 'wake-up strokes') then you should record a 'last-seen-well' time and hand this over to medical staff.

Oxygen should not be routinely administered to patients suffering a stroke and oxygen saturations kept between 94% and 98%, except in patients with COPD or at risk of hypercapnia.[1]

Take a look at your stroke pathways as they may specify which hospitals you should take acute stroke patients to, and whether you should take your patient straight to a HASU or the CT scanner. Don't forget to pre-alert the receiving hospital to minimise delay once you arrive.

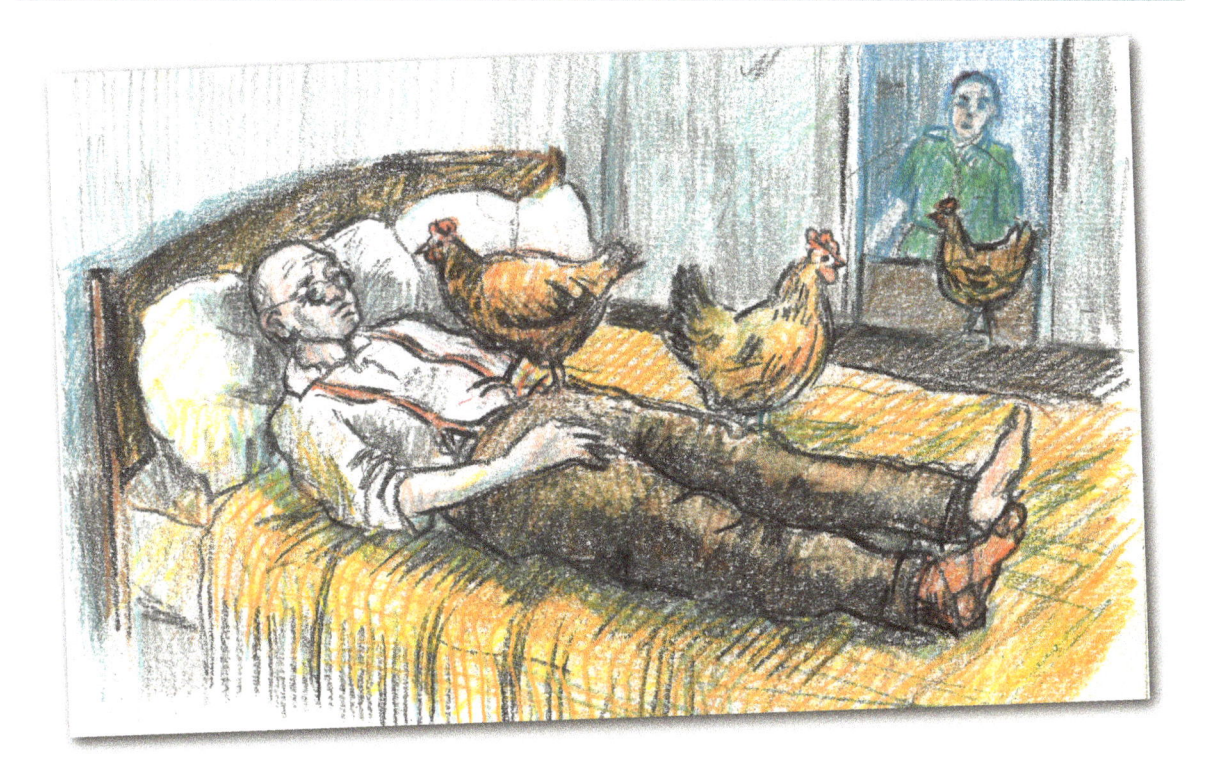

Transient Loss of Consciousness

You are on standby in a residential area, watching the early morning commuters scrape the ice off their cars and wondering what could be in their garage that is so precious that their executive cars are best left on the drive. You get a brief glimpse of one such garage as its owner opens it briefly to retrieve something. Most of the contents look like junk and certainly not worth more than the £20,000 car they have left unattended with the keys in the ignition and the engine running.

The MDT interrupts this chain of thought, passing you details of your next patient, an 85-year-old man who is suffering from palpitations and dizziness. As you arrive at the address the sun rises, bathing the street in light and reflecting rather nicely off the frost-covered lawn leading up to the patient's bungalow. Your attention is drawn to the back of the house, where you can see a chicken shed – at least you assume it is, judging by the chooks who are currently exiting and wandering freely down the garden. The fun doesn't stop outside either. As you enter the bungalow, you are greeted by at least three hens who have ventured inside the property, thanks to an open kitchen door. Despite the best efforts of Freda, the patient's wife, they are running amok through the rooms. Mind you, she is trying to chase them while walking with a Zimmer frame, so it's perhaps not surprising that she is not having much luck.

Chapter 3 Disability

You step over a hen and enter the bedroom where you find Leon, your patient, lying on the bed. He looks shocking, with central cyanosis and cold and shut-down peripheries. After introducing yourself, you enquire about events while your colleague prepares the oxygen for administration. Leon tells you that he was letting his beloved chickens out and escorting them into the run a bit further down the garden, when he experienced a sudden onset of palpitations. It made him feel dizzy, but he managed to struggle back to the house before he collapsed on the bed. You ask about any loss of consciousness, but he can't be sure as it all happened so fast.

Your colleague, having placed a non-rebreathe mask on the patient, is bending over to reach the oxygen cylinder on the floor, when a hen unwisely chooses to enter. She is just about to see it off with a swift kick of her steel toecap boots when you point out that Leon is rather fond of his chickens. She looks at the hen and says "Shoo." The hen eyes your colleague for a moment and then appears to decide that a tactical withdrawal is wise and instead heads off to explore the living room.

While your colleague exposes the patient's chest and starts applying chest leads for a 12-lead electrocardiogram (ECG), you obtain a set of observations:

Airway

Patent

Breathing

Respiratory rate: 20 breaths/min
SpO_2: unrecordable, poor signal
Good bilateral air entry

Circulation

Radial pulse palpable, but weak and thready, 28 beats/min
Blood pressure: 78/51 mmHg

Disability

(GCS Score: 15/15
Blood sugar: 4.6 mmol/l

Exposure/Environment

Temperature: 35.8°C.

Your colleague hands you the 12-lead ECG, which as you expect shows a very slow heart rate. It looks like the P waves are retrograde, which is interesting, and the QRS complexes are not as wide as you expected, since rates of below 30 beats/min you normally associate with complete heart block. A bit of head scratching doesn't help either, so you decide to crack on with some treatment. After gaining intravenous access, you administer a couple of rounds of atropine and two fluid boluses, and after 15 minutes or so, the patient is looking pinker and feeling better. You record another set of observations:

Airway

Patent

Breathing

Respiratory rate: 16 breaths/min
SpO_2: 100% with high-flow oxygen

Circulation

Heart rate: 50 beats/min
Blood pressure: 110/84 mmHg
12-lead ECG: Sinus bradycardia

Disability

GCS score: 15/15

Exposure/Environment

Temperature: 36.4°C.

You remove the oxygen mask and find that the patient's oxygen saturations remain above 94%. The patient states that he does not have any medical problems due to the fact that he has not seen his GP for 5 years. He does recall that the GP wanted to give him some medication, but he never bothered picking it up from the pharmacy.

Now the patient is feeling better, he turns his attention to his beloved chickens and the harm they may come to if they are allowed to roam free. Having mis-interpreted your colleague's restraint with the hen in the bedroom as being a fellow chicken-lover, he asks if she wouldn't mind rounding them up and placing them into the run. "They all love being stroked," he purrs. Your colleague's face drops, but fortunately she is saved by a neighbour who, having seen the ambulance and the very free range chickens, had popped over and managed to round them all up.

After an uneventful journey and hospital handover, you catch up with the doctor in resus at the local ED later on in the shift and discover that your patient was referred to cardiology and required temporary pacing, as his heart rate and blood pressure plummeted soon after you left.

Scale of the problem

Transient loss of consciousness (TLoC) is a state of real or apparent loss of consciousness with loss of awareness, characterised by amnesia for the period of unconsciousness, abnormal motor control, loss of responsiveness and a short duration. It is broadly divided into traumatic and non-traumatic TLoC.[16] We are going to focus on the non-traumatic group. It is very common, affecting around half of the UK population at some point in their lives and is due to a variety of causes with cardiovascular disorders being the most common.[17] Non-traumatic TLoC is subdivided into: syncope, epileptic seizures, psychogenic and rare causes.

It is important to realise that TLoC and syncope are not synonymous, since syncope is defined as TLoC due to transient global cerebral hypoperfusion characterised by rapid onset, short duration, and spontaneous complete recovery and so excludes conditions such as epilepsy, which TLoC does include.[16]

Syncopal TLoC

The syncopes are split into three categories, based on their pathophysiology: reflex syncope (the most common), syncope due to orthostatic hypotension and cardiac syncope (the most dangerous, Table 3.3).[16,18]

Reflex syncope

The overriding cause of the reflex syncopes is a vagal nerve-mediated bradycardia, or a reduction in sympathetic vasoconstriction, or both, giving rise to the term 'vasovagal'.[19] It is triggered by fear, pain, phobias and other forms of emotional distress, or anticipation of these. Situational subtypes, such as syncope caused by gastrointestinal stimulation induced by visceral pain, or syncope on micturition are thought to be caused by similar mechanisms as vasovagal syncope. However, the commonest, prolonged standing, may be caused by abnormal fluid shifts to the extremities, exacerbated by dehydration, with failure of the muscle pumps in the legs due to standing for prolonged periods.[18]

Carotid sinus syncope is rare in patients under 40 years of age and mainly occurs in the elderly. This is generally diagnosed during a medical examination with carotid sinus massage, but is rarely caused by direct mechanical manipulation of the carotid

Chapter 3 Disability

Table 3.3 Syncopal TLoC.

Types	Subtypes	Mechanism	Causes
Reflex syncope	Vasovagal	Inappropriate neural control over the circulation	Emotional distress: fear, pain, blood Orthostatic stress
	Situational		Cough, sneeze GI stimulation Micturition Post-exercise
	Carotid sinus syncope		Sick sinus syndrome
Syncope due to orthostatic hypotension	Primary autonomic failure	Insufficient vascular tone causing orthostatic hypotension	Multiple system atrophy Lewy body dementia
	Secondary autonomic failure		Diabetic neuropathy Spinal cord injuries
	Drug-induced		Alcohol, vasodilators, diuretics, phenothiazines, anti-depressants
	Volume depletion		Haemorrhage Diarrhoea and vomiting
Cardiac syncope	Arrhythmia	Insufficient pumping action of the heart	Paroxysmal SVT, VT, long QT syndrome
	Structural cardiac disease		Valvular disease Cardiomyopathy

Adapted from: Brignole et al., 2018; Saklani et al., 2013.

sinuses (such as caused by head movements or compression of the neck).

Syncope due to orthostatic hypotension

In autonomic failure (ANF), sympathetic efferent nervous activity is impaired, which leads to insufficient vasoconstriction, manifesting as orthostatic hypotension (OH), an abnormal decrease in blood pressure on standing, with either syncope, or pre-syncope.[16] Technically, there is no overlap between reflex syncope and ANF, but in reality, the clinical picture can be complicated making a differential diagnosis tricky. This has led to the use of the term 'orthostatic intolerance' when patients are symptomatic on moving to an upright position, and includes causes of reflex syncope.[16,20]

- Classical OH – A progressive and sustained systolic blood pressure drop of ≥20 mmHg or diastolic drop of ≥10 mmHg or decrease in systolic blood pressure to <90 mmHg **within 3 minutes of standing** from a supine position (this requires repeated blood pressure measurements during the 3 minute stand).
- Initial OH – An immediate drop in systolic blood pressure of >40 mmHg on standing,

but prompt resolution of hypotension and symptoms within 30 seconds.
- Delayed (progressive) OH – This is an age-related impairment of compensatory reflexes and stiffer hearts in elderly patients who are sensitive to the decrease in pre-load that occurs on standing, resulting in a slow progressive decrease in systolic blood pressure. There is typically no vagal-induced bradycardia, which differentiates this condition from reflex syncope.[21]
- Postural orthostatic tachycardia syndrome (POTS) – This usually affects young women (often with chronic fatigue syndrome). Characterised by a rise in heart rate (>30 beats/min increase or >120 beats/min) without hypotension, but with symptoms of orthostatic intolerance.[22]

ANF can be primary, that is, caused by a disease that directly targets the brain and nervous system, such as multiple system atrophy, or secondary, in that it is caused by a disease that primarily affects organs and tissues outside of the nervous system, such as diabetes.

Probably the most important causative factor in autonomic failure is prescribed medication, with drug groups such as anti-hypertensives, diuretics and anti-depressants being implicated.[19]

Finally, volume depletion, if severe enough, can cause OH and syncope by itself, although usually it plays a supportive role, exacerbating orthostatic intolerance due to reflex syncope or the types of OH.[16]

Cardiac syncope

Causes of cardiac syncope are generally divided into arrhythmias, the most common cause of cardiac syncope, and structural abnormalities. These causes of TLoC are more likely in elderly patients with a history of cardiac disease, so typically should only be considered in patients over 35 years of age. Of course, there are exceptions, and younger patients can be affected by cardiac syncope if they have long QT syndrome or cardiomyopathy. Arrhythmias cause TLoC by inducing haemodynamic impairment by critically reducing cardiac output and cerebral perfusion.

Structural abnormalities cause TLoC when circulatory demand increases, during exertion for example, and the impaired heart cannot provide the required rise in cardiac output. This typically occurs as a result of valvular disease, acute myocardial infarction, hypertrophic cardiomyopathy and, less commonly, in extrinsic causes such as pulmonary embolism, acute aortic dissection and pulmonary hypertension.[16]

Non-syncopal TLoC

Epileptic seizures

Epileptic seizures are similar to TLoC in that they are usually transient, of short duration and self-limiting. However, the key difference is in the underlying pathophysiology, in that epileptic seizures are caused by abnormally excessive or synchronised neuronal activity, and loss of consciousness does not always occur.[23]

Epileptic seizure types that are associated with TLoC are all generalised seizures and described on the basis of patient movement during the seizure, that is, clonic, tonic, tonic-clonic and atonic. Tonic refers to the body and limbs being held in a stiff position, usually with the limbs extended. Clonic movements are coarse, large-scale and powerful jerking movements of the arms and legs, which are usually synchronised over the body. Tonic-clonic movements are a combination of the two.[19] As the name implies, atonic seizures lead to a sudden loss of muscle tone and are sometimes referred to as 'drop attacks'.

Chapter 3 Disability

Psychogenic TLoC

Psychogenic pseudo-syncope (PPS) and psychogenic non-epileptic seizures (PNES) are generally bundled into the term psychogenic TLoC. As the name implies these have a psychological cause but should not be considered to be 'faking', although they not medical emergencies.[20,24]

Note that there is no evidence that psychogenic TLoC occurs more often in patients with a psychiatric history. In fact, there is good evidence that patients on medication to treat depression, schizophrenia and bipolar disorder are more likely to suffer from drug-induced OH.[19] The main groups of drugs responsible are phenothiazines, tricyclic anti-depressants and mono-amine oxidase inhibitors.

Rare causes

Transient ischaemic attacks (TIA), steal syndromes, subarachnoid haemorrhage and cyanotic breath holding spells can lead to TLoC by causing a temporary regional cerebral hypoperfusion. It is very uncommon for TIAs to cause a loss of consciousness unless it is a high vertebrobasilar TIA involving the thalamic structures. However, in these TIAs, the loss of consciousness is not transient and so does not commonly feature as a differential diagnosis.[25]

The subclavian steal syndrome can occur when the proximal subclavian artery (usually on the left) is sufficiently stenosed or occluded that the blood pressure post-occlusion drops significantly. This leads to a reversal in the blood flow of the vertebral artery on the same side in order to provide blood to the brachial artery. To do this, blood is 'stolen' from the vertebral artery and in turn the carotid artery and Circle of Willis. However, patients are often asymptomatic with the condition and TLoC is very rare.[26,27]

Subarachnoid haemorrhage can present with a short period of loss of consciousness, but the classical sudden onset of severe headache (sometimes referred to as thunderclap headache) provides the diagnostic clue as to the cause.[16]

Loss of consciousness due to cyanotic breath-holding spells is exclusive to infants. TLoC is caused by a cessation of expiratory respiration following an injury or the infant being startled. If the circulation becomes subsequently impaired, this can affect the brain, resulting in loss of consciousness.[20]

Assessment

Your initial evaluation will include taking a careful history, undertaking a thorough examination including the recording of orthostatic (lying/standing) blood pressures and a 12-lead electrocardiogram (ECG). There are four specific characteristics that define TLoC and all come from the history:[20]

1. Loss of consciousness of short duration (<5 minutes when measured, i.e. not estimated)
2. Abnormal motor control, for example, loss of postural control leading to a fall
3. Loss of responsiveness, for example, no response to voice or pain stimulus
4. Amnesia for the period of loss of consciousness.

The presence of all four of these is indicative of TLoC. TLoC can be excluded if any of the following are present throughout the episode:

- Motor control remains normal
- Patient remains responsive
- Patient can remember events.

Identifying the cause of TLoC

Events prior to TLoC

Find out what position the patient was in at the time of TLoC. Patients who were standing at the time of onset are more likely to have suffered from reflex syncope or autonomic failure, as opposed to those who were supine. Patients who were urinating, defecating or swallowing suggest reflex syncope, whereas exercise of the arms may indicate steal syndrome. Onset of TLoC during physical exercise, particularly cardiovascular, is more indicative of a cardiac cause, perhaps due to a structural defect. Finally, enquire about any predisposing factors. Reflex syncope and autonomic failure can be the cause of TLoC immediately following the cessation of exercise, in high temperatures and in cases of dehydration and/or diarrhoea. Reflex syncope can also be caused by stress but so can other non-syncopal causes of TLoC, such as epilepsy and psychogenic TLoC. Rapidly flashing lights and sleep deprivation are suggestive triggers for an epileptic seizure. Autonomic failure may occur during or following a meal, particularly in the elderly.

Onset of TLoC

Features of reflex syncope often include feeling hot/warm and/or nauseous, as well as experiencing vomiting, abdominal pain, pallor and sweating. Blurred vision and light-headedness are common to all causes of syncope (and part of the prodrome). The 'coat-hanger sign' of pain in the shoulders and neck due to local muscle ischaemia is a sign of autonomic failure. Features that suggest epilepsy as a cause include patient reports of a rising sensation from the abdomen, unpleasant smell or tastes in the mouth, déjà vu and other auras. Enquire about palpitations as this suggests that an arrhythmia may be the cause.

Events during TLoC

If the patient fell, enquire whether they were flaccid (that is, slumped to the ground) or were rigid and stiff, suggesting a tonic posture more indicative of epilepsy. The presence of myoclonus (brief involuntary twitching of muscles or muscle groups) is not always a sign that the patient has suffered from an epileptic seizure. However, movements that occur prior to the fall, which are symmetric and synchronous, last for more than 30 seconds and are associated with a lateral tongue bite (anterior bites are common in syncope), frothing at the mouth and with the patient's head consistently turned to one side, do suggest epilepsy as the cause. Incontinence is just as likely in syncopal causes as it is in epilepsy, as are open eyes throughout the episode. Movements that come and go in presence and intensity, pelvic thrusting and patients who forcibly keep their eyes closed suggest psychogenic pseudo-TLoC. Syncope is more likely in the presence of asynchronous myoclonic movements (often mistaken for epileptic seizure activity) and a duration of less than 15 seconds.

Events following TLoC

Patients with syncope usually recover almost immediately once consciousness is regained, whereas post-ictal confusion is common following epileptic seizures, as are complaints of aching muscles. Chest pain and palpitations predictably suggest a cardiac cause, as can facial flushing, although this is also associated with reflex syncope.

Relevant medical history

Ask the patient about any history of cardiac disease, neurological conditions such as Parkinsonism, epilepsy and narcolepsy, and metabolic disorders such as diabetes. Also enquire about any family history of sudden death, congenital arrhythmogenic heart diseases and fainting. If the patient is taking any prescribed medication, take note of any anti-hypertensive, anti-anginal, anti-depressant, anti-arrhythmic, diuretic and QT-segment prolonging agents. Alcohol consumption and illicit drug use should also be determined.

Chapter 3 Disability

12-lead ECG

All patients who experience TLoC should have a 12-lead ECG recorded. Take note of any of the following red flag signs:[17]

- Inappropriate persistent bradycardia
- Any ventricular arrhythmia (including ventricular ectopics)
- Long or short QTc interval (corrected QTc >450 ms or <350 ms)
- Brugada syndrome
- Ventricular pre-excitation (such as Wolff–Parkinson–White syndrome)
- Left or right ventricular hypertrophy
- Abnormal T-wave inversion
- Pathological Q waves
- Sustained atrial arrhythmias
- Paced rhythm.

Management

Convey all patients with TLoC to an ED in the presence of the following:[17]

- Any red flag sign on the 12-lead ECG
- Family history of sudden cardiac death in family members under 40 years of age
- Patients who have an inherited cardiac condition
- Patients over 65 years of age without prodromal symptoms prior to their TLoC
- Any history of new or unexplained breathlessness
- Heart failure (either clinical signs and symptoms or from the medical history)
- TLoC during exertion
- Presence of a heart murmur.

Other important co-morbidities that should be considered when making a transport decision include severe anaemia and electrolyte imbalances.[16]

Patients may be suitable to be left at home if you are confident that their TLoC is due to an uncomplicated faint or situational syncope. A diagnosis of uncomplicated faint should only be made in patients when there is nothing in the history or examination to suggest an alternative and there are features suggestive of an uncomplicated faint, typically summarised as the 3 P's:[1]

- Posture (prolonged standing)
- Provoking factors (such as pain, or a medical procedure)
- Prodromal symptoms (such as sweating or feeling warm/hot before TLoC).

Situational syncope can be diagnosed when there are no features from the initial assessment that suggest an alternative diagnosis and the TLoC is clearly and consistently provoked by straining during micturition (usually while standing) or by coughing or swallowing, for example.

If you are satisfied clinically and socially that the patient is safe to be left at home, advise the patient to take your patient care record (if possible) and the 12-lead ECG along to their GP.

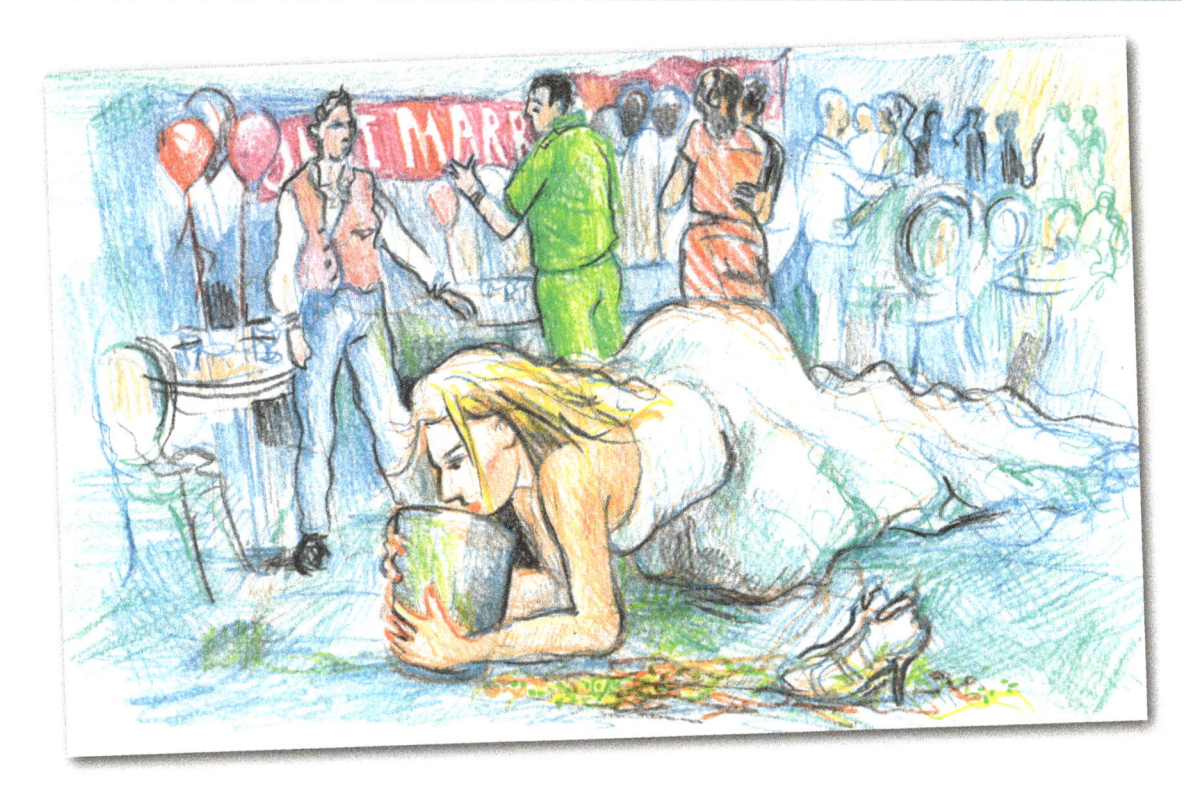

Headache

You are on standby early on Saturday evening, awaiting the onslaught of drunken revellers. However, you are well stocked with vomit bowls and have a medical student riding along with you, who is going to get some up-close and hands-on experience of anyone expelling bodily fluids.

Things start sedately enough, with a number of revellers who have clearly peaked a little too early, and have passed out due to excess alcohol consumption, prior to 22.00. After this, a prolonged on-scene negotiation with a suicidal patient brings you up to midnight. No sooner have you called clear than you are passed another job, which has been held for the past 30 minutes. The address is a rather swanky hotel on the edge of town. "Nice place for a wedding," enthuses the medical student. As the ambulance scrunches up the gravel drive of the hotel, it appears he is correct, as there is a sea of people in posh frocks and morning suits smoking outside the hotel entrance. Just in front of them, an exasperated limousine driver is trying to prevent a number of the wedding guests from decorating his vehicle with silly string and streamers.

You pull up alongside the limo and head into the hotel through the motley crowd. "I thought the strippers were firemen," quips one of the inebriated guests. "Classy crowd for a classy venue," mutters your colleague

Chapter 3   Disability

under his breath. Inside, the hotel manager greets you and directs you to the hotel ballroom, which is now resonating in time to the heavy bass from the large speakers next to the dance floor. Sat on the dance floor is the bride, with her head in a waste paper bin. The medical student seems keen to obtain a history, so you give him an encouraging nod and he tries talking to the bride. This does not go so well given that she has her head in a bin and the music is so loud, but undeterred, he pulls the groom to one side and tries again. The groom has clearly had a bottle or three of champagne and is not much use, but he does reveal that the bride has had a headache for most of the day and taken some of her 'pills'.

"What's up with her, doc?" the groom yells over the dance track. It's difficult to make out what the student is saying, and the groom doesn't seem to have a clue either. Just as there is a break in the music, the medical student, keen to make himself heard, manages to bellow out "Is there any history of brain cancer in the family?" "She's got brain cancer?" wails the groom to the dance floor. The bridesmaids hurry over, their eyes filling up with tears. Despite this, they manage to start texting and updating a popular social networking website with the news.

Your colleague's eyes shoot daggers at the medical student as he tries to allay the fears of the guests, giving you time to find the bride's ear under a large mop of her hair. You ask her if she suffers from migraines (she nods) and whether this feels like one now (again, she nods). On enquiring about medication, she points a shaky hand at a small purse on the dance floor. Inside you find some prochlorperazine and sumatriptan. She has taken her sumatriptan, but not the anti-emetic, and given her current condition, you ask her whether it might be a good idea to have this too, since she has a buccal preparation. She agrees and inserts it between her cheek and gum. "Can you walk?" you ask and she shakes her head. "Wobbly," she replies. You signal for a chair, which is swiftly fetched, and assist her into it. It takes all three of you to wheel her and the wedding dress onto the ambulance.

Once aboard, and with the lights dimmed due to her mild photophobia, you quietly obtain a history. The prochlorperazine seems to be doing its job and your patient is able to provide a good history, now that she is not retching so frequently. She tells you that her headache started this morning while having her hair and make-up done. It is mainly on the left side of her head, throbbing in nature and has been building up all day. She had forgotten her regular analgesia and so instead had taken a couple of co-codamol that the hairdresser had offered. She denies drinking alcohol, apart from a small toast of champagne, as she started feeling nauseous during the reception, and became more unsteady on her feet, having been dragged onto the dance floor by her drunk bridesmaids. Currently, her pain score is an 8/10 and she has not had any analgesia in over 12 hours.

What are you going to do: Administer **Opiates** (read on) or **Non-steroidal anti-inflammatory drugs (NSAIDS)** (skip the next paragraph)?

Opiates

Severe pain calls for serious analgesia and you head to the morphine safe. Just as you are trying to open it, the medical student speaks up, clearly intent on improving his standing with your colleague, who has not forgiven him for causing a ruckus on the dance floor. "I think opiates are discouraged when treating migraines," he says, wilting a little under your colleague's fierce gaze. However, a quick consultation of the JRCALC Guidelines, reveals that he is quite correct.

NSAIDs

You recall that opiates are generally not recommended for headaches due to worsening, potentially, her condition and/or hindering further assessment,[1] so elect to go for NSAIDs. It turns out that ibuprofen is the patient's drug of choice and she happily chows down on two 200 mg tablets now that she is feeling less nauseous. Having started to address the patient's symptoms, you have to decide what to do next. The patient's observations are mostly normal (she has a temperature of 37.5°C) and apart from the headache, mild photophobia, neck stiffness and ataxia, she is fine.

> What are you going to do: **Leave her at the hotel** (read on) or **Take her to hospital** (skip the next paragraph)?

Leave her at the hotel

The patient is not keen on going to hospital and you don't want to ruin her wedding night, so you excuse yourself from the ambulance to try and find someone sober enough to look after the patient. You spot the groom laughing with one of the bridesmaids and walk over to where they are standing. He jumps with a start when you cough your presence and looks guiltily in your direction as you enquire whether there is anyone who may be in a position to assist the bride. He suggests the bride's mother and wanders off into the hotel to find her, returning a few minutes later with the mother in tow. You usher the pair of them onto the ambulance. The mother is aware of her daughter's migraines, although mentions that she does not normally have neck stiffness or ataxia. The bride tries to stand, but she is not up to walking, since she cannot seem to co-ordinate her legs. "They have a mind of their own," she states.

Clearly she is not going to manage at the hotel.

Take her to hospital

You gently explain that although this is likely to be a migraine, some of her associated symptoms are of concern. "But it's my wedding night," wails the bride, before wincing at the pain caused by the noise she is making. On arrival at the ED, you explain the situation to the triage nurse who, despite the busy night, tries to get the bride seen promptly by one of the senior doctors. You catch up with the doctor later and find out that, although they think it was probably a migraine, the neurologists decided to admit her overnight.

Scale of the problem

Headache (cephalalgia, head pain) is common, with a lifetime prevalence in excess of 40%.[28] Around 4.4% of GP appointments and 0.8–2% of emergency department (ED) attendances are for headaches. Most are not life-threatening, although 13–18% of patients who attend the ED do have a serious underlying cause.[29] The trick is to spot them amongst the others!

Headaches are classified into primary and secondary types (Table 3.4). The causes of primary headaches are poorly understood, and, although they can be disabling (particularly migraines), are not going to kill your patient. The most common type of primary headache is the tension-type headache (TTH), followed by migraines, medication overuse headaches (MOH) and cluster headaches.[28]

Secondary headaches are caused by an underlying pathological cause, such as infection, vascular problem, intracranial tumour, or due to medication (most commonly drugs taken for a primary headache disorder).[30] They are far less common than primary headache disorders.

Primary headaches

From Table 3.4, it can be seen that there are three main types of primary headache (with the obligatory fourth category, other). None of these are fatal, although patients can be severely debilitated by these types of headaches, particularly migraines.[31]

Migraines

It has been suggested that migraine is a 'headache plus' syndrome since it is characterised by head pain plus other symptoms, such as nausea and vomiting, photophobia and phonophobia.[32] The pathophysiology of migraines is complex, with hypothalamic activation and alteration in thalamo-cortical circuits leading to trigemino-cervical complex activation in the brainstem, which in turn leads to transmission of pain to the upper cervical nerves resulting in neck and head pain.[33]

Migraines are classified according to the presence or absence of an aura. Auras affect around a third of migraine sufferers, usually preceding their headaches, although can occur during and after a headache. A typical aura consists fully reversible visual, sensory and/or dysphasic set of symptoms which

Table 3.4   Headache classification.

Type	Description	Example
Primary headaches	Migraine with and without aura	
	Tension-type headache	
	Cluster headache and other trigeminal autonomic cephalalgias	
	Other	
Secondary headaches	Headache attributed to head and/or neck trauma	
	Headache attributed to cranial or cervical vascular disorder	Subarachnoid haemorrhage, giant cell arteritis
	Headache attributed to non-vascular intracranial disorder	Idiopathic intracranial hypertension, intracranial tumour
	Headache attributed to a substance or its withdrawal	Carbon monoxide, alcohol, medication overuse headache
	Headache attributed to infection	
	Headache or facial pain attributed to disorder of cranium, neck, eyes, ears, nose, sinuses, teeth or mouth	Cervicogenic headache, acute glaucoma
	Headache attributed to psychiatric disorder	
	Cranial neuralgias, central and primary facial pain and other headaches	Trigeminal neuralgia

Adapted from: Brignole et al., 2018.

typically have an onset time of minutes, but last no longer than 60 minutes.[28] These can be positive (for example, seeing flickering lights, spots, zigzag lines or experiencing paraesthesia) or negative (for example, loss of vision, numbness).[34] Auras normally have a gradual onset over a period of more than five minutes and resolve within an hour.

Prodromal symptoms up to 24–48 hours before the migraine starts are common, and include changes of mood and behaviour. The classic presentation of a migraine headache is a single-sided, throbbing pain, which builds up over minutes to hours, with associated symptoms. The pain typically lasts for 4–24 hours, but can persist for up to 72 hours in severe cases.[35]

Tension-type headaches

Although TTH are the most common type of primary headache, they are also the least likely to lead to a visit to the GP or ED. Typically, these headaches are not as severe as a migraine, and the pain is bilateral, non-throbbing and described as a tightening or pressure.[30] It does not usually present with nausea or vomiting, or incapacitate the patient as is the case with migraine. However, photophobia or phonophobia (but not both) may be present.[36] They can be linked to stress and/or associated with neck or cranial musculoskeletal problems.

TTH are broadly split into two types, episodic and chronic. As the names suggest, episodic TTH occur with variable duration of frequency, and often co-exist with migraines without aura, whereas chronic TTH occur on more than 15 days per month for more than three months.[36]

Cluster headaches

Cluster headaches belong to a group of disorders known as the trigeminal autonomic cephalagias. They are much more common in men and patients are typically 30–50 years of age.[28] As the name suggests, they occur in blocks, which can last for weeks or months, following by a remission period lasting months to years.

The pain is severe, always unilateral, and focused in and around the orbits and/or temples. In the worst cases, the pain can be excruciating, with patients unable to lie down and classically resorting to pacing about.[36] During the cluster period, headaches will be in the same location each time. Associated symptoms include ipsilateral conjunctival injection, lacrimation, nasal congestion, rhinorrhoea, forehead and facial sweating, miosis, ptosis and/or eyelid oedema.[30]

Secondary headaches

Serious causes of secondary headaches are uncommon, but must not be missed! These include intracranial tumours, meningitis, giant cell (temporal) arteritis, carbon monoxide poisoning and subarachnoid haemorrhage.[30]

Medication overuse headache

The most common cause of secondary headaches is medication overuse headache (MOH), which is usually caused by the chronic overuse of analgesia and/or triptans (commonly used for migraines).[28]

Intracranial tumours

With the exception of pituitary tumours, intracranial tumours are unlikely to produce headaches until they are large, and often present with other neurological symptoms.[37] If headache is the only symptom, then idiopathic intracranial hypertension is more likely (particularly if your patient is obese).[38] If you are able to perform fundoscopy (and have the equipment to do so), then bilateral papilloedema (swelling of the optic disc) is a sign of raised intracranial pressure, although this will not indicate the cause. Headaches associated with raised intracranial pressure

Chapter 3   Disability

are normally worse when lying down and may awaken the patient from sleep.

Meningitis

This diagnosis may be straightforward in a systemically unwell patient with fever, neck stiffness, photophobia and nausea and vomiting. However, these signs are often absent in the early stages of the disease and some may be masked by over-the-counter medication. Headache in meningitis is commonly progressive, taking hours or longer to build and can be generalised or frontal. It sometimes radiates to the neck, and in the latter stages is associated with nausea and an altered level of consciousness.[39]

Giant cell arteritis

Giant cell arteritis (GCA) is an inflammatory disease of the medium and larger arteries, most commonly affecting the branches of the external carotid artery. Symptoms are caused by local ischaemia due to endovascular damage, and cytokine-mediated systemic illness.[40] It is not life-threatening but can cause irreversible blindness unless it is diagnosed and treated early, so these are not patients to leave at home with a couple of paracetamol. It is a disease of ageing and is virtually never seen in patients under the age of 50.[28] Most patients will complain of headache, with around 50% of headaches localised to the temples, which will also be tender on palpation.[41] Other symptoms such as visual disturbance and jaw claudication are less common, but increase the likelihood that the cause is GCA.[42]

Carbon monoxide (CO) poisoning

This is a rare, but likely under-reported, cause of headache and general illness, but is easily overlooked if not included as a differential diagnosis. In addition to headache, patients may complain of nausea and vomiting, giddiness, muscle weakness and dimming and double vision.[43] Multiple patients at the same address with the same or similar symptoms should raise suspicion.

Subarachnoid haemorrhage (SAH)

Around 70% of patients with SAH present with headache as the main symptom. Approximately 50% of these patients with headache will describe it in terms that are consistent with a thunderclap headache. However, only 11–25% will actually have a SAH.[44]

Headaches are described in terms of their mode of onset and severity, and thunderclap is the term usually used to describe a severe headache of sudden onset. Any headache which scores a 7/10 or more with an onset time of 1 min or less can be described as a thunderclap.[44] Patients often describe SAH headaches as their 'worst ever', but this is rather undermined by the fact that patients typically describe migraines using the same terminology, making it unhelpful for diagnostic purposes. Thunderclap headaches can occur spontaneously or as a result of a valsalva manoeuvre or physical effort.[36] They can also be primary or secondary in cause and there are no reliable features to differentiate between the two.

Assessment

The history is the most important aspect when trying to determine the cause of a patient's headache. The following provides some features that may help in differentiating between the types of headaches:[29,36]

- Onset: Sudden (instantaneous to several minutes) or gradual (several minutes to days)?
- Provoking: Made worse by lying down, coughing, straining, sitting, standing (in low pressure headaches)
- Palliating/relieving: Improved by lying down (in low pressure headaches) or taking analgesia/triptans

- Quality: Is the pain throbbing, stabbing or a tightening/pressure?
- Radiation: Common sites of radiation include the neck and jaw
- Severity: Migraines and thunderclap headaches may be described as the 'worst ever'. Enquire about previous episodes
- Timing/periodicity: Is the headache episodic, for example, several days between attacks or persistent? Some patients who have previously sought medical help may have been asked to keep a headache diary
- Associated symptoms: Note the presence of fever, nausea and vomiting, photophobia, neck stiffness, neurological or systemic symptoms
- Past medical history: Does the patient have a known primary headache syndrome or malignancy?
- Drug history: Is the patient's current medication likely to cause headache as a side effect, for example, oral contraceptives or dipyridamole. Note the use of over-the-counter analgesics and recreational drug use
- Social history: This may be relevant although most patients are stressed because they have a headache, not the other way around!
- Family history: Not that useful, but there is limited evidence that migraines and cluster headaches have a familial component. Family histories of brain tumours/haemorrhages do not increase the risk that your patient has either of these, but are sometimes mentioned by worried patients and relatives.

Review and exclude the following 'red flag' signs and symptoms:[28,30]

- New onset or change in headache in patients who are aged over 50 years
- Thunderclap: Rapid time to peak headache intensity (seconds to 5 minutes)
- Focal neurological symptoms (for example, limb weakness, aura lasting less than 5 min or more than 1 hour)
- Non-focal neurological symptoms (for example, cognitive dysfunction)
- Change in headache frequency, characteristics or associated symptoms
- An abnormal neurological examination
- Headache that changes with posture (orthostatic)
- Headache precipitated by physical exertion or valsalva manoeuvre (for example, coughing, laughing, straining)
- Jaw claudication, tongue pain or visual disturbance
- Neck stiffness
- Vomiting without any other obvious cause
- Worsening headache with fever
- New onset headache in a patient with a history of human immunodeficiency virus (HIV) infection
- New onset headache in a patient with a history of cancer
- Head injury within the past 3 months.

Figure 3.5 provides some guidance to determine a possible diagnosis, but further tests, such as a CT scan and lumbar puncture, may be required to determine this with confidence. Have a low threshold for referring patients to the ED.

Treatment

Analgesia and anti-emetics are typically the order of the day. The British Association for the Study of Headaches (BASH) guidance advises administering NSAIDs such as aspirin (note this is not an indication for administration in the *JRCALC Clinical Guidelines*) or ibuprofen as a first-line management of headaches.[36] Opiates are discouraged since they can worsen the patient's condition and/or hinder further assessment.[1] Administration of anti-emetics, such as prochlorperazine, are useful in treating nausea associated with headaches, and the patient may have these on prescription in a buccal preparation. Alternatively, your locally available anti-emetic can be administered,

Chapter 3 Disability

although these are typically only available in injectable forms.

There is evidence to suggest that high-flow oxygen may be beneficial in primary headaches.[45] However, it is detrimental in secondary headaches, so is not currently advocated by the *JRCALC Clinical Guidelines*.

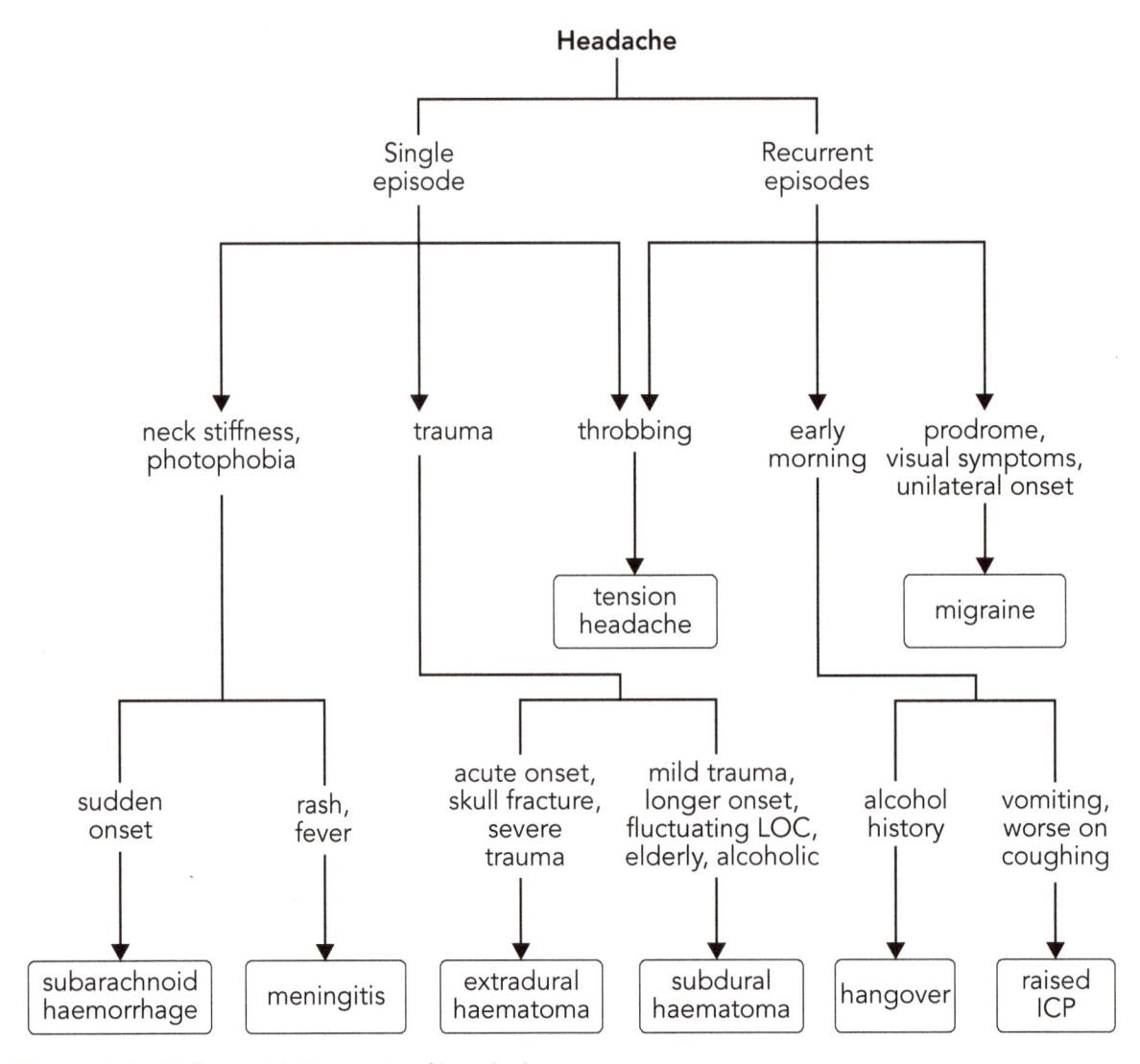

Figure 3.5 Differential diagnosis of headache.

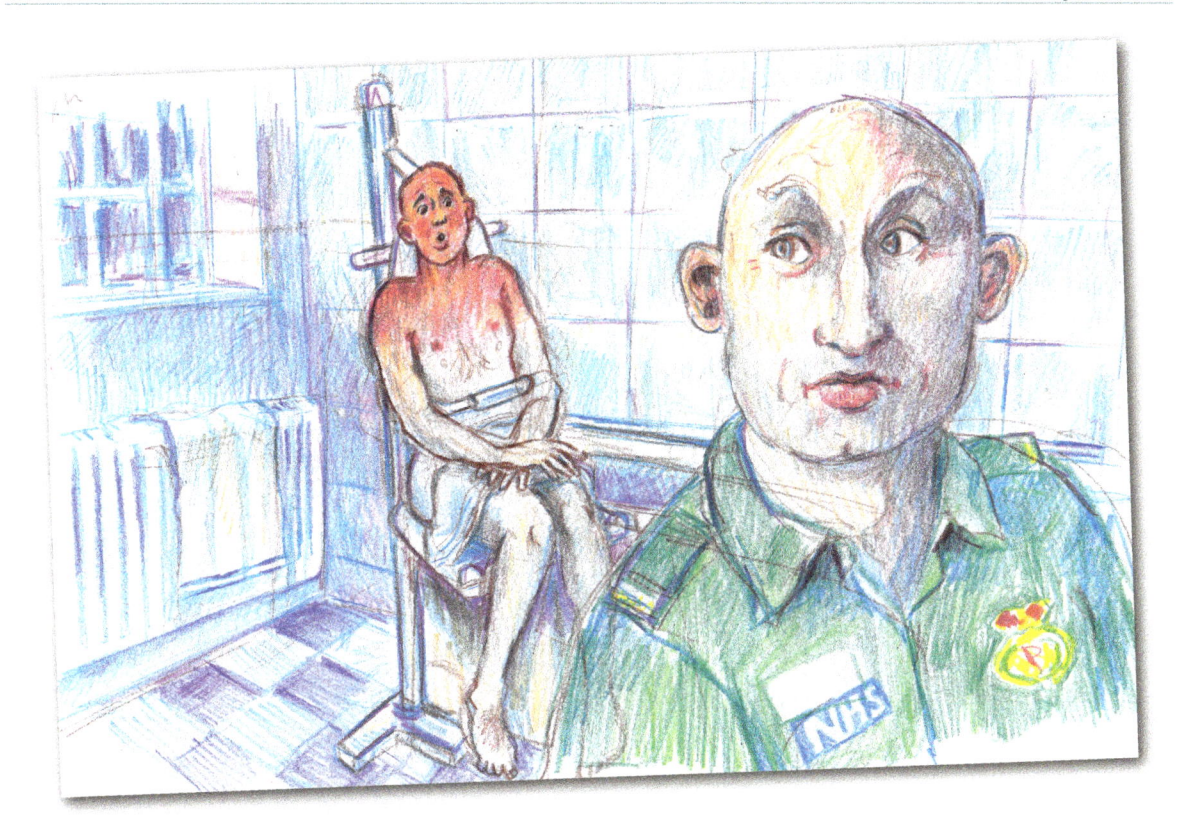

Autonomic Dysreflexia

You are on standby with Butch, the station weight-lifting champion. He has muscles, lots of muscles and he's tough, very tough. You are watching him devour a dozen pickled eggs, and dreading the toxic fumes that will soon be permeating through the cab, when you are passed details about your next emergency.

The call is for a 50-year-old male at a local spinal injuries rehabilitation centre. The details are scarce, but there is mention of a crush injury, which sounds traumatic. The call has been triaged as low priority, and you are instructed to make a cold response. However, the roads are quiet and within 20 minutes you pull up outside the address.

For a change there is a carer to meet you at the door, although he looks rather pale. You are directed to one of the bathrooms. As the door opens, you are greeted by quite a sight. The patient is suspended on a bath chair, with nothing but a small towel covering his modesty. You are struck by how flushed his skin is above his nipple line, but is very pale below. He is also profusely sweating. The carer quickly explains that the patient had suffered a T4 spinal cord injury several months ago and is at the centre for some additional therapy. The patient was being lowered into the bath using a seat-type hoist with a hole in the bottom. Unfortunately, it was being

Chapter 3 Disability

lowered by a rather inattentive carer who failed to notice that the patient's testicles had become squeezed between the edge of the chair-hoist and the bottom of the bath.

Since the patient has no sensation at that level, he did not notice at first either. However, the throbbing headache and blocked up nose that he experienced soon after told him something was wrong. "It's my AD," he says. The carer had started to raise the hoist, but the call-taker had told them not to move the patient, so he has been left suspended over the bath in the hoist. "How are they?" the patient enquires, looking forlornly down at his groin. You gingerly lift the towel and peer under the hoist-seat to see a grapefruit-sized scrotum. Butch whimpers, causing you to look at him. He has gone rather pale and looks like he might faint. To spare him his blushes you ask if he could fetch the ambulance trolley and he gratefully shoots out of the bathroom. With Butch gone, you turn your attention back to the patient and plan your next move.

> What are you going to do: **Tell a joke** (read on) or **Record his vital signs?** (skip the next paragraph)

Tell a joke

You think it might be a good idea to lighten the mood, but after pondering for a moment, you realise that you only know one joke pertinent to the current situation. However, 'what do you call a Russian with only one testicle?' is not the most professional thing to mutter now, so you decide to record some vital signs.

Record his vital signs

This is probably not the best time to be cracking jokes, so you set about trying to look professional while tittering to yourself about Ivor Bolokov and record the patient's baseline observations. You find the following:

Airway
Patent

Breathing
Respiratory rate: 24 breaths/min
SpO_2: 98% on air

Circulation
Heart Rate: 48 beats/min
Blood pressure: 220/110 mmHg

Disability
GCS score: 15/15
Pain score: 7/10 (due to headache)

Exposure/Environment
Skin: flushed and sweating above the nipple line. Pale and clammy below.

The patient asks for his pills and you think that some analgesia is a great idea. However, he rebuffs your offer of paracetamol and ibuprofen and instead chews on a nifidepine tablet. Butch returns with the ambulance trolley under his arm and you lower the patient gently onto it before wheeling him out to the ambulance.

En route to hospital, you recheck the patient's vital signs and see that his blood pressure has fallen slightly but is still elevated. You make a pre-alert call to the hospital and before long you are rolling up outside. After handing over the patient you return to the cab of the ambulance to find it a hazardous area. After leaving the doors open for five minutes, it is safe to enter ... for now.

The scale of the problem

Spinal cord injury (SCI) is rare, although the exact incidence is not known. Even in high risk groups (patients trapped following a road traffic collision (RTC), for example), the incidence is less than 1%.[46] The most common cause is a fall, although, significantly, a third of these are falls of LESS than 2 m in height. Falls are closely followed by RTCs and the other, much rarer causes, such as sports injuries and shootings. SCI due to a falls of less than 2 m in patients over 65 years appear to be on the increase, reflecting the pattern for major trauma generally.[47]

People with SCI can suffer from a range of autonomic dysregulation-related problems. One that primarily affects those with an injury at T6 or above is autonomic dysreflexia. Untreated, it can lead to intracranial haemorrhage, convulsions, myocardial ischaemia and even sudden death. The most common causes are bladder and bowel irritation.[48]

Anatomy and physiology

As you may recall from your anatomy and physiology classes, the autonomic nervous system (ANS) is divided into three parts (yes, three, not two). These are the sympathetic, parasympathetic and enteric nervous systems. They are called autonomic because it was originally believed that they functioned completely independently from the central nervous system (CNS). However, it is now known that the hypothalamus and brain stem regulate ANS activity.[7]

The enteric division is an extensive network of neurons which reside within the walls of the gastrointestinal (GI) tract, pancreas and gall bladder. It has a sensory nervous function enabling the monitoring of the mechanical state of the alimentary canal and the chemical status of the stomach and intestines. In addition, it can output motor signals to modify the motility and secretions of the gut, as well as controlling the diameter of local blood vessels.[11]

Although classed as a separate arm of the ANS, the enteric division is influenced by the sympathetic and parasympathetic nervous systems, which are most relevant to autonomic dysreflexia and so will be the focus from here on.

The sympathetic and parasympathetic divisions of the ANS are often thought of as being at either end of a see-saw. This is true in some organs such as the heart, but in reality this is rather a simplistic view. Some parts of the body only receive inputs from one division, whereas in others, the effects of the sympathetic and parasympathetic divisions are similar. However, their actions are carefully controlled and co-ordinated by the hypothalamus.

Sympathetic division

This is often referred to as the fight-or-flight division as its actions prepare the body to respond to stress, facilitating sudden strenuous exercise and increased vigilance. In addition, it helps control blood pressure, thermoregulation, and gut and urogenital function.

The cell bodies of efferent, motor neurons of the sympathetic nervous system are found in the lateral horns of the spinal cord and extend from T1 to L2. They connect with a chain of ganglia located outside the CNS, but close to either side of the vertebral column and are called sympathetic chain or paravertebral ganglia (Figure 3.6).[7] The neurons connecting the spinal cord to each ganglion are known as preganglionic neurons and they do not just connect to one ganglion, but can ascend and descend the ganglion chain, resulting in rapid and simultaneous sympathetic nervous system stimulation throughout the body.

The post-synaptic neurons are known as postganglionic neurons. They consist of unmyelinated axons which pass into their target organs. However, some preganglionic

Chapter 3   Disability

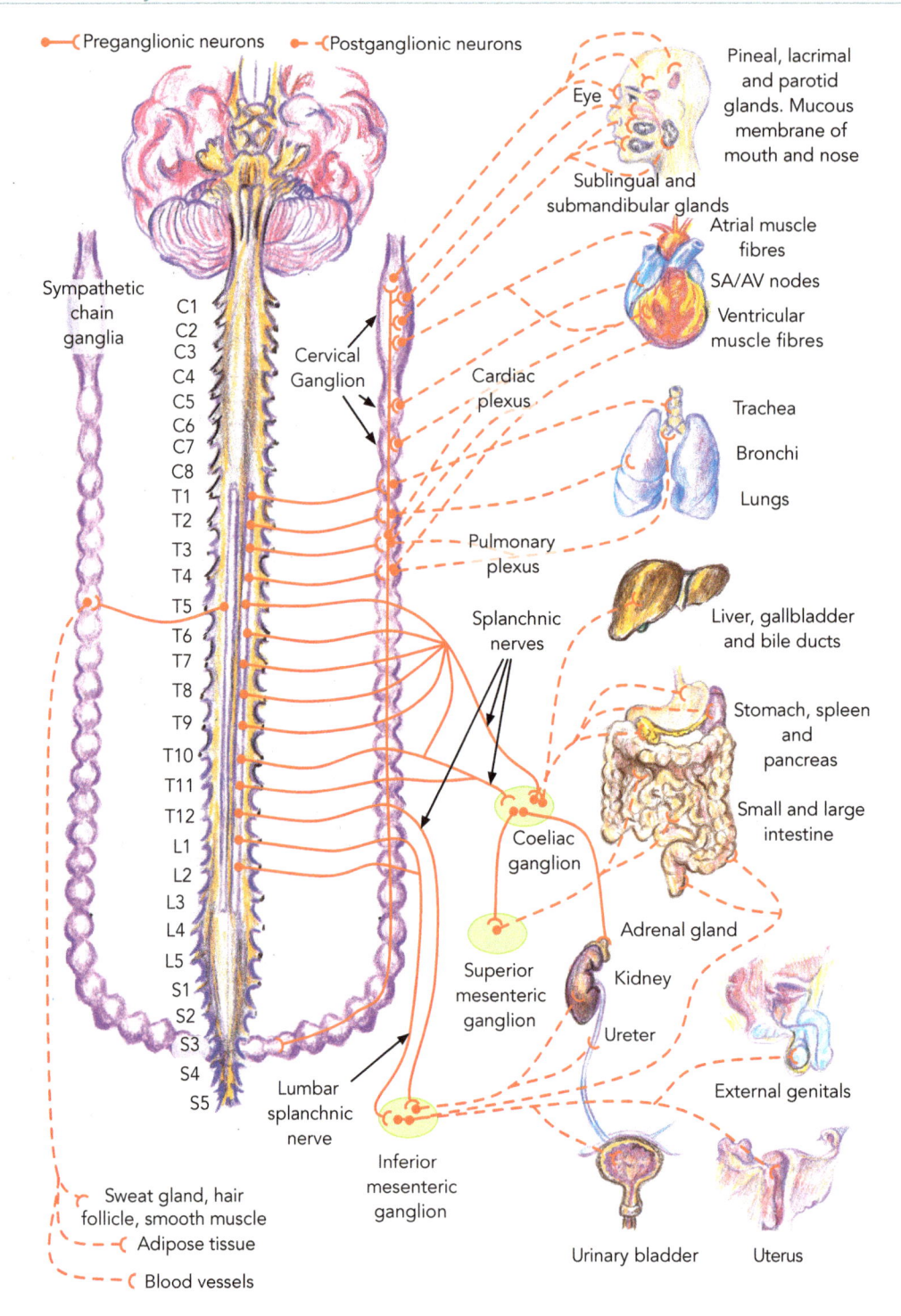

Figure 3.6   The sympathetic division of the autonomic nervous system.

neurons do not synapse in the paravertebral ganglia, but continue closer to the target organs via the splanchnic nerves, including neurons that innervate the adrenal medulla, causing the release of adrenaline and noradrenaline.

In contrast to the efferent, motor neurons just described, afferent sensory nerves pass through the paravertebral ganglia without synapsing and their cell bodies reside in the dorsal root ganglia.

The sympathetic division innervates both cardiac and vascular smooth muscle and dominates in times of stress, leading to raised heart rate and blood pressure.[48] Innervation to the heart and upper extremity blood vessels originates above T6 (usually T1–T5), leaving the larger vasculature of the gut and lower extremities to be signalled by nerves originating from T6–L2, which becomes significant in SCI around the T6 level, if communication with higher brain function is reduced or lost.

Parasympathetic division

The parasympathetic division is often referred to as the rest-and-digest division. Actions of the parasympathetic division include antagonising some effects of the sympathetic division, for example heart rate, gut motility and bronchiole diameter, and controlling many body functions in non-stress states such as GI secretion to aid digestion, micturition and defaecation. Another important difference between the sympathetic and parasympathetic divisions is their structure (Figure 3.7). Parasympathetic neurons are clustered at either end of the spinal cord.

One cluster originates from the brainstem, using the third, seventh and ninth (III, VII and IX) cranial nerves to serve structures in the head and the vagus nerve (cranial nerve X) for the thorax and abdomen. The other cluster forms the sacral portion of the parasympathetic division and is served by the pelvic splanchnic nerves which exit from S2–S4 of the spinal cord.

The preganglionic neurons of the parasympathetic division are long and do not synapse until very close, or within their target organ.[7] Since these nerves originate from the brainstem, they are usually unaffected by any SCI, but, in adults, the parasympathetic nervous system has no effect on cardiac or vascular smooth muscle, only the heart rate.

Pathophysiology

Key to the maintenance of homeostasis within the ANS is the cerebral cortex and hypothalamus, which provide appropriate excitatory and inhibitory inputs to various areas in the medulla, which plays a crucial role in cardiovascular control. This relies on feedback from afferent sensory impulse from central and peripheral baroreceptors. Thus, it is not difficult to see that SCI, depending on the level and completeness of the injury and cord interruption, can dramatically affect the body's ability to keep control of the ANS.[49]

Despite the common use of words like transection, cutting and severing of the spinal cord after a traumatic injury, in reality a spinal cord lesion (abnormality or damage) is primarily caused by ischaemic necrosis. Traumatic injury mechanisms include displacement of one or more vertebral bodies causing compression and/or stretching of the cord, which may result in no visible disruption, but leads to oedema and vascular disruption. However, not all SCI is due to trauma. Other causes include spinal tumours, transverse myelitis, vascular thrombosis or haemorrhage, and infection and abscesses caused by tuberculosis or meningitis.[50]

It's very cosy within the vertebral canal and an oedematous spinal cord is soon compressed. This disrupts blood and oxygen flow, resulting

Chapter 3 Disability

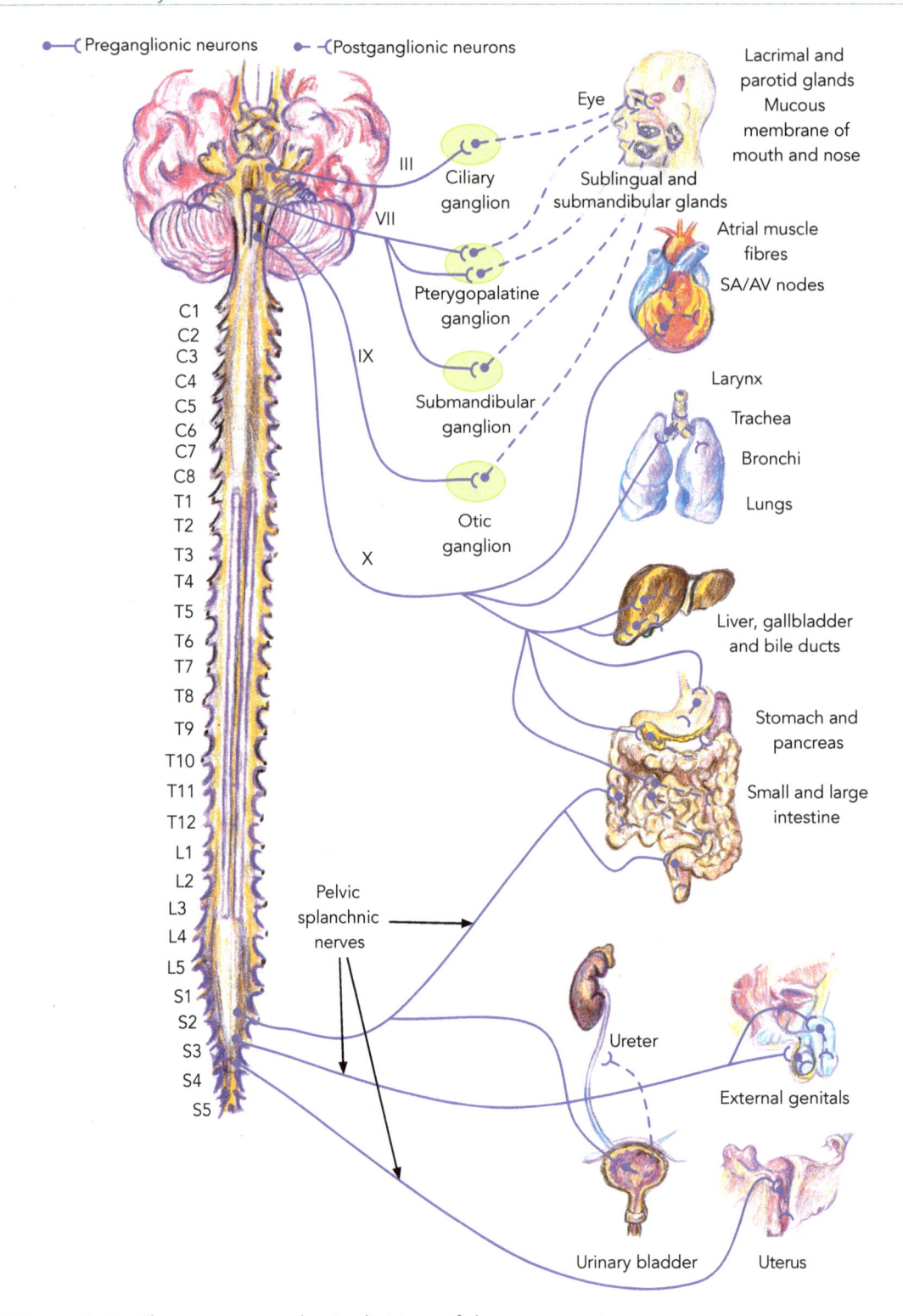

Figure 3.7 The parasympathetic division of the autonomic nervous system.

in ischaemic tissue, and ultimately, necrosis. The rapid cessation of signal transmission that this process causes leads to a range of signs and symptoms, which are termed 'spinal shock'. Note that this is not to be confused with the haemodynamic effects of SCI (such as hypotension) which are referred to as neurogenic shock.[51]

As previously mentioned, nerves originating from T1 to T5 are responsible for most heart and vascular control and injuries below this level typically do not have such a dramatic effect on the ANS. However, an injury at T6 or above can lead to interruption of sympathetic division control from the brain. Parasympathetic innervation of the heart arises from the brain and so is typically unaffected, making the parasympathetic division dominant (Figure 3.7).

The resulting signs and symptoms also depend on the completeness of the SCI. The classic picture in complete SCI is vasodilation and flaccidity of muscles below the injury, as well as loss of temperature regulation mechanisms such as vasodilation and sweating. This can lead to a poikilothermic state, where the body adopts the temperature of the surrounding environment (whether hot or cold). Depending on how high the SCI injury is, the blood pressure can dramatically fall to 80 mmHg systolic in high cervical injuries, for example, but there is no compensatory tachycardia, since the sympathetic signals are blocked. In fact, parasympathetic division dominance leads to bradycardia, further reducing cardiac output. In an incomplete SCI, there is a mixed picture of paralysis and paraesthesia, but not profound hypotension or bradycardia, making the absence of these signs unreliable in excluding SCI in unconscious patients.[51]

Neurogenic shock can last for days to weeks following injury and although there is usually some improvement, cardiovascular control does not typically return to normal. The fact that it improves at all provides some insight to contradict the notion that an SCI is irreversible. It turns out that the nervous system is capable of effecting repairs thanks to its neuroplasticity.

Neuroplasticity

Following SCI, the body undergoes a variety of changes in response to the insult. This occurs within the spinal cord, brain and ganglia outside the CNS. There are a range of strategies employed, including structural regeneration of injured nerves and collateral growth of nearby intact nerve fibres. In addition, changes in gene expression affect neurotransmitters and associated receptor function as well as alteration of ion channels within cell membranes. This has the potential to promote recovery and regain pre-injury function, but the process is not perfect, and can result in a number of unpleasant complications, including:[52]

- Muscle spasticity
- Neuropathic pain
- Autonomic dysreflexia
- Bowel and bladder dysfunction
- Cardiac arrhythmias
- Sexual dysfunction.

Autonomic dysreflexia

Autonomic dysreflexia occurs in patients with SCI at T6 or higher. It is typically triggered by a noxious stimulus which leads to sympathetic division activation that the brain cannot override as it occurs below the level of the cord injury.[48] Common causes of autonomic dysreflexia include:[49]

- Bladder and bowel distension
- Ingrowing toenail or fracture below the SCI
- Pressure sores, contact burns, scalds and sunburn
- Urinary tract infection, bladder spasm
- Kidney stones

Chapter 3   Disability

- Pregnancy, uterine contractions and childbirth
- Deep vein thrombosis and pulmonary embolism.

These noxious stimuli send afferent sensory signals to the spinal cord, which in turn generate reflex sympathetic impulses. Above the injury, the parasympathetic division can react to the changes in physiology and attempts to compensate, resulting in a blend of signs and symptoms, sometimes with a clear demarcation, particularly in skin signs, above and below the level of cord injury. This parasympathetic compensatory response leads to nasal congestion and skin flushing. Other signs and symptoms of autonomic dysreflexia include:[48,53]

- Severe hypertension rising at least 20–40 mmHg above an adult's pre-injury blood pressure (although this is often not known)
- Pounding headache
- Vasodilation above injury, vasoconstriction
- Profuse sweating above the injury
- Piloerection (goosebumps)
- Blurred vision
- Bradycardia, cardiac arrhythmias including atrial fibrillation.

Management

This is a medical emergency and should be treated as such. Remember that your patient and their carers are likely to be much more knowledgeable about their condition, so listen and act on their instruction. Patient management can be divided into non-pharmacological and pharmacological interventions.[48,49,54]

Non-pharmacological interventions

- If supine, sit the patient upright, dangling their legs if possible and loosen tight clothing. This may allow blood to pool in the lower extremities and help reduce blood pressure.
- Recheck blood pressure and heart rate every 2–5 minutes.
- Remove the noxious stimulus if possible. Most commonly this is related to bladder distension or bowel impaction. Check a catheter if it is in situ, particularly the presence of kinks in tubing. If skilled help is available, then replacement of a catheter and a rectal examination may have already been attempted. Don't forget other potential causes including pressure sores, ingrown toenails and crushed testicles, for example.

Pharmacological interventions

- If the non-pharmacological methods fail and the systolic blood pressure remains at 150 mmHg or higher, then nifedipine or nitrates are generally advocated.[48,55] You are likely to only carry one of these, GTN, but the *JRCALC Clinical Guidelines* do not indicate the use of this (or any) drug for autonomic dysreflexia.[1] However, a typical regimen would be 10 mg nifedipine sublingual or chewed or GTN spray 1–2 sprays, repeated every 20–30 min as required.[56]
- Patients with high SCI may well already have a management plan, including the use of drugs, so ask the patient or a carer what to do. If that is not possible (for example the patient is unconscious), then check for an autonomic dysreflexia card, which the patient may carry.

References

1. Joint Royal Colleges Ambulance Liaison Committee, Association of Ambulance Chief Executives. JRCALC Clinical Guidelines. Cited from JRCALC Plus (Version 1.2.13) [Mobile application software]. Bridgwater: Class Publishing Ltd; 2021.
2. Morrison L. Advanced prehospital stroke triage in the era of mechanical thrombectomy. *Journal of Paramedic Practice*, 2019 Apr 2;11(4):144–152.
3. Intercollegiate Stroke Working Party. National clinical guideline for stroke [Internet]. 2016. Available from: https://www.strokeaudit.org/SupportFiles/Documents/Guidelines/2016-National-Clinical-Guideline-for-Stroke-5t-(1).aspx
4. Stroke Association. Stroke statistics [Internet]. Stroke Association. 2020. Available from: https://www.stroke.org.uk/what-is-stroke/stroke-statistics
5. NHS England. NHS Stroke action will save hundreds of lives [Internet]. 2019. Available from: https://www.england.nhs.uk/2019/05/nhs-stroke-action-will-save-hundreds-of-lives/
6. Drake RL, Vogl W, Mitchell AWM, Gray H. *Gray's anatomy for students*, 3rd edition. Philadelphia: Churchill Livingstone/Elsevier; 2015.
7. Marieb E, Hoehn K. *Human anatomy & physiology*, 11th edition. Pearson; 2019.
8. Stroke Association. Are you at risk of stroke? [Internet]. Stroke Association. 2015. Available from: https://www.stroke.org.uk/what-is-stroke/are-you-at-risk-of-stroke
9. O'Donnell MJ, Xavier D, Liu L, Zhang H, Chin SL, Rao-Melacini P, et al. Risk factors for ischaemic and intracerebral haemorrhagic stroke in 22 countries (the INTERSTROKE study): a case-control study. *The Lancet*, 2010 Jul;376(9735):112–123.
10. Rodgers H, Greenaway J, Davies T, Wood R, Steen N, Thomson R. Risk factors for first-ever stroke in older people in the north east of England: a population-based study. *Stroke*, 2004 Jan 1;35(1):7–11.
11. Ross J, Horton-Szar D. *Crash course nervous system*, 4th edition. Smith C, editor. London: Mosby; 2015.
12. Saver JL. Time is brain–quantified. Stroke. 2006 Jan 1;37(1):263–266.
13. Harbison J, Hossain O, Jenkinson D, Davis J, Louw SJ, Ford GA. Diagnostic accuracy of stroke referrals from primary care, emergency room physicians, and ambulance staff using the face arm speech test. *Stroke*, 2003 Jan 1;34(1):71–76.
14. National Institute for Health and Care Excellence. Stroke and transient ischaemic attack in over 16s: diagnosis and initial management [Internet]. NICE; 2019. Available from: https://www.nice.org.uk/guidance/ng128
15. McClelland G. Paramedic identification of stroke mimic presentations: development and preliminary evaluation of a pre-hospital clinical assessment tool. Newcastle: PhD Thesis; 2018.
16. Brignole M, Moya A, de Lange FJ, Deharo J-C, Elliott PM, Fanciulli A, et al. 2018 ESC Guidelines for the diagnosis and management of syncope. *European Heart Journal*, 2018 Jun 1;39(21):1883–1948.
17. National Institute for Health and Care Excellence. Transient loss of consciousness ('blackouts') in over 16s [Internet]. NICE; 2014. Available from: https://www.nice.org.uk/guidance/cg109
18. Saklani P, Krahn A, Klein G. Syncope. *Circulation*, 2013 Mar 26;127(12):1330–1339.
19. Thijs RD, Bloem BR, Dijk JG. Falls, faints, fits and funny turns. *Journal of Neurology*, 2009 Feb;256(2):155–167.
20. Brignole M, Moya A, de Lange FJ, Deharo J-C, Elliott PM, Fanciulli A, et al. Practical instructions for the 2018 ESC Guidelines for the diagnosis and management of syncope. *European Heart Journal*, 2018 Jun 1;39(21):e43–80.
21. Gibbons CH, Freeman R. Delayed orthostatic hypotension: a frequent cause of orthostatic intolerance. *Neurology*, 2006 Jul 11;67(1):28–32.
22. Fedorowski A. Postural orthostatic tachycardia syndrome: clinical presentation, aetiology and management. Journal of Internal Medicine, 2019;285(4):352–366.
23. Berg AT, Berkovic SF, Brodie MJ, Buchhalter J, Cross JH, van Emde Boas W, et al. Revised terminology and concepts for organization of seizures and epilepsies: Report of the

Chapter 3 Disability

ILAE Commission on Classification and Terminology, 2005–2009. *Epilepsia*, 2010 Apr;51(4):676–685.
24. Brown RJ, Reuber M. Psychological and psychiatric aspects of psychogenic non-epileptic seizures (PNES): a systematic review. *Clinical Psychology Review*, 2016 Apr 1;45:157–182.
25. Nadarajan V, Perry RJ, Johnson J, Werring DJ. Transient ischaemic attacks: mimics and chameleons. *Practical Neurology*, 2014 Jan 2;14(1):23–31.
26. Alcocer F, David M, Goodman R, Jain SKA, David S. A forgotten vascular disease with important clinical implications. Subclavian steal syndrome. *American Journal of Case Reports*, 2013 Feb 25;14:58–62.
27. Osiro S, Zurada A, Gielecki J, Shoja MM, Tubbs RS, Loukas M. A review of subclavian steal syndrome with clinical correlation. Medical Science Monitor: International Medical Journal of Experimental and Clinical Research, 2012 May 1;18(5):RA57–63.
28. British Association for the Study of Headache. National headache management system for adults [Internet]. 2019. Available from: https://www.bash.org.uk/downloads/guidelines2019/02_BASHNationalHeadache_Management_SystemforAdults_2019_guideline_versi1.pdf
29. Moragas-Garrido M, Davenport R. Acute headache. *Medicine (Baltimore)*, 2013;41(3):164–168.
30. National Institute for Health and Care Excellence. Headaches in over 12s: diagnosis and management [Internet]. NICE; 2015. Available from: https://www.nice.org.uk/guidance/cg150
31. Mayans L, Walling A. Acute migraine headache: treatment strategies. *American Family Physician*, 2018 Feb 15;97(4):243–251.
32. Davenport R. Headache. *Practical Neurology*, 2008 Oct 1;8(5):335–343.
33. Charles A. The pathophysiology of migraine: implications for clinical management. *The Lancet Neurology*, 2018 Feb 1;17(2):174–182.
34. Bounes V, Edlow JA. Migraine: diagnosis and pharmacologic treatment in emergency department. The European Review for Medical and Pharmacological Sciences, 2011;15(2):215–221.
35. Karsan N, Goadsby PJ. Biological insights from the premonitory symptoms of migraine. Nature Reviews Neurology, 2018 Dec;14(12):699–710.
36. International Headache Society. Headache Classification Committee of the International Headache Society (IHS): The International Classification of Headache Disorders, 3rd edition. *Cephalalgia*, 2018 Jan;38(1):1–211.
37. Gondim JA, Almeida JPC de, Albuquerque LAF de, Schops M, Gomes É, Ferraz T. Headache associated with pituitary tumors. The Journal of Headache and Pain, 2009 Feb;10(1):15–20.
38. Subramaniam S, Fletcher WA. Obesity and weight loss in idiopathic intracranial hypertension: a narrative review. Journal of the North American Neuro-Ophthalmology Society, 2017 Jun;37(2):197–205.
39. Giamberardino MA, Affaitati G, Costantini R, Guglielmetti M, Martelletti P. Acute headache management in emergency department. A narrative review. Internal and Emergency Medicine, 2020 Jan 1;15(1):109–117.
40. Koster MJ, Matteson EL, Warrington KJ. Large-vessel giant cell arteritis: diagnosis, monitoring and management. *Rheumatology*, 2018 Feb 1;57(suppl_2):ii32–42.
41. Hassan N, Dasgupta B, Barraclough K. Giant cell arteritis. *British Medical Journal*, 2011 May 23;342(may23 1):d3019–d3019.
42. Dejaco C, Duftner C, Buttgereit F, Matteson EL, Dasgupta B. The spectrum of giant cell arteritis and polymyalgia rheumatica: revisiting the concept of the disease. *Rheumatology*, 2016 Aug 1;kew273.
43. Adams R, Bennett A, Jackson G. NPIS Carbon Monoxide Poisoning Surveillance Project - CO Exposure Monitoring Using NPIS Resources July 2015 to June 2016 (year one). *Gas Safety Trust*; 2016.
44. Ducros A, Bousser M-G. Thunderclap headache. *British Medical Journal*, 2013 Jan 9;346(jan08 15):e8557–e8557.
45. Ozkurt B, Cinar O, Cevik E, Acar AY, Arslan D, Eyi EY, et al. Efficacy of high-flow oxygen therapy in all types of headache: a prospective, randomized, placebo-controlled trial. *American Journal of Emergency Medicine*, 2012 Nov;30(9):1760–1764.

References

46. Nutbeam T, Fenwick R, Smith J, Bouamra O, Wallis L, Stassen W. A comparison of the demographics, injury patterns and outcome data for patients injured in motor vehicle collisions who are trapped compared to those patients who are not trapped. Scandinavian Journal of Trauma, Resuscitation and Emergency Medicine, 2021 Dec;29(1):17.
47. Beck B, Cameron PA, Braaf S, Nunn A, Fitzgerald MC, Judson RT, et al. Traumatic spinal cord injury in Victoria, 2007–2016. *The Medical Journal of Australia*, 2019;210(8):360–366.
48. Eldahan KC, Rabchevsky AG. Autonomic dysreflexia after spinal cord injury: systemic pathophysiology and methods of management. Autonomic Neuroscience: Basic and Clinical, 2018 Jan;209:59–70.
49. Krassioukov A. Autonomic dysreflexia. Clinical Journal of Sport Medicine, 2012 Jan;22(1):39–45.
50. Gupta A, Taly AB, Srivastava A, Murali T. Non-traumatic spinal cord lesions: epidemiology, complications, neurological and functional outcome of rehabilitation. *Spinal Cord*, 2009 Apr;47(4):307–11.
51. Eckert MJ, Martin MJ. Trauma: spinal cord injury. *Surgical Clinics of North America*, 2017 Oct;97(5):1031–1045.
52. Brown A, Weaver LC. The dark side of neuroplasticity. *Experimental Neurology*, 2012 May;235(1):133–141.
53. Sharif H, Hou S. Autonomic dysreflexia: a cardiovascular disorder following spinal cord injury. *Neural Regen Res*, 2017 Sep;12(9):1390–400.
54. Consortium for Spinal Cord Medicine. *Acute management of autonomic dysreflexia: individuals with spinal cord injury presenting to health-care facilities*, 2nd edition. Washington: Paralyzed Veterans of America; 2001.
55. Royal College of Physicians. Chronic spinal cord injury [Internet]. RCP London. 2008. Available from: https://www.rcplondon.ac.uk/guidelines-policy/chronic-spinal-cord-injury
56. Royal National Orthopaedic Hospital. Autonomic Dysreflexia [Internet]. Available from: https://www.rnoh.nhs.uk/services/spinal-cord-injury-centre/medical-management-advice/autonomic-dysreflexia

4   Exposure

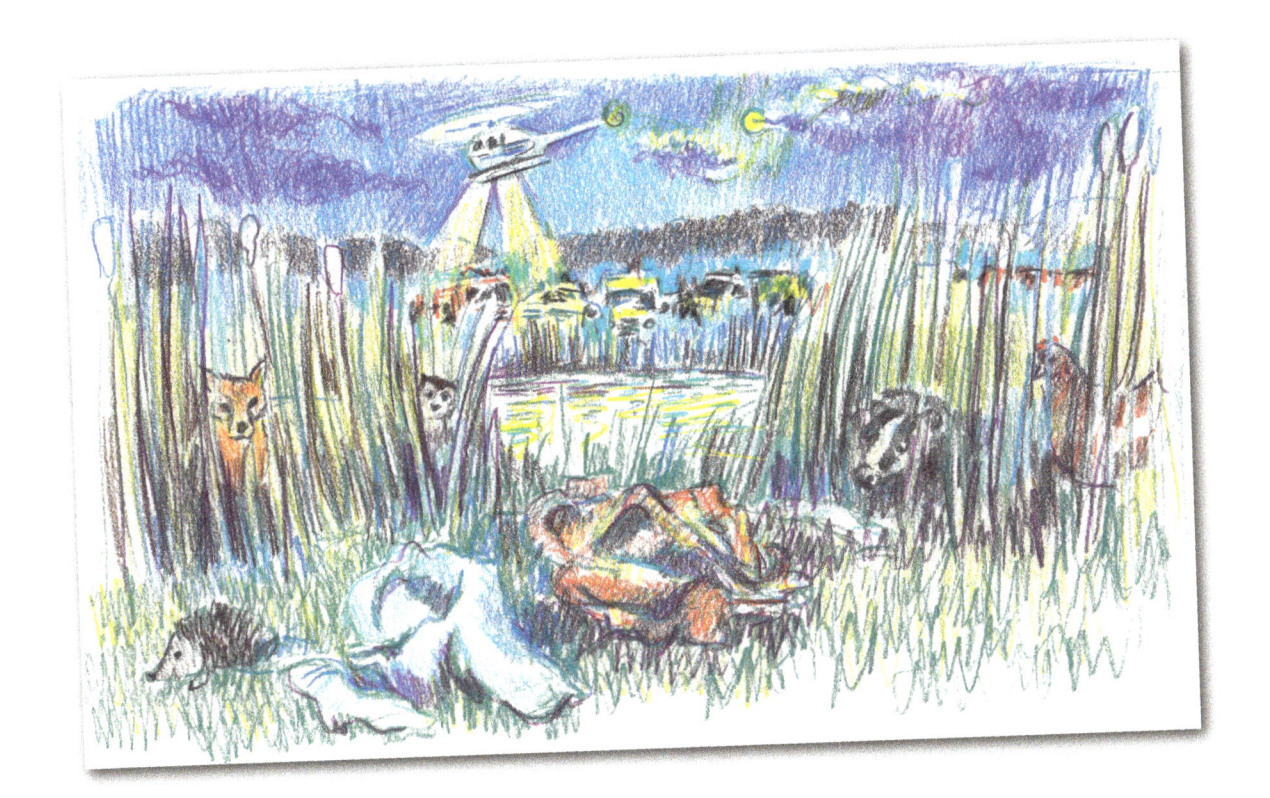

Drowning

You are sat on standby gazing at the full moon as it breaks through some light cloud. The shift has been hectic and the last patient, a young man who thought he was a werewolf ("Look at the hair on the palms of my hands," he kept insisting), has prompted your colleague to adopt a bizarre howling speech.

At the suggestion of a drink he responds with, "You want a cup of coffee, do yoooooou?" Having been amusing initially, it is now getting rather tedious and you are glad when the MDT passes details of the next job. "What are we off toooooo?" asks your colleague. You check the MDT, "a pile of clothes found discarded next to a pond," you reply and your colleague lets out a triumphant howl. "Child's clothes," you add and the smile drops from his face. "Oh, right." Instead, he settles for making the ambulance's engine scream en route to the incident location.

Chapter 4   Exposure

As you arrive on scene, it is clear by the large number of flashing blue lights in the distance, that many other emergency vehicles are already on scene. To reach them, you need to negotiate a rough track that runs around a field. It's only just wide enough for the ambulance and you cannot see if there is room to turn around.

> What are you going to do: Advise your colleague to continue driving **Forwards** or **Reverse** in? (Remember your answer)

Having negotiated your way up the rough track, your colleague adds the ambulance's blue lights to the impressive array already present. There are two fire tenders, a major incident support vehicle, several senior fire officer cars, two police cars and an ambulance rapid response vehicle (RRV). You are informed over the radio that the hazardous area response team (HART) are on their way, although it is hard to hear the transmission over the noise from the police helicopter circling overhead.

After asking for directions, you head off across a paddock, which is adjacent to a sloping field. At the bottom of the field is a fishing lake. It is surrounded by bushes on three sides and is full of reeds. Close to the shore are a set of children's clothes and a pair of shoes that look like they were discarded in a hurry.

> What are you going to do: **Wade in** (read on) or **Wait on the shore** (skip the next paragraph)?

Wade in

A child could be in that lake and everyone just seems to be stood on the bank doing nothing. Before anyone can object, you stomp off into the water. The good news is that it is only waist deep. The bad news is that there is a lot of silt at the bottom and you only make it a couple of metres from the shore before getting well and truly stuck. Now you are in the water, you can make out some rescuers in dry suits searching the far side of the lake. After having your photo taken by representatives from all the emergency services present, you suffer the indignation of being rescued by the fire service and being told, "Next time, leave it to the professionals."

Wait on the shore

The lake doesn't look that deep and is clear, which should make the child fairly easy to find. In addition, having looked carefully, you can make out some rescuers in dry suits who have appeared from behind a bunch of reeds. Your colleague is having fun poking a long stick into the water. "The silt at the bottom looks a bit sticky," he muses, prophetically as it turns out. No sooner have the words left his mouth when one of the rescuers gets stuck and requires assistance from several colleagues on the shore to pull him out. However, your amusement is short-lived as you are yelled at by a fire officer for being too close to the edge of the lake without a life-vest.

With the RRV paramedic guarding your kit, you stroll back up to the vehicle to greet the HART who have just arrived, and brief them on the situation. They gear-up and accompany you back to the pond to assist with the search. "Lucky it's fresh water, better for drowning survivors," your colleague mutters as you return to the pond.

> What are you going to reply: **Mmm, yes** (read on) or **I'm not sure you're right** (skip the next paragraph)?

Mmm, yes

You murmur in agreement, but are contradicted by a HART operative who has overheard your conversation. "Actually, I think you'll find that the tonicity of the water makes no difference," she states before strolling off into the darkness. A quick-draw of smartphones ensues as you and your colleague Google for an answer.

I'm not sure you're right

"I don't think it makes a difference," you reply while plucking out your smartphone to search for an answer. Wikipedia, that bastion of evidence-based research, supports your position. "Whatever," your colleague mutters sulkily.

After an hour and a half, your feet are cold and both of you are very bored. However, there is good news. The police trace the clothes to a child who was spotted running naked through a nearby town the day before and have confirmed that he is safe and well. You head back to the ambulance, stow your kit and prepare to leave.

> Which way did you come down the track: **Forwards** (read on) or **Reversing** (skip the next paragraph)?

Forwards

Although driving down the track was easy, reversing out, with the lights of the other emergency service vehicles still flashing, makes things difficult for your colleague. He asks you to see him back. The track is narrow and you gingerly make your way around to the back of the ambulance. Unfortunately, you slip into a drainage ditch, which although not deep contains the most foul-smelling material. After clambering out and watching your colleague reverse, you get into the cab and the pair of you retch your way back to station.

Reversing

Although it was a pain reversing down the track, it is a trivial process getting out. This is fortunate, because a drainage ditch just where you parked seems to contain some offensive-smelling material. "Lucky you didn't fall down there," says your colleague.

The scale of the problem

The definition of drowning has been complicated in the past and so in 2002 (at the World Congress on Drowning in Amsterdam) a single definition was agreed. As a result, drowning is now defined as a process resulting in primary respiratory impairment from submersion/immersion in a liquid.[1] Whether the victim lives or dies after this process is not important, they have still drowned. If they do not survive, then they have fatally drowned.[2] The differentiation between submersion and immersion is less concrete. However, submersion is generally said to have occurred when the patient's airway goes below the surface of the liquid medium to differentiate it from immersion.[3]

In the UK, there has been a reduction in deaths from drowning over the past decade. For example, there were approximately 650 deaths from drowning in 2010, which had reduced to 344 in 2019.[2] The vast majority of these were accidental, although in nearly a quarter of cases, the nature of the drowning was not recorded. However, many more are involved in non-fatal events that, without intervention from rescuers, for example, Royal National Lifeboat Institution (RNLI) lifeguards, may have resulted in a fatal drowning.[4]

Chapter 4 Exposure

Pathophysiology

Most drownings occur in water that is not thermoneutral (that is, water temperature where heat loss is equal to heat production) and is the focus of this section. Immersion in cold water produces large and rapid reductions in skin temperature, which in turn leads to a cold shock response consisting of: gasping, hyperventilation, increased cardiac output and hypertension.[5] This can occur in water less than 25°C, peaking at water temperatures of 10–15°C. Cold shock is thought to be caused by stimulation of cutaneous cold thermoreceptors, which result in an excessive sympathetic nervous system response. The magnitude of the cold shock response is reduced by the victims' clothing, their habituation to cold (regular winter swimming in just your Speedos, for example) and orientation on immersion (for example, intentionally diving into the water … in winter … in your Speedos).[6]

A significant consequence of cold shock is the effect on breath-holding, which can be reduced from approximately 45 seconds in warm water to less than 10 seconds when the cold shock response is evoked. Intoxication and deliberate aspiration of liquid (such as occurs in suicide) also reduce breath-holding time.[5] During submersion, once the inspiratory drive is too high to resist, the victim will take a breath and water will be aspirated into the airways. Laryngospasm may occur, but this is rapidly terminated by cerebral hypoxia and active ventilation, with aspiration of water, will resume.

Whether due to laryngospasm or breath-holding with no gas exchange the victim becomes increasingly hypoxaemic, hypercarbic and acidotic. Unless they are rescued, the victim will succumb to hypoxaemia, leading to loss of consciousness and apnoea. The cardiac rhythm deteriorates, usually following a sequence of tachyarrhythmias, bradyarrhythmias, pulseless electrical activity (PEA) and asystole.[7]

If the victim is fully submerged in cold water, the diving response may be activated, although its importance as a protective mechanism in drowning is unclear. It is likely to be less important than rapid selective cooling of the brain and heart caused by aspiration and ingestion of ice-cold water, for example.[5] It also is less commonly found in adults compared to infants. However, it is caused by cooling of the cold thermoreceptors on the face, which are innervated by the ophthalmic and maxillary division of the trigeminal nerve. This results in a profound sinus bradycardia due to parasympathetic nervous system stimulation of the heart, an expiratory apnoea due to inhibition of central respiratory neurons, and sympathetic nervous system mediated vasoconstriction of the trunk and limbs. A similar response is also possible by stimulation of vagal receptors in the pharynx and larynx.[8]

It has been suggested that this simultaneous stimulation of both sympathetic and parasympathetic pathways of the autonomic nervous system results in an 'autonomic conflict', leading to life-threatening arrhythmias that may result in death in susceptible individuals (Figure 4.1).[6]

As if everything mentioned so far wasn't bad enough, an additional problem is that as muscles cool (particularly the arms), superficial muscle fibres become impaired and at temperatures of <20°C, nerve conduction is slowed sufficiently to effectively result in peripheral paralysis. Note that this can occur, even in cases where core body temperature is above 35°C, that is, the patient is not hypothermic.[5]

Although the tonicity of the water (for example, sea water versus fresh water) was once thought to be important, the effect on the lungs is ultimately the same, although with a different osmotic gradient. The fragile alveolar-capillary membranes are disrupted, leading to increased permeability and movement of

Drowning

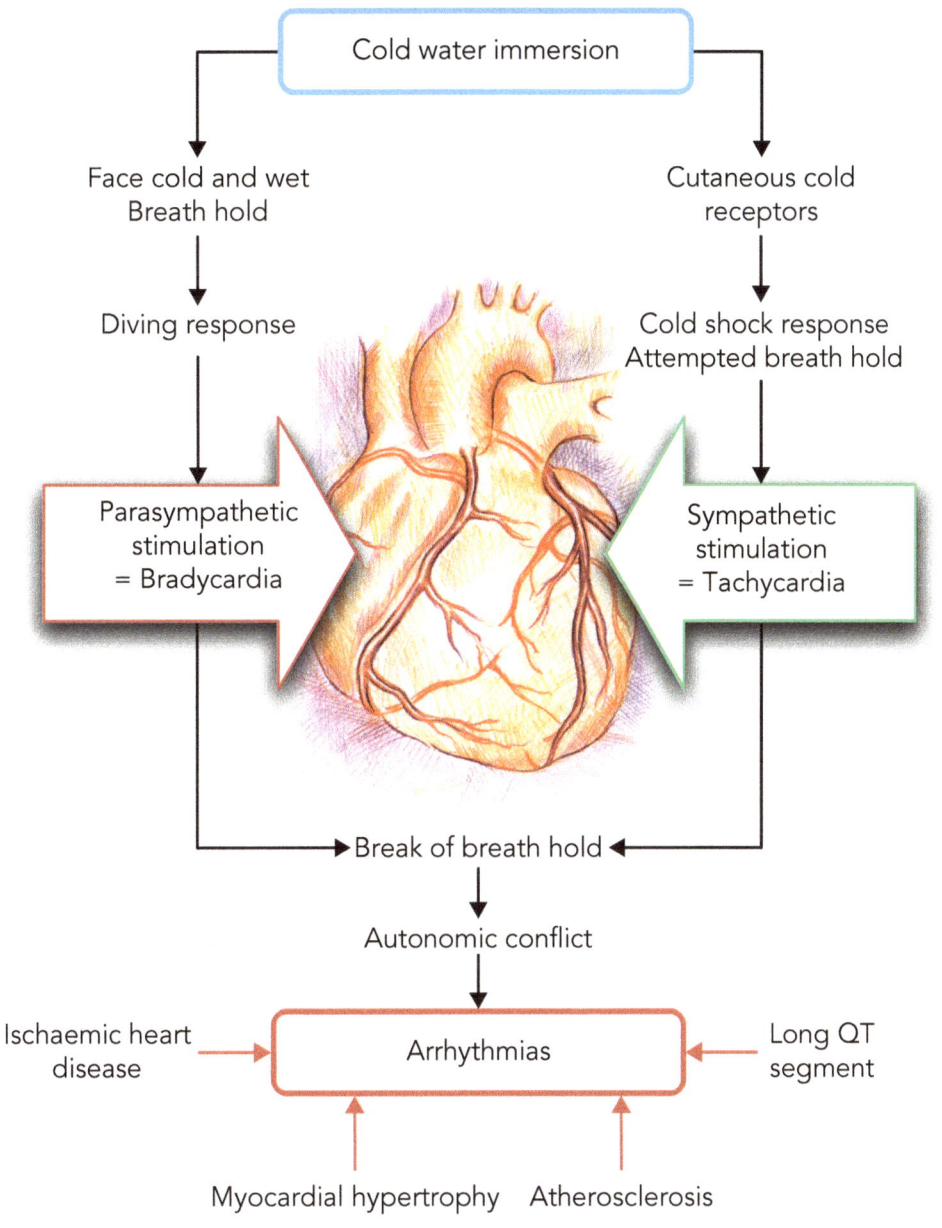

Figure 4.1 Autonomic conflict.

fluid, plasma and electrolytes.[9] Clinically, this leads to significant amounts of blood-stained pulmonary oedema and decreasing gaseous exchange of oxygen and carbon dioxide. In addition, the presence of plasma in the alveoli may generate foam, further decreasing pulmonary efficiency. Following drowning, the presence of additional fluid and/or plasma in the lungs and the loss of surfactant lead to increasing areas of the lungs becoming regions of low or no ventilation and perfusion (pulmonary shunting), and there is widespread atelectasis and bronchospasm.[7] Similarly, the haemodynamic and cardiovascular effects seen in drowning are not related to tonicity either, but primarily as a consequence of anoxia.[9]

Management

Undertake a dynamic risk assessment to determine whether rescue is feasible and appropriate. In cases of submersion, submersion duration is the best available prognostic indicator (although it is not great) for making decisions about whether to treat the incident as a rescue or recovery.[10]

Try to avoid getting wet. You should only go into the water to rescue a drowning victim as a last resort and only if you are adequately trained and equipped. Many victims who are drowning can help themselves with firm coaching, or will have already been rescued by bystanders or professional rescuers, who can have a dramatic impact on the victim's outcome.

If you need to rescue the victim, remember to 'call, reach, throw, wade and row'. As previously mentioned, encourage victims to self-rescue first. Next, try to reach them with an object such as a pole, tree branch or even items of clothing. Consider throwing something that is buoyant, ideally a rescue ring with a lifeline attached. Wading into the water is the next possibility as long as someone on the shore has hold of you, the water is shallow enough to stand in and the victim is within reach. Alternatively, use a boat, if available.

In-water resuscitation should only be performed by highly trained rescue teams and limited to up to 1 minute of ventilation in patients who are unconscious and not breathing.[11] Chest compressions are futile in deep water, so wait until the patient is on a firm surface, such as the shore or deck of a boat.[12] The incidence of spinal injuries is very low (around 0.5%) and delays effective resuscitation, so only immobilise the spine when there is a clear mechanism of injury that could cause spinal injury (such as diving into shallow water or water skiing).[13,14]

Get the victim out of the water as soon as possible and place them supine (on their back), with head and torso at the same level and check for breathing. If they are breathing but unconscious, provide high-flow oxygen via non-rebreathing mask as per clinical guidelines and place them in the recovery position. Victims of prolonged immersion in water (typically 30 minutes or more, but less as water temperature decreases), may also suffer the added complication of circum-rescue collapse.[15] This is due to the increased hydrostatic pressure from the water on the victim's legs and torso increasing venous return and cardiac output. Central baroreceptors mistake this for hypervolaemia resulting in increased diuresis. In addition, peripheral vasoconstriction will occur as the water is cold relative to the body, which magnifies this response.[16] Once the victim is removed from the water, the hydrostatic pressure is lost, exacerbating the hypovolaemia. This can also be compounded by hypothermia and physical effort if the victim attempts to remove themselves from the water, for example. The sudden drop in venous return can reduce coronary perfusion enough to induce cardiac arrest. For this reason, it is advised to remove victims horizontally from the water if possible.[13]

Hypothermia is likely to occur and wet clothes should be cut off to minimise movement. Hypothermic patients (doesn't seem right to call them victims anymore, now that there is a highly trained healthcare professional by their side!) are at risk of cardiac arrhythmias, including ventricular fibrillation, even with minor movement.[17] Get the patient covered with blankets and in a warm ambulance as soon as possible.

If your patient is not breathing or is breathing abnormally, administer five rescue breaths via a bag-valve-mask connected to high-flow oxygen. Note that this is different from the usual CAB approach that the current resuscitation guidelines advocate for adults, but reflects that correction of hypoxia is the most important aspect in the management of the drowned patient. It can be difficult to differentiate post-arrest gasping from initial respiratory efforts of the drowning patient, so if you are unsure, administer ventilations and start CPR. Pulse checks are unreliable, so try to utilise other diagnostic tests if available, such as electrocardiogram (ECG) and end tidal carbon dioxide ($EtCO_2$) monitoring. If in doubt, commence chest compressions with ventilations at a ratio of 30:2. Compression-only CPR is not advocated. Perform tracheal intubation if this can be undertaken safely.[11]

Advanced life support follows the normal algorithm, unless the patient is hypothermic (core body temperature less than 30°C). In this case, only administer a maximum of three shocks if the patient is in VF or pulseless VT, and do not administer any adrenaline until you have them warmed up. Once the core body temperature is over 30°C you can give intravenous drugs, but double the time interval between each administration. Once the patient is over 35°C, resuscitate the patient as normal (for example, shock them until your batteries run out and give adrenaline every 3–5 minutes).

Do not stop resuscitation efforts unless it is clear that it would be futile to continue (for example, due to the patient sustaining massive traumatic injuries). There are no completely accurate prognostic indicators in drowning, although duration of submersion is correlated with risk of death or severe neurological impairment.[18] In water above 6°C, survival after submersion for more than 30 minutes is unlikely. At 6°C or below, survival time can be extended up to 90 minutes, although this is more likely to apply to children immersed in ice-cold water.[19] As with hypothermia, the general rule is your patient is not dead, until they are warm and dead.

Chapter 4 Exposure

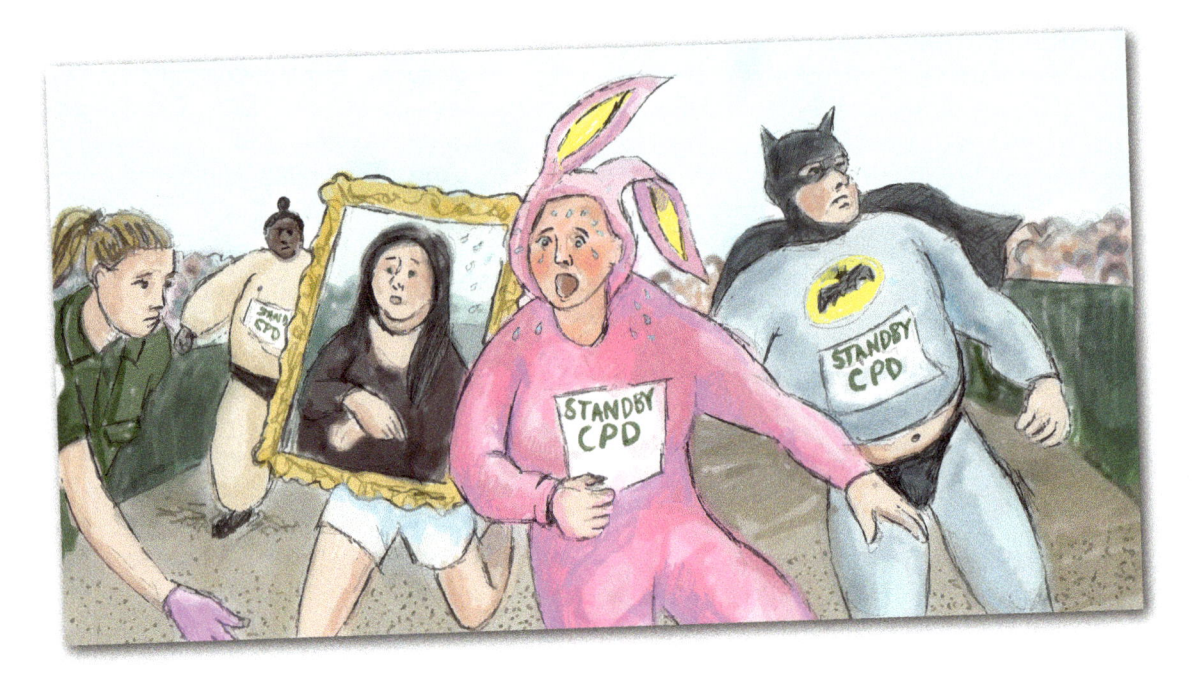

Heat-Related Illness

You are on standby at a local 'fun run', which according to your colleague is a contradiction in terms. Spring has sprung and the weather is good. Very good. In fact, the sun has some real warmth, which is making your standby very pleasant indeed. "Not so good for the runners though," your colleague points out. In particular, a number of the runners who are wearing some serious fancy-dress gear. Highlights include a woman wearing a painting complete with frame, superheroes, a chap in an inflatable sumo suit and someone dressed for batting in cricket, complete with pads and helmet. "I wonder if he's wearing a box too," laughs your colleague. However, it looks like your new favourite fancy-dress runner has just staggered over the hill and is meandering towards your location. The woman is wearing a pink rabbit onesie. She does not have a typical runner's habitus either. "She looks hot," says your colleague dryly. Certainly, her face is as red as a beetroot and you don't like the look of her running/staggering style. She is certainly gaining the attention of the crowd and other runners which is fortunate, because just as she comes alongside your position, she stumbles towards the ground. A couple of runners nearby come to her aid and help her to the edge of the road.

You nod to the security staff and they move a barrier so you can get to the woman. You introduce yourself to her, but she appears to be having trouble talking, although she does manage to tell you her name is Sheena, or Sheila, you're not quite sure. However, security note her race number and quickly come back with her details. It turns out her name is Sylvia and she is 50 years old.

Your colleague finishes assembling the carry chair and you assist Sylvia onto it and head for the ambulance. Sylvia's head is starting to loll about in a rather alarming fashion and you are keen to get her onto the ambulance trolley. Your primary survey reveals the following:

Airway

Patent

Breathing

Respiratory rate: 28 breaths/min
SpO_2 : 100% on air
Good bilateral air entry

Circulation

Flushed, sweaty skin, hot to touch
Heart rate: 140 beats/min
Blood pressure: 104/50 mmHg

Disability

GCS score: 12/15
Pupils: PEARRL
Blood sugar: 4.7 mmol/l

Exposure/Environment

Temperature: 40.7°C
Peripheral oedema
No rash

> What are you going to do: **Calculate the NEWS** (read on) or **Take off the onesie** (skip the next paragraph)?

Calculate the NEWS

Working out the national early warning score is an important part of a patient's clinical management, as you'll be able to work out an appropriate response to Sylvia's current clinical condition. Your colleague watches you trying to add up using your fingers, tuts, tells you the NEWS and suggests that action is better than maths right now. "How about we skin the bunny?" she suggests.

Take off the onesie

Working out the NEWS can wait, it is clear that Sylvia is very unwell. Although you can't quite recall the difference between heat exhaustion and heat stroke, it is clear that Sylvia is suffering from a heat-related illness and cooling her down is a priority. You unzip the onesie and coax Sylvia out of it. She has some running gear underneath, which you also remove.

"How are we going to cool her down?" asks your colleague. That is a good question. You look around the ambulance for inspiration.

> Which cooling method are you going to use: **Cold-water immersion** (read on) or **Evaporative cooling** (skip the next paragraph)?

Cold-water immersion

You recall from your scholarly reading while on a previous standby, that cold-water immersion is the optimal field treatment to achieve rapid temperature reduction in heat stroke.[20] However, you don't have a handy cold-water bath or convenient body of water such as a pond or lake to utilise. You realise that evaporative cooling is probably the best option.

Chapter 4 Exposure

Evaporative cooling

Since you don't have a cold bath handy, you elect to spray the patient with water and fan her vigorously. A knock at the ambulance door reveals a first-aider from a nearby first-aid point. They have bottles of water and some chemical cold packs. You thank them for their gifts and spread the cold packs liberally over Sylvia's body.

Another knock at the door reveals another paramedic who offers assistance. You elect to have them travel with you (who is going to keep up with water sprinkling and fanning otherwise?). With the other paramedic taking over fanning duties (although they claim that to maintain optimal performance, fanners should swap every two minutes), you quickly obtain intravenous access in the time it takes for your colleague to exit the vehicle, get into the driver's seat and prepare to leave the scene.

You take over fanning duties and the other paramedic sets up an IV line, administering a 250 ml bolus while making a pre-alert call to the local emergency department. You arrive 15 minutes later with another 250 ml bolus administered and the patient's level of consciousness has improved slightly.

The resus team are impressed that the patient almost completed the fun run while wearing a pink rabbit onesie, but that does not stop them inserting a rectal temperature probe. Thanks to your cooling efforts, the patient's temperature is 39.2°C and they set about continuing the cooling process, while you try to figure out a way to dry out the back of the ambulance, which is now awash with litres of water.

Scale of the problem

Heat-related illnesses can occur as a result of external factors such as the sun, or internal factors such as drugs and exercise. It presents on a continuum, with heat stress the least serious heat-related illness, through to multi-organ dysfunction and even death at the other extreme.[13]

Heat-related illnesses are common worldwide, and although the UK does not seem to have long hot summers, climate change models predict that the exceptional heatwave that occurred in the summer of 2003 may become the norm by 2040. During that summer, there were over 71,000 fatalities throughout Europe, with approximately 2,000 deaths occurring between the 4th and 13th August in England.[21]

Although there is no definition of a 'heatwave', excess deaths are known to occur when the ambient temperature exceeds 24.5°C. In addition, escalation of the Department of Health heat plan occurs when target day and night temperatures are reached. These vary throughout regions, but are on average 30°C during the day and 15°C at night, with higher threshold temperatures for the south-east and London, and lower threshold temperatures for Yorkshire and the north-east.[21] The plan also identifies higher-risk groups who are more likely to suffer from heat-related illness (Table 4.1).

Table 4.1 Groups at higher risk of heat-related illness, stratified by place of residence.

Community	Care home or hospital
Over 75 years	Over 75 years
Female	Female
Severe physical or mental illness	Severe physical or mental illness
Multiple medications	Multiple medications
Babies and young children	Babies and young children (hospitals)
Urban areas	Frailty
Living on own and isolated	

South-facing top flat	
Alcohol and/or drug dependency	
Homeless	

Source: GOV.UK, 2014.

Physiology

Humans are homeotherms, maintaining their temperature around 37°C thanks to feedback mechanisms that are co-ordinated by the hypothalamus. The body uses two main mechanisms to control body temperature:[22]

- Autonomic
- Behavioural.

Autonomic

As the name implies, autonomic control is involuntary and includes sweating, increasing cardiac output and redirection of blood to the skin (peripheral vasodilation). However, these responses can be diminished or delayed in older people and other vulnerable groups such as patients with chronic illnesses and in those taking some groups of medication, such as diuretic and anti-cholinergic drugs.[23]

Behavioural

In contrast to autonomic mechanisms, behavioural mechanisms are under conscious control and include:

- Fan cooling
- Turning on air conditioning
- Seeking shade
- Removing clothes.

However, conscious control means that these mechanisms can be ignored, exacerbating heat-related illness. For example, older people may not have or want to use air conditioning, due to concerns about the cost, and athletes or military personnel may continue to undertake high levels of physical activity even in hot weather.

Heat exchange

There are four methods of heat exchange:[22,24]

- Conduction
- Convection
- Evaporation
- Radiation.

Conduction

Conduction occurs if part of the body surface is in contact with a solid object. Heat exchange is dependent on the thermal conductivity of the object, as well as the surface area of the skin exposed. Conductive heat transfer occurs across the body's tissues too, although the subcutaneous fatty layers are poor conductors of heat.

Convection

Dry heat transfer occurs when air or water passes over the skin, but the rate of this heat exchange is dependent on the temperature gradient between the environment and the skin, thermal currents, exposed body surface area and bodily movements. Within the body, convection causes heat transfer between the blood vessels (especially capillaries) and other body tissues.

Evaporation

Evaporation can lead to significant heat loss, even when environmental temperature is the same as (or higher than) skin temperature, or when body temperature is raised, for example as a result of exercise. Evaporative cooling occurs thanks to sweat being vaporised from

Chapter 4   Exposure

the skin surface but is sensitive to humidity and wind velocity.

Radiation

Heat transfer can also occur via the exchange of electromagnetic energy. It is unaffected by ambient temperature or air velocity, but clothing can reduce transmission of radiant heat from the skin.

Pathophysiology

Heat stress

This is a mild form of heat-related illness and is the body's response to a hot environment, particularly during physical activity. It is characterised by:[11,20,24]

- Normal temperature or mild temperature elevation
- Heat oedema: Swelling of feet and ankles as a result of hydrostatic pressure, vascular leak and peripheral vasodilation
- Heat syncope: Vasodilation causes hypotension
- Heat cramps: Depletion of salts leads to muscle cramps.

Heat exhaustion

This is a more severe form of heat-related illness, with symptoms mostly occurring as a result of fluid loss and electrolyte imbalances:[20]

- Systemic reaction to prolonged heat exposure (hours to days)
- Core body temperature normal or over 37°C but less than 40°C
- Headache, dizziness, nausea and vomiting, tachycardia, hypotension, sweating, muscle pain, weakness and cramps
- Can progress quickly to heat stroke.

Heat stroke

Heat stroke is a severe heat illness characterised by a triad of severe hyperthermia (that is, core temperature >40°C), neurological abnormality (such as altered level of consciousness) and exposure of environmental heat or strenuous exercise.[11,20] It comes in two types: non-exertional heat stroke, which is caused by high external temperatures and/or high humidity, and exertional heat stroke, which is caused by excess heat production as a result of physical exercise. Non-exertional heat stroke tends to occur in the elderly, very young and chronically ill, whereas exertional heat stroke is more typical in active groups such as athletes, manual workers and military recruits.[13] Risk factors for heat illness are summarised in Table 4.2.[24,25]

Table 4.2   Risk factors for heat illness.

Individual	Environment	Medication and drug use	Chronic conditions
Age	High ambient temperature	Alcohol	Viral infection
Obesity	High humidity	Amphetamines	Inflammation
Poor physical fitness	Lack of air flow	Anti-cholinergics	Skin disorders
Lack of heat acclimatisation	Lack of shelter	Anti-depressants	Cardiovascular disease

Dehydration	Heatwave	Anti-histamines	Diabetes mellitus
		Anti-psychotics	Malignant hyperthermia
		Benzodiazepines	Sickle cell trait
		Beta-blockers	
		Calcium channel blockers	
		Diuretics	
		Laxatives	
		Neuroleptics	
		Phenothiazines	
		Thyroid agonists	

Adapted from: Auerbach, 2016.

Once core body temperature rises above a critical level (clinically defined as >40°C, although this is likely to vary between individuals), a cascade of cell and systemic responses occur, which if left unchecked result in a systemic inflammatory response syndrome (SIRS) similar to that seen in sepsis.[25]

Small rises in blood temperature (<1°C) lead to the hypothalamus activating a sympathetic-mediated increase of blood flow to the peripheries in an attempt to dissipate the extra heat to the environment. This can result in blood flows delivered to the peripheries as high as 8 l/min, which requires diversion of blood away from the kidney and mesentery (that is, blood flow to the gut).[20] However, this can cause ischaemia of the gut, which in turn makes the endothelial lining of the gut porous allowing endotoxins to enter the systemic and portal circulations. Toll-like receptors (TLRs) detect their presence and activate an immune response causing release of both pro- and anti-inflammatory cytokines (Figure 4.2).

In parallel to this response, heat-shock proteins (HSPs) are released by organs that find heat toxic (such as the gut, kidneys and spleen). These proteins provide some level of protection against hyperthermia, but may also contribute towards the SIRS response. In addition, it has been theorised that at some critical level of hyperthermia HSPs are overcome, allowing apoptosis (programmed cell death) and necrosis to occur.[26]

Management

The key aim of management of the patient with heat-related illness is rapid reversal of hyperthermia.

Minor heat-related illness

For less severe heat-related illness, simple first-aid measures are effective:[20]

- Remove patient from source of the heat. For example, place patient in the shade or an air-conditioned ambulance.
- Heat cramps are not due to neuromuscular fatigue and so will not improve with passive stretching. Instead, patients require oral rehydration and electrolyte replacement. Salt tablets are not suitable, however.
- Heat oedema can be reversed by elevating the extremities or placing compression stockings on the patient, assuming you have those squirrelled away in your response bag.

Chapter 4 Exposure

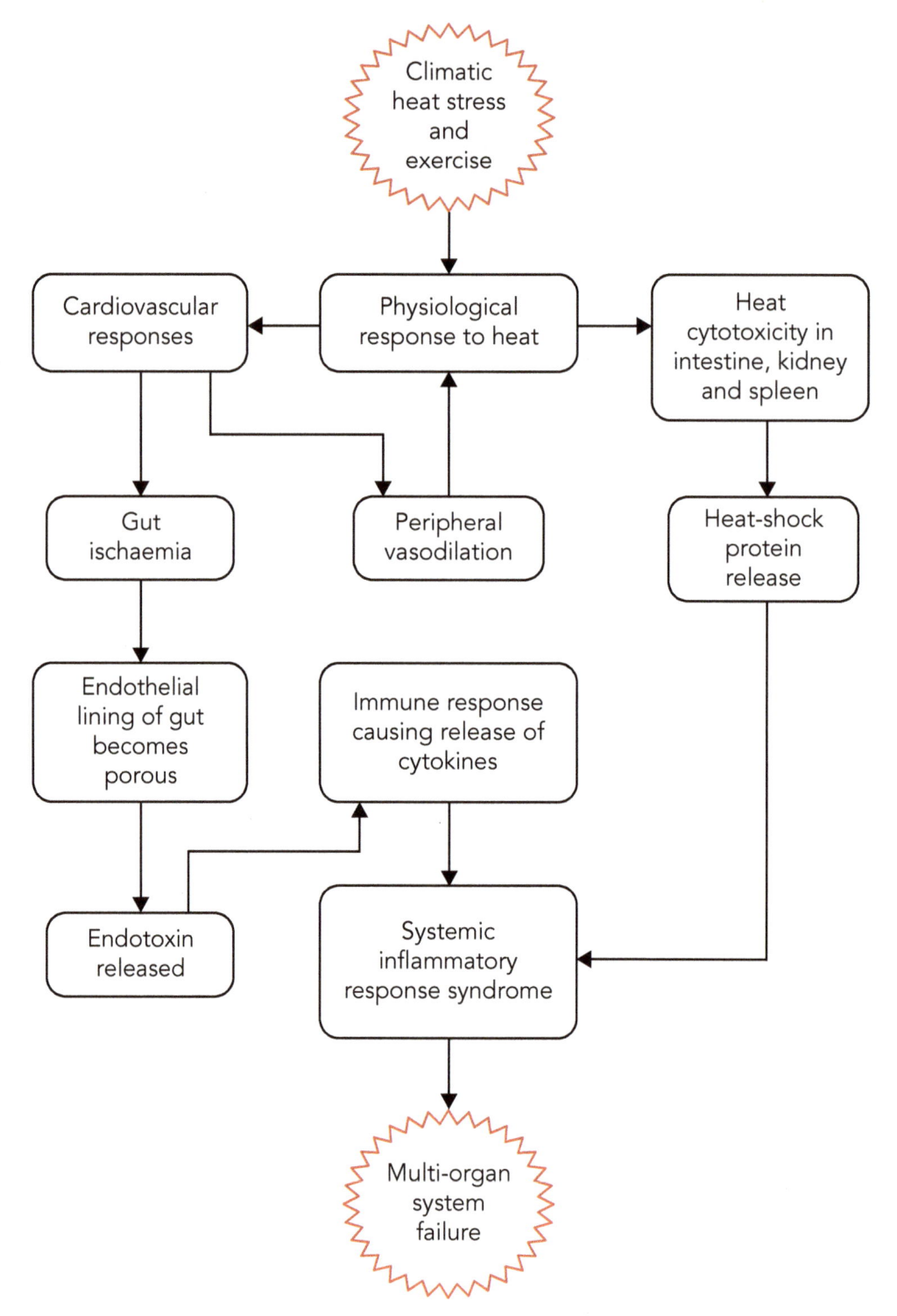

Figure 4.2 Pathophysiology of heatstroke.

- Heat syncope should be treated with oral fluid replacement and passive cooling (that is, place them in the shade with or without air conditioning). Don't forget to consider other causes of syncope.

Heat exhaustion

Heat exhaustion requires more aggressive intervention and active cooling methods to avoid heat stroke:[13,20]

- Remove patient from source of the heat.
- Commence evaporative and convective cooling by loosening/removing patient's clothing, spraying or splashing them with water and fanning vigorously. Note that it might be necessary to massage the skin if peripheral vasoconstriction occurs.
- Oral rehydration should be possible, but give IV fluids if the oral route is not possible.

Heat stroke

Heat stroke is the most serious heat-related illness. Management includes:[11,13,20]

- Manage airway, breathing and circulation.
- Start cooling immediately. Cold-water immersion (CWI) is the most effective method of cooling and, if possible, should be commenced at scene. This might warrant increasing your on scene time (by 20 minutes, for example) before rapidly transporting the patient to the emergency department (ED).[27]
- CWI is best achieved by removing the patient's clothes and submersing their trunk and limbs into a cold-water bath or convenient body of water, such as a lake or pond. Obviously, the patient should not be left and their head kept above water at all times!
- In situations where CWI is not possible and/or the patient's clinical condition warrants prompt removal from scene, undertake evaporative and convective cooling en route to the ED.
- Ice packs are also helpful, although they are better spread liberally all over the patient and not just the neck, axillae and groin. One study found that placing cold packs on the glabrous (hairless) areas of the body, such as the cheeks, palms and soles of the feet was effective in reducing core body temperature.[28]
- Note that anti-pyretic drugs are not effective in heat-related illness and should not be administered.

Chapter 4   Exposure

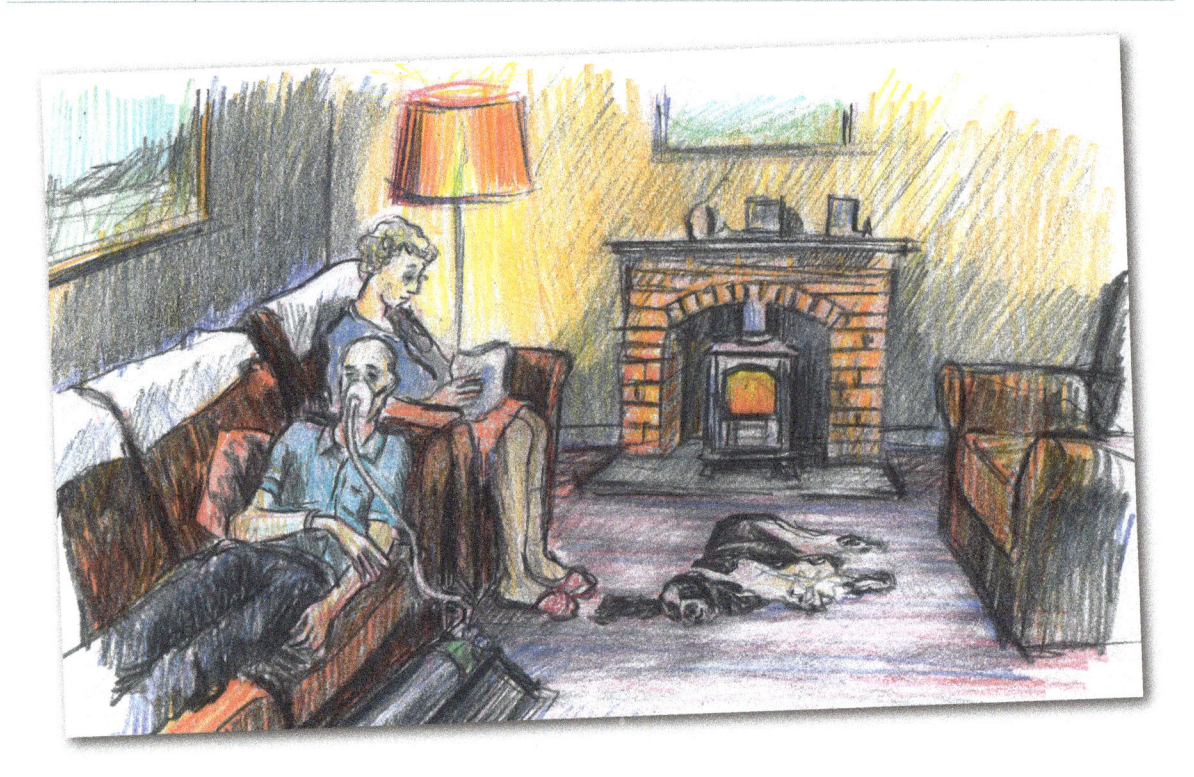

Carbon Monoxide Poisoning

You are on standby totting up the number of stomach bugs and flu-like symptoms you have seen over the past few weeks, when the MDT passes you details of a 69-year-old male who appears to be having a stroke. There is an RRV on scene who is requesting immediate backup, which sounds promising, and you have had a number of good experiences recently, utilising the hyperacute stroke pathway.

It's a little after midnight when you turn into the patient's street. Predictably, you cannot see a single house number. To make things worse, due to the recent bad weather, all of the wheelie bins seem to have been secured out of sight. Fortunately, as you round a corner, you can just spot the RRV parked up in between a couple of vans.

You are greeted at the door by a neighbour, the patient's daughter, and a strong smell of sulphur. The daughter explains that the smell is due to her parents burning cheap coal in the solid fuel stove, but the neighbour rolls his eyes, making it clear that he does not think that this is normal.

Your patient is lying on the sofa and has an oxygen mask hissing away on his face. The RRV paramedic explains that the patient suffered a head injury four days previously. Since he is on warfarin for a previous pulmonary embolism,

Carbon Monoxide Poisoning

he was taken to the local emergency department (ED) for a computerised tomography (CT) scan, which was clear. He was discharged the following day and had been well, initially. However, since yesterday, he had been feeling generally unwell, as have other members of the family. The wife has diarrhoea and vomiting, and the dog, a Springer Spaniel, is slumped by the fire and struggles to manage a half-hearted tail wag.

The emergency call was prompted by the daughter, who had been staying with her parents to look after her father, as her mother was struggling to cope. She had just nipped to the garage and on returning, could not rouse her father and so dialled 999. The RRV paramedic reports that the patient was only responding to pain on his arrival, but had since improved with oxygen, and now has a Glasgow Coma Score of 13/15. However, he has an obvious unilateral limb weakness and is slurring his speech. Recognising that the patient was FAST positive, the RRV paramedic had checked the patient's blood sugar and found it to be 8.8 mmol/l. The patient is also pyrexic and there is no history of epilepsy or any reports of convulsions recently.

> What are you going to do: **Use the stroke pathway** (read on) or **Chat to the daughter** (skip the next two paragraphs)?

Use the stroke pathway

Time is brain, so you instruct your colleague to help you lift the patient onto the carry chair and transfer him to the ambulance as quickly as possible. The daughter goes to open the back door, but is moving rather slowly, and fumbles with the lock. Your colleague tuts, and the daughter mumbles an apology, stating that she has been suffering from a bad headache. You eventually manage to get through the door and suggest she take some paracetamol. You set off for the local ED and make a pre-alert call, noting the patient's improving Glasgow Coma Scale (GCS), but highlighting the fact that he is still FAST positive.

On arrival at the ED, you explain the story about the recent head injury and the doctor mutters something about a sub-dural haemorrhage. You make a quip about how all of the family are ill, even the dog, which piques the attention of the nurse and doctor in resus. They ask you about the family's symptoms and become even more concerned. "Did you consider carbon monoxide poisoning?" they ask. No, you hadn't, and there are still two people and a dog in the house. You contact the Emergency Operations Centre (EOC) and find that there are no ambulances available, so you offer to return to the house. After arriving on scene, you knock at the door and the daughter answers (read on).

Chat to the daughter

You decide to find out more from the daughter, but it soon becomes clear that she is having trouble speaking and is complaining of a severe headache. You ask if she has headaches often, or suffers from migraines, but she denies this, stating that she only became unwell after staying over with her mother and father.

You take a minute to review the story so far. Three adults in the same property are ill, albeit with a mixture of symptoms. They are as sick as the dog, you think to yourself, and have a little titter at your wit. As sick as the dog…

> What are you going to do: **Contact a vet** (read on) or **Ask the neighbour** if he will take the dog (skip the next three paragraphs)?

Contact a vet

The fire in the living room is roaring, thanks to the daughter giving it a good stoke, and you

Chapter 4 Exposure

decide that what everyone needs is a good cup of tea, except for the dog, who could do with a vet. Your colleague puts the kettle on, while you thumb through the local telephone directory.

After 20 minutes of searching, you are still struggling to find a vet who will see to the dog. In fact, it is getting hard to see the text as it seems to swim around the page. The nausea and banging headache are not helping either. Your colleague is attempting to answer the radio as the EOC are trying to get in touch with you, but he seems to have forgotten which button to press.

Fortunately, after an hour or so, the neighbour pops back round to see why the ambulance is still parked outside the house. He leaves immediately and returns to his house to make a 999 call. He contacts the Fire and Rescue Service and informs them the next door family and an ambulance crew called to help them are all unconscious in the living room. He also tells them about the smell of sulphur and his concern about the solid fuel stove. You and your colleague have to be rescued and you are the butt of stations jokes for the next 6 months. If only you had spoken to the neighbour.

Ask the neighbour

Then it dawns on you. A solid fuel stove and multiple unwell patients equals carbon monoxide poisoning. You realise that you should not have entered the house, but it's a bit late for that. Instead, you quickly arrange for the prompt removal of everyone in the house. With a lot of encouragement, the dog manages to drag himself out of the living room and into the arms of the neighbour who agrees to look after him until the family return home.

Predictably, there are no ambulances available, so you set off with all of the family on high-flow oxygen and make a pre-alert call en route. In resus, all three family members are found to have elevated levels of carboxyhaemoglobin, but make a full recovery, as does the dog.

Scale of the problem

Carbon monoxide (CO) is a colourless, odourless and flammable gas formed by incomplete combustion of carbon-containing products. Although faulty flues belonging to gas appliances in the home are a common source of poisoning, any stove, heater or portable burner is a potential source, if there is an inadequate supply of oxygen or removal of waste combustion.[29] Other sources of CO poisoning have been reported, including water pipe smoking (shisha, narghile, hookah, hubble-bubble) and the use of barbecues in confined spaces, such as tents.[29,30]

CO poisoning is responsible for the accidental death of around 30 people each year in the UK. The peak months for incidents are, perhaps not surprisingly, November to January and the most common location, the home.[31]

Pathophysiology

CO is not all bad, and in small physiological quantities, endogenous CO produced by enzymatic heme degradation functions as a neurotransmitter. At these levels, CO is also thought to control inflammation, apoptosis (programmed cell death), cell proliferation and the creation of mitochondria within cells.[32,33]

However, as CO levels increase, tissue hypoxia and direct cellular changes occur, which result in poisoning. This is achieved through a variety of mechanisms including:[32]

- CO binding to intracellular proteins
- Nitric oxide generation resulting in peroxynitrite production
- Apoptosis
- Immune-mediated injury
- Delayed inflammation.

CO enters the blood after being inhaled, diffusing rapidly across the alveolar and capillary membranes, the plasma and red blood cell membranes. Approximately 80–90% of the CO binds with haemoglobin in the same way as oxygen does, forming carboxyhaemoglobin (COHb). This decreases the oxygen-carrying capacity of the haemoglobin, particularly as the affinity for CO is 245 times higher than for oxygen.[29] In addition, once it is bound to the haemoglobin, the oxyhaemoglobin dissociation curve is shifted to the left, further reducing the rate at which oxygen is delivered to the cells. This can lead to inadequate cellular respiration and tissue hypoxia. The association between air CO concentration and blood COHb is shown in Table 4.3.

In the brain, hypoxia leads to an increase in the level of circulating excitatory amino acids, which in turn increases brain nitrite levels causing nerve cell damage. Brain hypoxia also causes oxidative stress, necrosis and apoptosis of nerve cells, contributing to inflammation and injury. Although CO is primarily bound to haemoglobin, it also binds to other haem proteins, leading to increasing cytosolic haem levels, further increasing oxidative stress, and leading to the production of reactive oxygen species (ROS, sometimes called free radicals), which exacerbate neuronal necrosis and apoptosis (Figure 4.3).[33]

Impaired cellular respiration produces a stress response, activating hypoxia-inducible factor 1a, which is neuro- and cardio-protective at low levels of CO, but causes inflammation via a multitude of pathways at higher, non-physiological levels, which results in neurological and cardiovascular injury.

Other mechanisms of CO-mediated injury include platelet-to-neutrophil aggregation and neutrophil adhesion to endothelial cells, which cause the release of myeloperoxidase and other enzymes, as well as ROS. These ROS steal electrons from lipids in cell membranes, including myelinated neurons, degrading their structure and triggering an immune response, increasing microglia activation and ultimately causing more neurological damage (Figure 4.3).

Assessment

Carbon monoxide is a mimic, with chronic exposure to low levels of CO presenting as flu or food poisoning. Symptoms are often non-specific, but the most common is a headache followed by symptoms involving the nervous and/or gastrointestinal systems (Table 4.4).[34] Public Health England has suggested using the mnemonic COMA to aid recognition of CO poisoning.[35]

- **C** – Cohabitees/companions. Is anyone else in the property affected?
- **O** – Outdoors. Do symptoms improve or resolve when the patient is out of the building?
- **M** – Maintenance. Are fuel-burning appliances and vents properly maintained?
- **A** – Alarm. Does the patient have a CO alarm?

Table 4.3 CO concentration in air and related COHb values.

CO concentration (ppm)	COHb concentration (%)
10	1.6
15	2.4
20	3.2
25	3.9
30	4.7
40	6.1
50	7.6
100	14.0

Source: Public Health England, 2016.

Chapter 4   Exposure

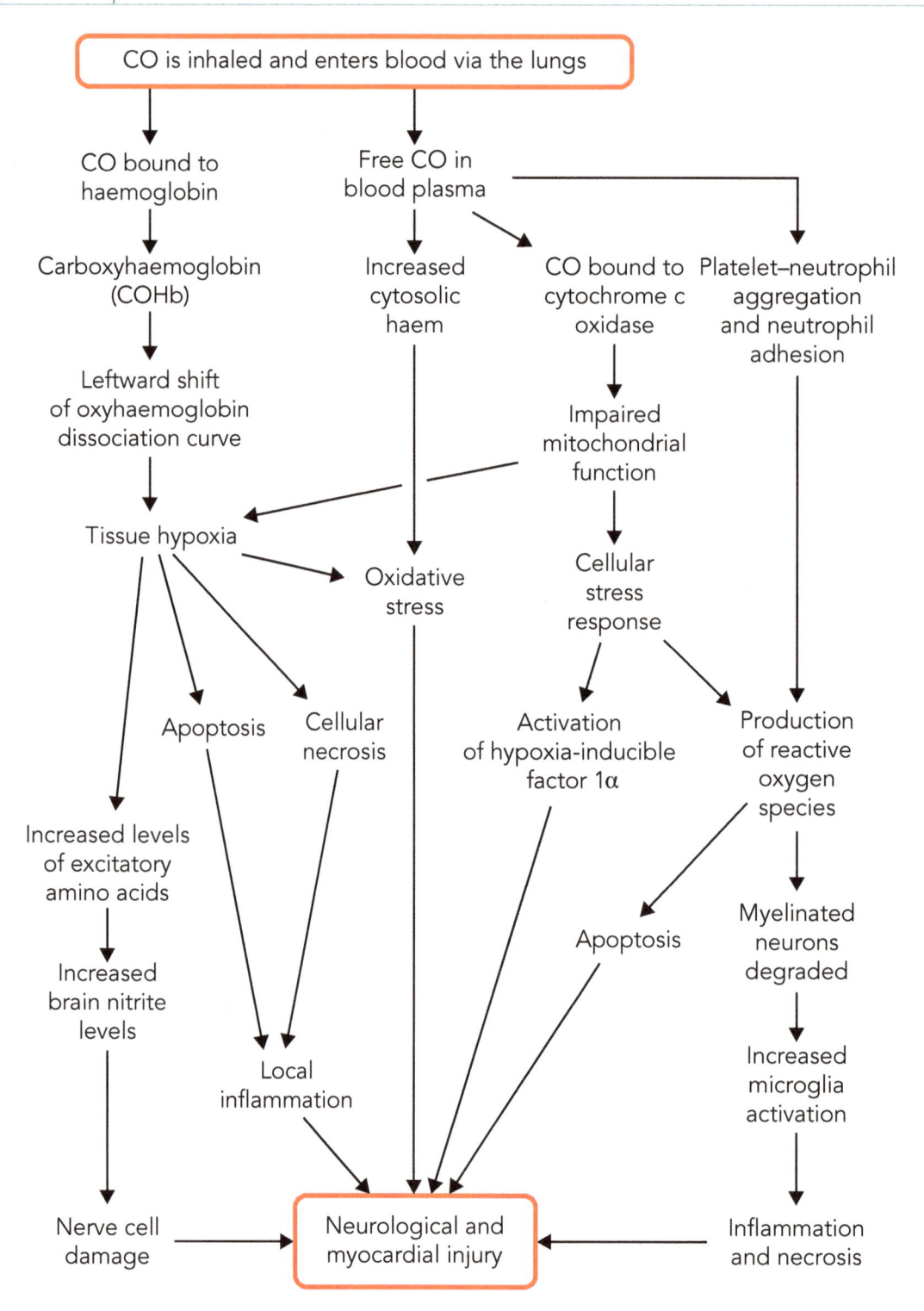

Figure 4.3   Pathophysiology of carbon monoxide poisoning.

Carbon Monoxide Poisoning

Table 4.4 Common signs and symptoms of carbon monoxide poisoning and their approximate incidence.

Signs and symptoms	Incidence (%)
Headache	90
Nausea and vomiting	50
Vertigo	50
Altered level of consciousness	30
Subjective weakness	20

Source: National Poisons Information Service, 2021.

Additional questions to ask in the history include:[36]

- Recent installation of heating/cooking appliances
- Use of gas oven/stove for heating as well as cooking
- Change in ventilation in the home, for example installation of double glazing
- Presence of sooty stains around appliances or an increase in condensation
- Any exposure to smoke, fumes or motor vehicle exhausts at work
- Whether the place of residence is semi-detached, terraced, flat, bedsit or hostel as CO can leak from another property.

Given that organs with a high oxygen uptake are most affected, it is no surprise that the brain and heart are susceptible to CO poisoning. It is important therefore to undertake a neurological examination, including testing co-ordination (such as finger-nose test and heel-to-toe walking) and performing a mini-mental test examination to highlight short-term memory loss, for example.[37]

Electrocardiogram (ECG) monitoring is important as in severe cases arrhythmias can occur and myocardial ischaemia can be severe enough to cause injury and infarct. Patients with chronic angina are particularly sensitive, even to low levels of CO exposure.[29]

Direct measurement of CO is possible in the community using breath analysis, which is sometimes carried by GPs and midwives involved with smoking cessation and antenatal clinics, respectively. However, unless you have been called to a practice or clinic, these are unlikely to be immediately at hand for you to use.

Another non-invasive test is CO-oximetry, which uses a finger probe similar to pulse oximetry to calculate levels of COHb. Pulse oximetry should not be used in cases of CO poisoning as oxygen and CO have similar light-absorbency, resulting in artificially high pulse oximetry readings. Baseline COHb should be around 0.5%, although in pregnancy and haemolytic anaemia this can be as high as 5%. Cigarette smokers also have a chronically raised level of COHb; in some cases this can be as high as 10%.[29]

The cherry red skin colour that has often been mentioned in medical texts is only observed when COHb exceeds 20%, and is only seen in around half of patients, even in cases of fatal exposures to CO.[32]

Management

Scene safety

If it is clear that the patient is in a high-concentration CO environment, such as a house fire or industrial setting, do not enter without breathing apparatus. Since this is not standard kit, you are likely to require the Fire and Rescue Service or Hazardous Area Response Team. However, it is more likely that CO poisoning will only become apparent once you have entered the scene and obtained a history. You will have to decide whether you can safely and quickly extract the patient(s), or leave immediately.[38] Do not become a victim!

Chapter 4 Exposure

Airway and breathing

Maintain a clear airway. Administer high-concentration oxygen until COHb is normal (typically under 3%).[32] Do not rely on SpO_2 to guide oxygen administration. The half-life of COHb is approximately 320 minutes, which can be reduced to 74 minutes with the administration of 100% oxygen.[29] Hyperbaric oxygen administered at twice normal atmospheric pressure reduces this further to 23 minutes; however, there is still some debate over the effectiveness of hyperbaric oxygen therapy and it is not routinely recommended.[34]

Circulation

Perform serial 12-lead ECGs and monitor closely en route. Correct arrhythmias and hypotension according to clinical guidelines. This is likely to exclude drugs such as sodium bicarbonate for QRS widening and magnesium for QT prolongation,[34] but atropine for symptomatic bradyarrhythmias and sodium chloride for hypotension may be appropriate.

Acknowledgement

Thanks to Gareth Morris for providing the inspiration behind the case study.

References

1. Idris AH, Berg RA, Bierens J, Bossaert L, Branche CM, Gabrielli A, et al. Recommended Guidelines for Uniform Reporting of Data From Drowning The "Utstein Style." *Circulation*, 2003 Nov 18;108(20):2565–2574.
2. National Water Safety Forum. 2019 Annual Fatal Incident Report [Internet]. 2020. Available from: https://www.nationalwatersafety.org.uk/waid/annual-reports-and-data/
3. Szpilman D, Bierens JJLMMD, Handley AJ, Orlowski JP. Drowning. *New England Journal of Medicine*, May 31. 2012;366(22):2102–2110.
4. Royal National Lifeboat Institution. RNLI Operational Statitics 2019 [Internet]. 2020. Available from: https://rnli.org/about-us/how-the-rnli-is-run/annual-report-and-accounts
5. Bierens JJLM, Lunetta P, Tipton M, Warner DS. Physiology of drowning: a review. *Physiology*, 2016 Mar;31(2):147–166.
6. Shattock MJ, Tipton MJ. 'Autonomic conflict': a different way to die during cold water immersion? *Journal of Physiology*, 2012;590(14):3219–3230.
7. Layon AJ, Modell JH. Drowning: update 2009. *Anesthesiology*, 2009;110(6):1390–1401.
8. Datta A, Tipton M. Respiratory responses to cold water immersion: neural pathways, interactions, and clinical consequences awake and asleep. *Journal of Applied Physiology*, 2006 Jan 6;100(6):2057–2064.
9. Orlowski JP, Abulleil MM, Phillips JM. The hemodynamic and cardiovascular effects of near-drowning in hypotonic, isotonic, or hypertonic solutions. *Annals of Emergency Medicine*, 1989 Oct;18(10):1044–1049.
10. Olasveengen Theresa M., Mancini Mary E., Perkins Gavin D., Avis Suzanne, Brooks Steven, Castrén Maaret, et al. Adult Basic Life Support: 2020 International Consensus on Cardiopulmonary Resuscitation and Emergency Cardiovascular Care Science with Treatment Recommendations. *Circulation*, 2020 Oct 20;142(16_suppl_1):S41–91.
11. Lott C, Truhlář A, Alfonzo A, Barelli A, González-Salvado V, Hinkelbein J, et al. European Resuscitation Council Guidelines 2021: Cardiac arrest in special circumstances. *Resuscitation*, 2021 Apr 1;161:152–219.
12. Szpilman D, Soares M. In-water resuscitation—is it worthwhile? *Resuscitation*, 2004 Oct;63(1):25–31.
13. Joint Royal Colleges Ambulance Liaison Committee, Association of Ambulance Chief Executives. JRCALC Clinical Guidelines. Cited from JRCALC Plus (Version 1.2.13) [Mobile application software]. Bridgwater: Class Publishing Ltd; 2021.
14. Watson RS, Cummings P, Quan L, Bratton S, Weiss NS. Cervical spine injuries among submersion victims. *Journal of Trauma*, 2001 Oct;51(4):658–662.
15. Golden FStC, David GC, Tipton MJ, University of Surrey, Great Britain. Health and Safety Executive. Review of rescue and immediate post-immersion problems : a medical/ergonomic viewpoint. Sudbury: HSE Books; 1997.
16. Lord SR, Davis PR. Drowning, near drowning and immersion syndrome. *J-R ARMY Med CORPS*, 2005;151(4):250.
17. Althaus U, Aeberhard P, Schüpbach P, Nachbur BH, Mühlemann W. Management of profound accidental hypothermia with cardiorespiratory arrest. *Annals of Surgery*, 1982;195(4):492.
18. Hooper AJ, Hockings LE. Drowning and immersion injury. *Anaesthesia and Intensive Care Medicine*, 2011 Sep;12(9):399–402.
19. Tipton MJ, Golden FStC. A proposed decision-making guide for the search, rescue and resuscitation of submersion (head under) victims based on expert opinion. *Resuscitation*, 2011 Jul;82(7):819–824.
20. Lipman GS, Gaudio FG, Eifling KP, Ellis MA, Otten EM, Grissom CK. Wilderness Medical Society Clinical Practice Guidelines for the Prevention and Treatment of Heat Illness: 2019 Update. *Wilderness & Environmental Medicine*, 2019 Dec 1;30(4):S33–46.
21. United Kingdom. Heatwave Plan for England [Internet]. 2014. Available from: https://www.gov.uk/government/publications/heatwave-plan-for-england
22. Adams T, Stacey E, Stacey S, Martin D. Exertional heat stroke. *British Journal of Hospital Medicine*, 2012 Feb 1;73(2):72–78.

Chapter 4 Exposure

23. Hajat S, O'Connor M, Kosatsky T. Health effects of hot weather: from awareness of risk factors to effective health protection. *The Lancet*, 2010 Mar 12;375(9717):856–63.
24. Auerbach PS, Cushing TA, Harris NS. *Wilderness medicine*, 7th edition. Philadelphia: Elsevier; 2016.
25. Pryor RR, Bennett BL, O'Connor FG, Young JMJ, Asplund CA. Medical evaluation for exposure extremes: heat. Wilderness & Environmental Medicine, 2015 Dec 1;26(4):69–75.
26. Epstein FH, Bunn HF. Pathogenesis and treatment of sickle cell disease. *New England Journal of Medicine*, 1997 Sep 11;337(11):762–769.
27. Casa DJ, Armstrong LE, Kenny GP, O'Connor FG, Huggins RA. Exertional heat stroke: new concepts regarding cause and care. Current Sports Medicine Reports, 2012;11(3):115–123.
28. Lissoway JB, Lipman GS, Grahn DA, Cao VH, Shaheen M, Phan S, et al. Novel application of chemical cold packs for treatment of exercise-induced hyperthermia: a randomized Controlled Trial. Wilderness & Environmental Medicine, 2015 Jun 1;26(2):173–179.
29. Public Health England. Carbon Monoxide: Toxicological Overview [Internet]. 2016. Available from: https://assets.publishing.service.gov.uk/government/uploads/system/uploads/attachment_data/file/571154/carbon_monoxide_toxicological_overview.pdf
30. Fisher DS, Bowskill S, Saliba L, Flanagan RJ. Unintentional domestic non-fire related carbon monoxide poisoning: data from media reports, UK/Republic of Ireland 1986–2011. *Clinical Toxicology*, 2013 Jun;51(5):409–416.
31. The Carbon Monoxide and Gas Safety Society. Statistics of Deaths and Injuries [Internet]. 2020. Available from: https://www.co-gassafety.co.uk/information/co-gas-safetys-statistics-of-deaths-and-injuries/
32. Hampson NB, Piantadosi CA, Thom SR, Weaver LK. Practice recommendations in the diagnosis, management, and prevention of carbon monoxide poisoning. *American Journal of Respiratory and Critical Care Medicine*, 2012 Dec;186(11):1095–1101.
33. Weaver LK. Carbon Monoxide Poisoning. *New England Journal of Medicine*, 2009 Mar 19;360(12):1217–1225.
34. National Poisons Information Service. TOXBASE – poisons information database for clinical toxicology advice [Internet]. 2021. Available from: https://www.toxbase.org/
35. Public Health England. Carbon monoxide (CO): algorithm to diagnose poisoning [Internet]. GOV.UK. 2015. Available from: https://www.gov.uk/government/publications/carbon-monoxide-co-algorithm-to-diagnose-poisoning
36. Public Health England. Diagnosing Poisoning: Carbon Monoxide [Internet]. 2013. Available from: http://www.hpa.org.uk/webc/HPAwebFile/HPAweb_C/1236845874045
37. Whitson C, Lim R, Poonai N. Carbon monoxide poisoning: a comprehensive review for prehospital specialists. *Journal of Paramedic Practice*, 2012;4(2):84–89.
38. Roth D, Krammel M, Schreiber W, Herkner H, Havel C, Laggner AN. Unrecognized carbon monoxide poisoning leads to a multiple-casualty incident. Journal of Emergency Medicine, 2013 Oct;45(4):559–561.

5   Medical Emergencies

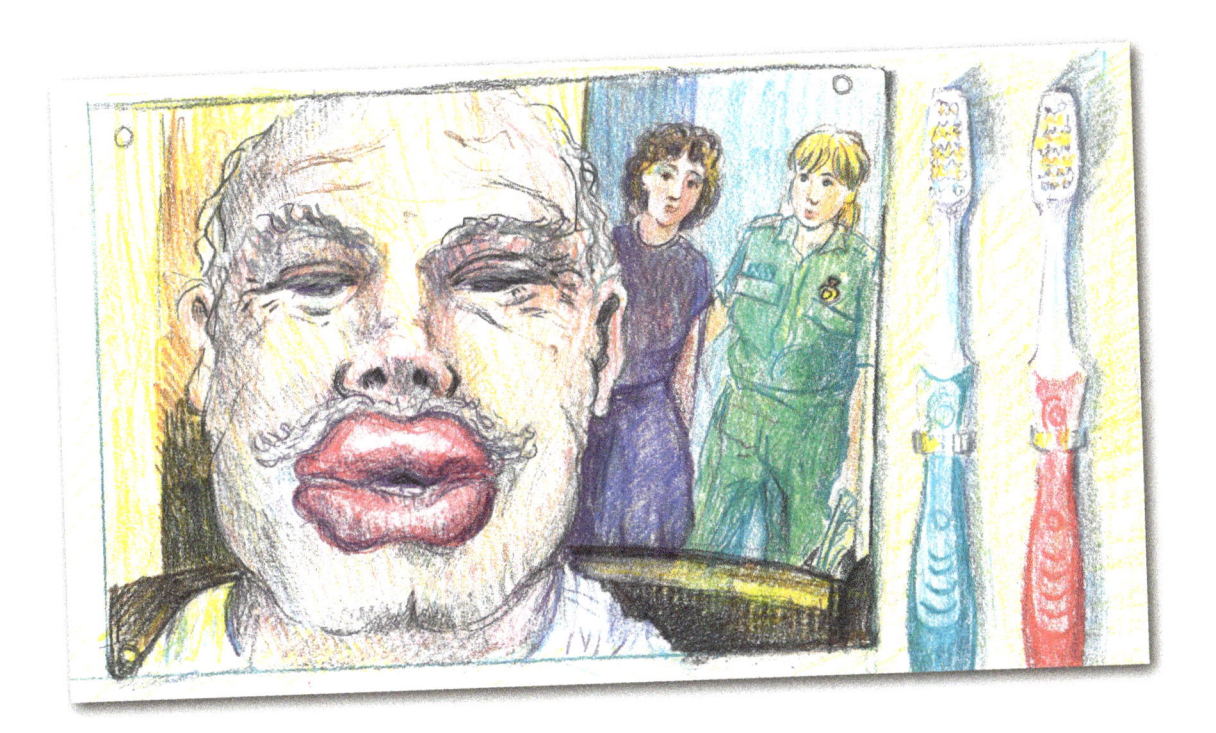

Anaphylaxis

You are on standby listening to your stomach growling. It's been a busy morning and lunch is rather overdue. Resisting the temptation to hassle the dispatcher about this, you are rewarded with a return to base message on the MDT. You begin to daydream about the culinary delight you are going to consume once you are back on station. The excess salivation is so severe, you could soon be drooling!

The station comes into view and you indicate to turn in. Just then, your luck runs out. An emergency call has come in for an elderly male with an allergic reaction. Minutes later, you pull up outside the patient's house and are waved inside by the daughter. She explains that her father is suffering from an allergic reaction due to toothpaste. This is a new one on you, but she sounds convincing as she outlines her father's history of four unwitnessed collapsing episodes after brushing his teeth. On discovering this, the daughter had taken her father to the dentist

135

Chapter 5 Medical Emergencies

this morning. They had recommended the leading brand of toothpaste for sensitive teeth as the answer.

Once home, she had insisted that her father try some while she was present. He had dutifully placed a pea-sized blob on his lower lip and within a minute, a rash had appeared and his face had swollen. "He seems to be having trouble with his breathing and won't talk to me now," she says. "I think he might be cross with me."

The patient is in the bathroom, with his back to the door. You enter and introduce yourself but he does not respond. You come around to face the patient, who is sat on a chair that appears to have come from a nearby bedroom. It is clear that the patient is not talking to you or the daughter because he is semi-conscious, probably due to cerebral hypoxia. You can see a raised rash on his chest consistent with urticaria, and on shouting his name he opens his eyes and briefly focuses on you, but does not speak spontaneously, or in response to any of your questions. He does, however, localise to pain.

> **What is the patient's GCS?**
> (Read on to find out!)

Your colleague wheezes up the stairs with the carry chair and surveys the patient. "Hmm, eyes opening to voice, not speaking and localising to pain?" he enquires. You nod and he continues, "That'll be a GCS of 3+1+5, which is 9 then," he calculates using his fingers. You agree (because that's what you worked it out as too, right?) and apply oxygen as your colleague obtains some observations. He relays his findings to you:

Airway

Patent ... at the moment, but lips and tongue are swollen

Breathing

Respiratory rate: 30 breaths/min with audible stridor
SpO$_2$: 86% on air

Circulation

Thready and rapid radial pulse at a rate of 130 beats per minute
Blood pressure: 86/45 mmHg

Disability

GCS score: 9/15
Blood sugar: 7.0 mmol/l

Exposure/Environment

Temperature: 36.4°C

He has angioedema, which makes his lips rather startling, but at least cleaning off the remnants of the toothpaste is much easier. Stridor is audible without a stethoscope, but on auscultation you can hear a widespread wheeze with reasonable, bilateral air entry.

> **What do you want to administer now: Salbutamol** (read on) or **Adrenaline** (skip the next paragraph)?

Salbutamol

Wheeze equals a nebuliser, right? You even remember to ask your colleague to undertake a pre-treatment peak flow, although they look at you as if you are an idiot. Still, you are too busy loading up the nebuliser chamber with a couple of 2.5 mg ampoules of salbutamol to notice. The bang of the patient hitting the floor does succeed in distracting you and that's when it becomes apparent that the patient is not breathing. You look forlornly at your nebuliser, realising that although salbutamol is useful in the treatment of bronchospasm in anaphylaxis, it should be administered after adrenaline. Despite your best efforts at resuscitation, the patient never regains an output. Next time, you will definitely give adrenaline first…

Adrenaline

An allergic history, short onset of symptoms, hives, angioedema, signs of shock and a reduced level of consciousness can only mean one thing … anaphylaxis!

You draw up 500 mcg of adrenaline and administer it intramuscularly. Your colleague applies a non-rebreathe oxygen mask and cranks up the flow rate. He then sets up the carry chair and you load the patient onto it for the trip downstairs. Once in the ambulance, you place the patient on the trolley and recheck the patient's observations.

En route, you manage to gain IV access and administer a couple of 250 ml boluses of normal saline. The patient's condition improves, with his blood pressure rising to 100 mmHg systolic as you make a pre-alert call to the local emergency department (ED). The patient requires more adrenaline and a lot of fluid in hospital but makes a full recovery. You catch up with him on a ward several days later and he tells you it appears that he is allergic to the mint additive in toothpaste. "I'm wondering about whether dentures might be less trouble," he says with a grin.

Scale of the problem

Anaphylaxis is a serious allergic reaction that is rapid in onset and may cause death.[1] Its hallmark is rapidly developing life-threatening airway/breathing/circulation (or any combination of the three) problem(s) and may occur without associated skin and mucosal changes or circulatory shock being present.[2] The exact incidence of anaphylaxis is unknown as many episodes are not reported, but it is thought to be around 1 in 1,300 of the population having an anaphylactic reaction at some point in their lives.[3] Mortality from anaphylaxis is rare, with an estimated 20–30 deaths per year in the UK, although this is likely to be an underestimate.[4]

The most common causes (triggers) are food, medication and insect stings. In children, food is the most common cause of allergy, whereas in older adults, it is medication.[5,6] Death is unlikely more than 4 hours after exposure to a trigger, but cardiac arrest can occur in minutes, particularly if the trigger is medication that has been administered intravenously. Envenomation typically causes cardiac arrest within 15 minutes, and food takes a little longer on average, at around 30 minutes.[7]

Pathophysiology

The list of potential triggers that can cause anaphylaxis is vast. The most common are peanuts, tree nuts, shellfish, fish, milk and eggs,[8] but there is one documented case of anaphylaxis caused by toothpaste.[9]

Triggers fall into three basic categories: immunological mechanisms involving immunoglobulin E (the most common); other immunological mechanisms such as activation of the complement and coagulation systems; and non-immunological causes. Non-immunological causes are not well understood but include exposure to cold air or water and exercise. Figure 5.1 summarises the pathophysiological changes that take place. Some triggers, such as insect venom, may act through more than one mechanism.[8,10]

Two types of cells are instrumental in the chain of events that can lead to anaphylaxis: basophils and mast cells. Basophils are granular leukocytes (a type of white blood

Chapter 5 Medical Emergencies

cell) which migrate to sites of inflammation, leaving the capillaries and entering the tissues where they release heparin, histamine and serotonin, intensifying the inflammatory reaction.[11] Mast cells are connective tissue cells found in high numbers near tissues that are exposed to the outside world. Examples include the skin, oral mucosa (which includes the lips and tongue), conjunctiva, the lungs and digestive tract.[12]

Most triggers lead to anaphylaxis due to the production of the immunoglobulin E (IgE) antibody, which cross-links with an antigen to activate high-affinity IgE receptors (FcεRI) on mast cells and basophils. Due to the high affinity of cross-linked IgE to FcεRI,

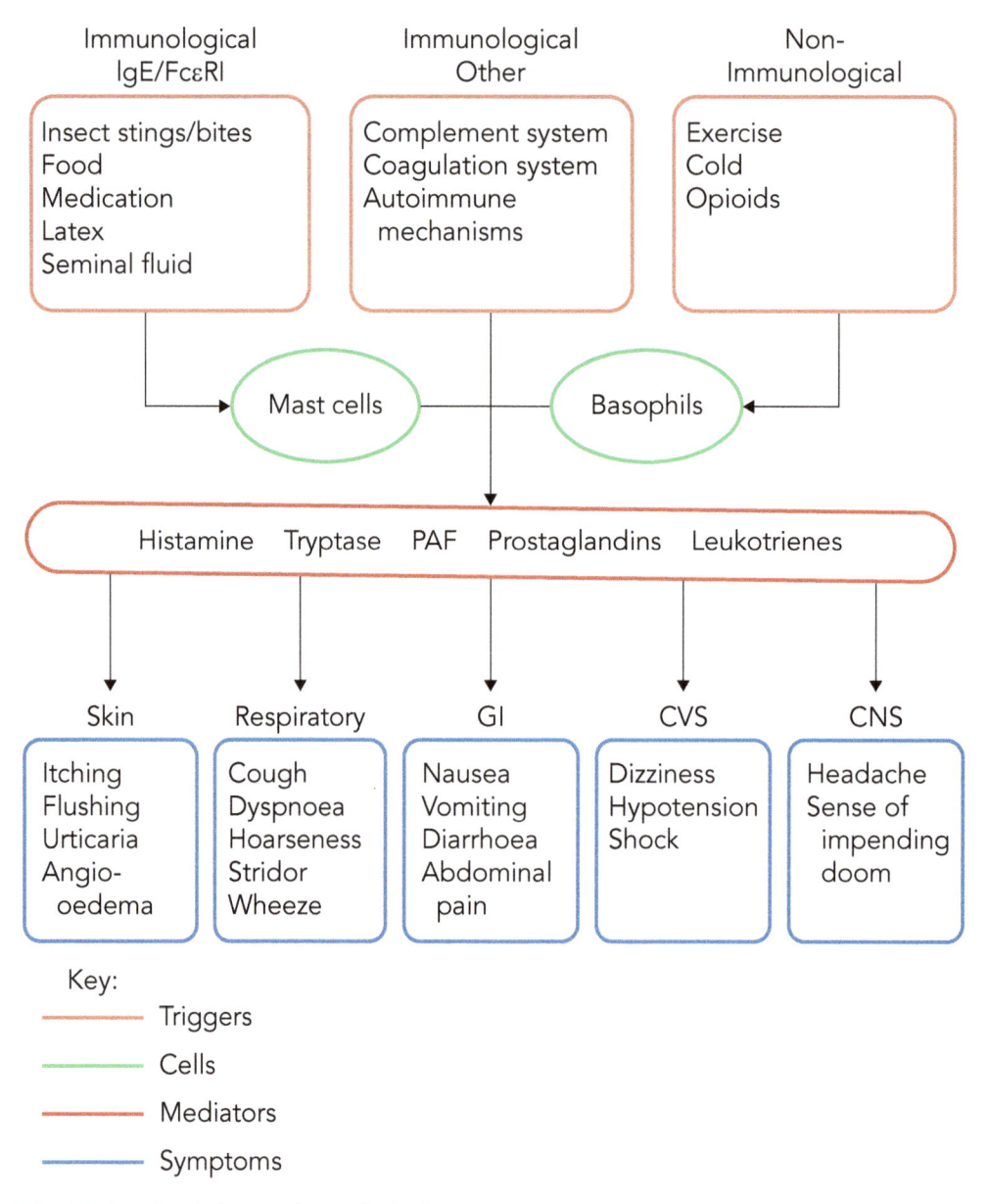

Figure 5.1 Pathophysiology of anaphylaxis.

Table 5.1 Actions of specific mediators.

Mediator	Actions
Histamine	Vasodilation Increased vascular permeability Increased heart rate and contraction Increased glandular secretion
Prostaglandin D2	Bronchoconstriction Pulmonary and coronary vasoconstriction Peripheral vascular dilation
Leukotrienes	Bronchoconstriction Increased vascular permeability
Platelet Activating Factor (PAF)	Severe bronchoconstriction Increased vascular permeability

Adapted from: Lee, 2011.

this process is essentially irreversible and initiates a series of cellular events, leading to activation of tyrosine kinase and an influx of calcium into basophils and mast cells.[13] The result is a rapid release of preformed mediators such as histamines, prostaglandins, leukotrienes and platelet activating factor (there are over 100 in total!). The action of several mediators is summarised in Table 5.1.

Of particular concern in fatal cases of anaphylaxis is the activation of human heart mast cells. These are located between myocardial muscle and around blood vessels. Low doses of preformed mediators can cause coronary artery spasm, myocardial injury and arrythmias.[14]

Recognition

Anaphylaxis is likely if a patient exposed to a trigger develops a sudden illness (that is, within minutes of exposure) with rapidly progressing, life-threatening A, B or C problems. The reaction is usually unexpected and typically associated with rapidly progressing skin changes, although these are absent in up to 20% of anaphylaxis cases.[4] Patients with severe anaphylaxis resulting in significant hypotension may not exhibit any cutaneous symptoms until their blood pressure is restored.[13]

Differential diagnoses

Just to make life a little more difficult for the ambulance clinician, there are a number of other disease processes that can mimic the signs and symptoms of anaphylaxis. Common differentials of anaphylaxis include acute asthma, anxiety attacks and foreign body aspiration. Table 5.2 provides a summary of many others.[2]

Table 5.2 Differential diagnoses for anaphylaxis.

Category	Differential diagnosis
Common diagnostic dilemmas	Acute asthma[a] Anxiety/panic attack Acute generalised urticaria[a] Aspiration of a foreign body Cardiovascular (myocardial infarction[a], pulmonary embolus) Neurological events (seizure, cerebrovascular event)
Post-prandial syndromes	Scombroidosis[b] Pollen-food allergy syndrome[c] Monosodium glutamate Sulphites Food poisoning
Excess endogenous histamine	Mastocytosis/clonal mast cell disorders Basophilic leukaemia
Flush syndromes	Peri-menopause Carcinoid syndrome Autonomic epilepsy Medullary carcinoma of the thyroid

Chapter 5 Medical Emergencies

Table 5.2 *(Continued)*

Category	Differential diagnosis
Shock	Hypovolaemic Cardiogenic Distributive[d] Septic
Non-organic disease	Vocal cord dysfunction Hyperventilation Psychosomatic episode
Other	ACE inhibitor-associated angioedema Systemic capillary leak syndrome Red man syndrome (vancomycin) Phaeochromocytoma (paradoxical response)

a: Acute asthma symptoms, acute generalised urticaria or myocardial infarction symptoms can also occur during an anaphylactic episode.
b: Histamine poisoning from fish, for example, tuna that has been stored at an elevated temperature; usually, more than one person eating the fish is affected.
c: Pollen-food allergy syndrome is elicited by fruits and vegetables containing various plant proteins that cross-react with airborne allergens. Typical symptoms include itching, tingling and angioedema of the lips, tongue, palate, throat and ears after eating raw, but not cooked, fruits and vegetables.
d: Distributive shock may be due to anaphylaxis or to spinal cord injury.

Source: Cardona et al., 2020.

Management

Having conducted your standard ABCDE assessment and determined that your patient is likely to be suffering from anaphylaxis, you should identify the trigger and remove it if possible (for example, stop any drug infusions, remove bee stings). However, if this is not possible, then do not delay treatment.

If you suspect food-induced anaphylaxis, encouraging the patient to vomit is NOT recommended.[4]

Patients with A or B problems are likely to be more comfortable sat up, whereas those with C problems are best managed recumbent with or without legs raised. It is important not to make patients sit or stand if they feel faint as this can cause cardiac arrest!

Administer intramuscular (IM) adrenaline as soon as possible. Patients who still have a pulse should not have adrenaline administered intravenously (IV), except by those who use vasopressors in their normal clinical practice (for example, critical care paramedics, anaesthetists). The preferred route is IM into the anterolateral thigh as there is a greater margin of safety, it is quick to administer (versus gaining IV access) and the peak plasma concentration is higher when adrenaline is administered in the thigh compared to the deltoid.[15] In the event of a cardiac arrest however, the patient should receive their adrenaline IV.[4] Doses of adrenaline can be repeated every 5 minutes depending on patient condition.

Once the first dose of adrenaline has been administered, ensure the airway is patent and then provide high-flow oxygen. Apply physiological monitoring, including pulse oximetry, ECG and serial blood pressure measurement.

If the patient is hypotensive or has a poor response to adrenaline, gain IV access and administer 500–1000 ml of a non-glucose containing crystalloid in adults and a bolus of 10 ml/kg in children.[4] These can be repeated as necessary.

Antihistamines, such as chlorphenamine, and steroids are no longer recommended as part of the initial management of anaphylaxis. Bronchodilators can be administered in addition to adrenaline but not instead of.[4]

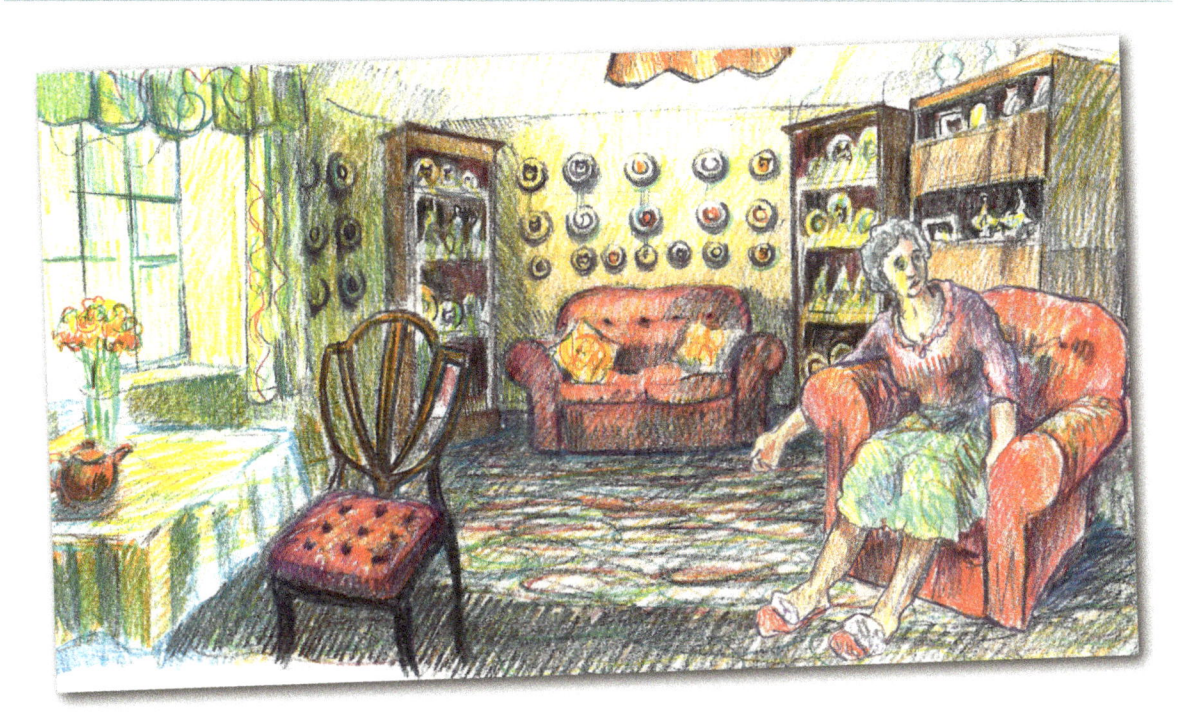

Hypoglycaemia

You are on standby, being bored to death by a colleague who is droning on about his recent conflict resolution training.

He is lamenting about the lack of teaching on restraining and subduing techniques. "It was all about break-away techniques," he moans, "now, if we had a Taser …" You zone out of the conversation and find yourself eyeing loose objects in the cab that you could batter him with.

Fortunately, any thoughts of assault and battery are interrupted by the MDT, which is passing details of a 65-year-old woman who is having a stroke. You ignore your colleague karate chopping the air and set off for the address.

As you pull up on scene, you recognise the impeccable frontage, recall the patient's name (Betty) and the cat plates in the living room (Chapter 3). Betty's husband greets you at the door like an old friend and directs your colleague to the living room. He lumbers through the door while you pause for a moment to chat to the husband and enquire about his wife's medication.

He explains that a new doctor at the practice has altered her medication, which is causing confusion. He also mentions that he forgot to tell the call handler that he had checked Betty's blood sugar and found it to be 1.8 mmol/l.

Chapter 5   Medical Emergencies

Betty's current medication consists of:

- Metformin
- Gliclazide
- Aspirin
- Amlodipine
- Bendroflumethiazide
- Atorvastatin
- Insulin (NovoMix® 30)

Further analysis of the medication is interrupted by a loud shout of "Pish osh!" This appears to have emanated from Betty, in response to your colleague's initial questioning. You enter the living room to find him reprimanding Betty for swearing. She is sat in an armchair and slumped to the right, with an obvious right-sided facial droop and arm weakness. However, her left leg is functioning perfectly, and she demonstrates this with a swift kick to your colleague's groin.

Your immense professionalism limits the reflex belly laugh to a minor shoulder judder and smirk, as your colleague rolls around the carpet.

A 65-year-old woman has incapacitated your colleague. You need to take over.

> What should you treat Betty for first: **Stroke** (read on) or **Hypoglycaemia** (skip the next paragraph)?

Stroke

You've been dying to try out the new stroke pathway, and although Betty is taking a swing at everyone who approaches her left side, including her husband, you are happy that she is FAST positive and make the call. Things go well until the stroke nurse asks for the blood sugar. They suggest that you treat the hypoglycaemia first, since hypoglycaemia is a stroke mimic. Feeling foolish, you hang up and open the drugs bag.

Hypoglycaemia

You know that hypoglycaemia can mimic the signs of a stroke and since the patient's blood sugar is only 1.8 mmol/l this needs addressing straight away. You rule out intravenous glucose, as coming close to Betty's swinging arm with a cannula is likely to end in tears.

> What drug are you going to administer: **40% glucose oral gel** (read on) or **Glucagon** (skip the next paragraph)?

40% glucose oral gel

Oral glucose seems the safest option, as there is no need for sharp needles. You try to explain to Betty the treatment plan, but she cannot comprehend what you are saying. Instead, you elect to adopt the 'insert and squirt' technique and then quickly step outside the range of her flailing left arm. However, Betty just spits and dribbles the glucose onto her dress and the carpet. You are going to have to use glucagon.

Glucagon

Getting close to Betty with a needle is not ideal, but you manage to work your way around to her right side and inject her arm with the glucagon. After 10 minutes, Betty's hemiparesis resolves and she reverts to her usual self. She enquires politely about your colleague who is still clutching his groin and looking like a wounded animal. He mumbles something and shuffles out of the room. You explain what has happened and encourage Betty to take some oral carbohydrates. Over the next 30 minutes, Betty appears to make a full recovery and her blood sugar rises to 6.8 mmol/l.

Hypoglycaemia

> ❓ What should you do with Betty: **Leave her at home** (read on) or **Take her to hospital** (skip the next paragraph)?

Leave her at home

After ensuring that there have been no recent episodes of hypoglycaemia, you elect to leave her at home. Betty and her husband are gushing with thanks and praise at the marvellous job you have done, and you feel pleased with yourself. That dissipates the day after when you spot Betty's name on the local ED board. It turns out that Betty suffered another bout of hypoglycaemia overnight, which led to hypoglycaemic encephalopathy. You spot her husband looking at his unconscious wife on the trolley with a look of despair on his face and wonder if you should have taken her to hospital the day before.

Take her to hospital

Everything seems back to normal, but Betty is a type 2 diabetic on sulfonylureas (Gliclazide), and you are concerned about the risk of another episode of hypoglycaemia. You take Betty to hospital and she is admitted overnight. Thanks to an observant nurse, an episode of nocturnal hypoglycaemia is recognised and treated. Your colleague suffers no lasting damage but continues to flinch when offered mints or is asked to pass a walking stick, by any woman over 60 years of age, for the next couple of weeks.

The scale of the problem

There are around 4.5 million people living with diabetes in the UK[16] and around 35% suffer at least one episode of hypoglycaemia each year, with type 1 diabetic patients being at a higher risk.[17]

Anatomy

The pancreas is a mixed endocrine and exocrine gland, situated posterior to the stomach, and extends across the posterior abdominal wall from the duodenum on the right to the spleen on the left (Figure 5.2). It is retroperitoneal, apart from its tail.[18]

Around 99% of the cells in the pancreas are involved in the production of pancreatic enzymes. The cells are organised into clusters called acini. Amongst the acini are collections of endocrine tissue called pancreatic islets, or islets of Langerhans after the German scientist, Paul Langerhans, who first described them.[19]

There are five types of cells in the pancreatic islets, which have a range of functions, including regulation of blood glucose (Table 5.3).[11,20,21]

Physiology

The brain consumes over 50% of the body's glucose and since it can only store a few minutes supply of glucose in the form of glycogen, it requires a constant supply from the blood. Once blood sugar drops to around 2.8–3.1 mmol/l (in healthy patients), brain function is affected.[22]

Falling blood glucose levels normally activate a series of glucose counter-regulatory processes to prevent, or quickly correct, hypoglycaemia. This is crucial, given that the brain's demand for glucose is fairly constant and the intake of (exogenous) glucose from eating is intermittent. This is accomplished by the dynamic control of endogenous production of glucose by the liver (and to a lesser extent, the kidneys) and reduction of glucose consumption by non-neural tissue, such as muscle.[23]

Hormonal control of blood glucose is largely dependent on the endocrine pancreas via the hormones insulin and glucagon. Insulin increases transport of glucose across cell

Chapter 5 Medical Emergencies

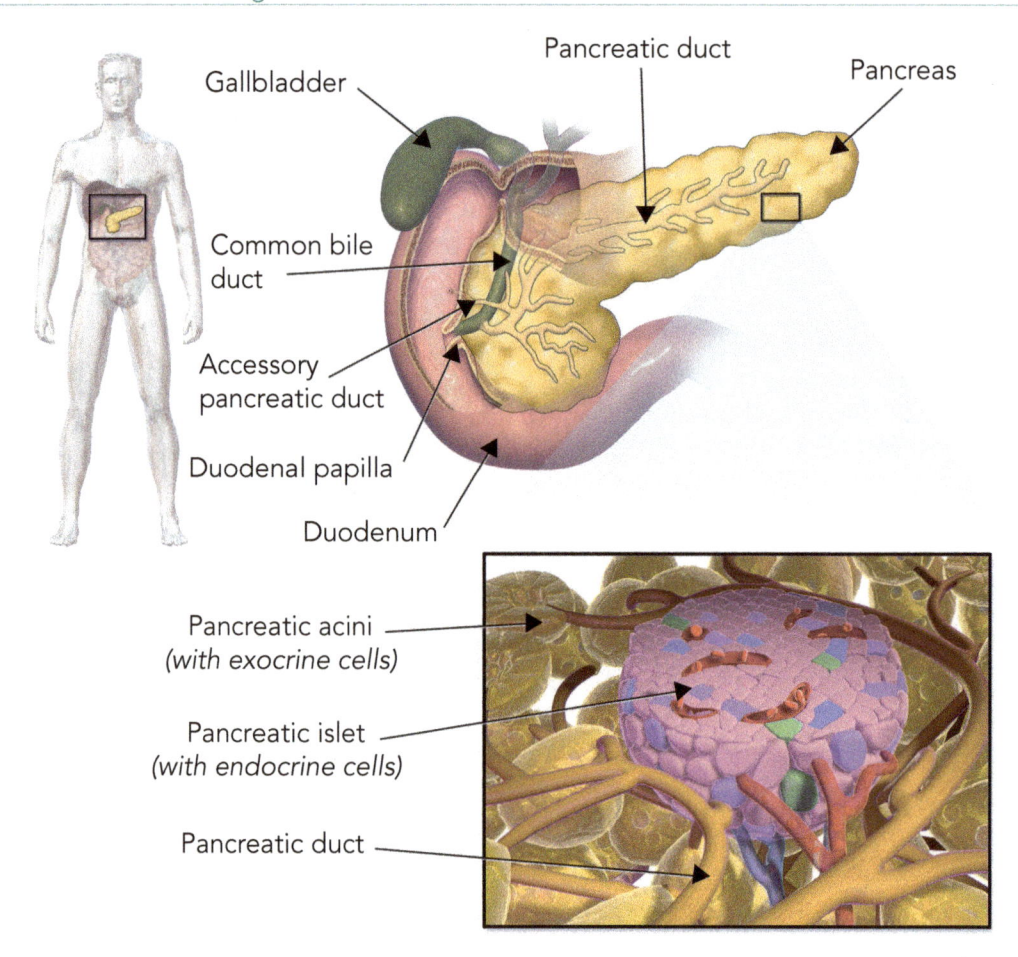

Figure 5.2 Pancreatic cells.
Source: Blausen.com staff (2014). 'Medical gallery of Blausen Medical 2014'. WikiJournal of Medicine 1(2). CC BY 3.0, via Wikimedia Commons.

membranes and is released by the beta cells. It targets the muscle, fat and liver cells causing gluconeogenesis and synthesis of triglycerides, fatty acids and proteins.[11]

Glucagon targets the liver, promoting conversion of glycogen into glucose and the creation of glucose from lactic and amino acids. This results in increased glucose release by the liver, into the blood. Glucagon release is inhibited by insulin and increased by falling blood glucose levels.

Insulin and glucagon are inhibited by somatostatin, which acts as a local negative feedback mechanism, to prevent uncontrolled insulin and glucagon release. Amylin also inhibits insulin and glycogen, but also somatostatin release as well.[24]

Defence against hypoglycaemia (also called glucose counter-regulation) can be broadly classified into physiological and behavioural responses. As blood glucose falls (although still within 'normal' limits), insulin secretion from the beta cells is reduced, leading to increased glucose production by the liver and virtual cessation of glucose use by tissue sensitive to insulin.[23]

Table 5.3 Cells of the pancreatic islets.

Cell	Hormone	
Alpha	Glucagon	Increases blood glucose
Beta	Insulin, amylin	Insulin: reduces blood glucose. Amylin: delays gastric emptying, inhibits insulin
Delta	Somatostatin	Inhibits glucagon and insulin release
PP (or F)	Pancreatic polypeptide	Inhibits somatostatin secretion, gallbladder contraction and secretion of pancreatic digestive enzymes
Epsilon	Ghrelin	Stimulates hunger

Source: Marieb and Hoehn, 2019.

When blood glucose falls below 4 mmol/l, glucagon release is increased from the alpha cells, further increasing glucose production and decreasing insulin release. In addition, adrenaline release from the adrenal medulla is increased by the sympathetic nervous system. Adrenaline has similar effects on the liver as glucagon, but can also stimulate renal production of glucose and plays a role in reducing insulin-stimulated glucose uptake.[24]

If blood glucose continues to fall, a more intense sympathetic mediated adrenaline release causes a behavioural response in the form of hunger, as well as other autonomic symptoms, such as palpitations, sweating and pallor.[25]

Pathophysiology

Hypoglycaemia in diabetics commonly occurs due to a relative excess of insulin in the blood and a compromised physiological and behavioural response to falling blood glucose levels. Since injected insulin and hypoglycaemic drugs such as sulphonylureas are not perfect pharmacokinetically, there are typically periods where there is an excess of insulin in the blood and falling blood glucose levels. The performance of the counter-regulatory defences is crucial in determining whether the patient will develop significant hypoglycaemia.

If the beta cells do not release insulin, such as occurs in type 1 and end-stage type 2 diabetes, glucagon release is usually impaired and the physiological defence relies completely on the nervous system response to falling blood glucose levels.[22] However, there are a number of factors that can dampen this response and cause a hypoglycaemia-associated autonomic failure (Figure 5.3).

The three main causes of hypoglycaemia-associated autonomic failure are previous episodes of hypoglycaemia, prior exercise and sleep. The mechanisms are not well understood, but repeated episodes of hypoglycaemia impair the mechanisms responsible for increased adrenaline release and hypoglycaemic symptoms, in both diabetics and non-diabetics in subsequent falls in blood glucose.[26] Strenuous exercise causes a late hypoglycaemic response up to 15 hours after the event and often at night. Sleep further dampens the nervous and adrenal response to falling blood glucose and patients have reduced arousal from sleep.[22] Thus, not only is the physiological defence potentially overcome, but the behavioural defence is also affected by an impaired awareness of hypoglycaemia. This is compounded by old age, patients with long-standing diabetes, the consumption of alcohol and very tight glycaemic control.[26]

Recognition

The 11 most common signs and symptoms of hypoglycaemia form part of a scoring system

Chapter 5 Medical Emergencies

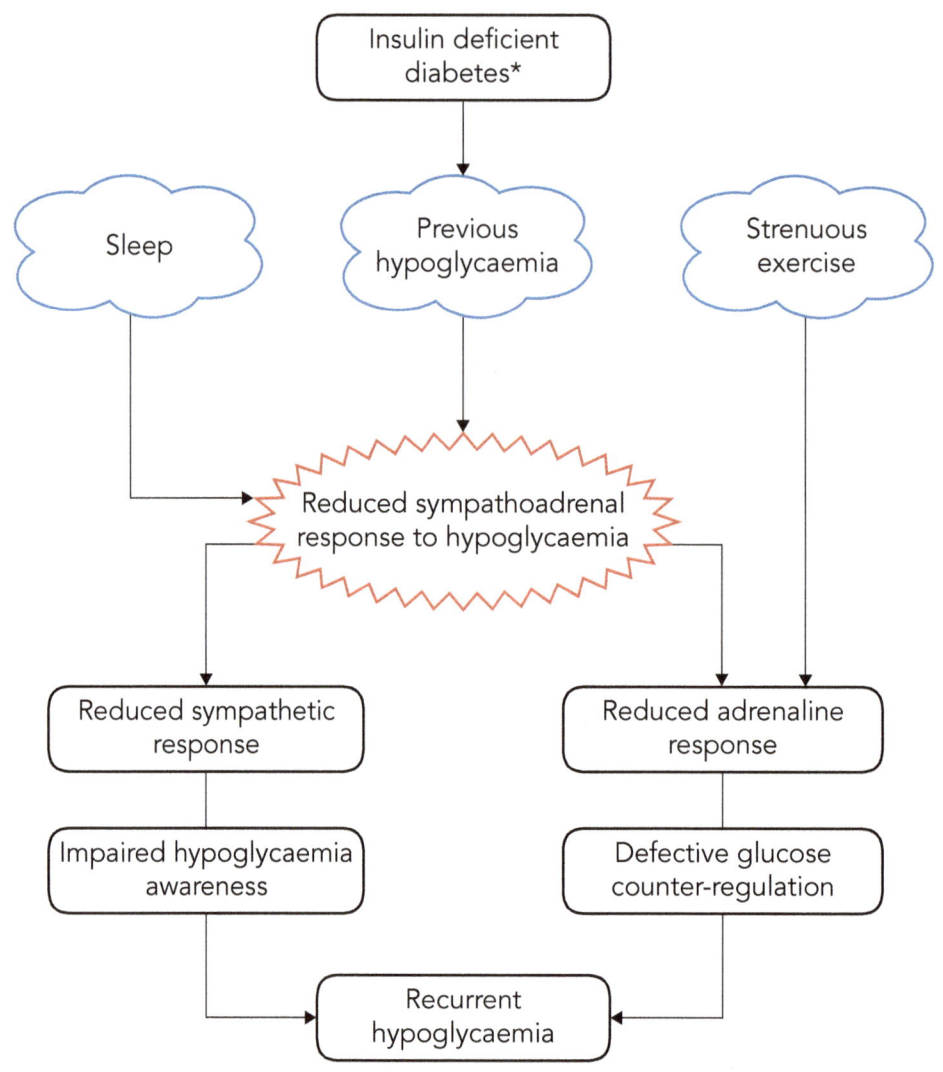

```
         Insulin deficient
           diabetes*
                │
                ▼
  Sleep    Previous      Strenuous
          hypoglycaemia   exercise
                │
                ▼
    Reduced sympathoadrenal
    response to hypoglycaemia
        │              │
        ▼              ▼
  Reduced sympathetic   Reduced adrenaline
      response              response
        │                     │
        ▼                     ▼
  Impaired hypoglycaemia   Defective glucose
     awareness            counter-regulation
              │        │
              ▼        ▼
              Recurrent
             hypoglycaemia
```

* There is no insulin decrease or glucagon increase, when blood glucose levels fall due to exogenous insulin administration

Figure 5.3 Hypoglycaemia-associated autonomic failure.

known as the Edinburgh Hypoglycaemia Scale (perhaps to keep up with Glasgow!) and is summarised in Table 5.4.[27] The threshold of onset for these symptoms can be altered by a variety of factors including duration of diabetes, tightness of glycaemic control and recent episodes of hypoglycaemia. In addition, symptoms diminish with advancing age and drugs such as beta-blockers not only reduce the counter-regulatory response but can also mask symptoms of hypoglycaemia.[28]

Management

The management of hypoglycaemia will be familiar to most ambulance staff. If the patient

Table 5.4 Common signs and symptoms of hypoglycaemia.

Autonomic (sympathetic nervous system mediated)	Neuroglycopaenic (direct brain effects of insufficient glucose)	General malaise
Sweating	Confusion	Headache
Palpitations	Drowsiness	Nausea
Shaking	Odd/aggressive behaviour	
Hunger	Speech problems	
	Incoordination	

Adapted from: Deary, 1993.

is still conscious and able to take oral glucose, then administer 15-20 g of glucose.

10 g of glucose is found in:[29]

- 5–7 Dextrosol tablets (or 4–5 Glucotabs)
- 1–2 tubes of 40% glucose gel
- 3–4 teaspoons of sugar.

Administration of oral glucose can be repeated after 10–15 minutes, if required.

If the patient is unable to take oral glucose due to impaired consciousness, is uncooperative or there is a risk of aspiration, then either IM glucagon or IV glucose should be administered. This decision will be a judgement call by the practitioner and will depend on whether IV access can be obtained.

The most common presentation of IV glucose for ambulance staff is a 500 ml bag containing 10% glucose. This replaced earlier pre-filled syringes of 50% glucose as it was found to be just as effective and possibly more beneficial to the patient, since lower doses are required, resulting in lower post-treatment glucose levels.[30] 10 g of glucose equates to 100 mls of the 10% solutions and 50 ml of the 20%. The maximum recommended dose in UK ambulance guidelines is 30 g, with repeated doses being administered 5 minutes apart (the 3rd occurring en route to hospital).[29]

Where it is not possible to administer IV glucose, then glucagon can be administered IM. The adult dose is 1 mg and can take up to 15 minutes to demonstrate an effect. Note that glucagon may not be effective in patients with inadequate stores of glycogen such as those who are intoxicated, alcoholic, anorexic and non-diabetic.[29]

Diabetic patients who suffer an episode of severe hypoglycaemia will often fully recover and can be discharged at scene safely as long as their blood sugar is above 4mmol/l and they consume a starchy snack such as a slice of toast or 200–300 ml of milk. It is recommended that patients are referred onto a diabetes specialist, as their treatment regimen may need to change.[31,32]

However, patients should be encouraged to attend hospital in the following circumstances:[29]

- Elderly (although no specific age range is cited in the literature)
- Previous treatment within the last 48 hours
- Not returned to normal mental status within 10 minutes of treatment
- Not diagnosed as diabetic
- Taking oral hypoglycaemic agents (mainly sulphonylureas such as glibenclamide or gliclazide)
- Blood glucose <5 mmol/l after treatment
- Treated with glucagon
- Co-morbidity (for example, renal failure/dialysis, chest pain, arrhythmias, alcohol consumption, dyspnoea, convulsions or focal neurological signs)
- Signs of illness/infection.

Chapter 5   Medical Emergencies

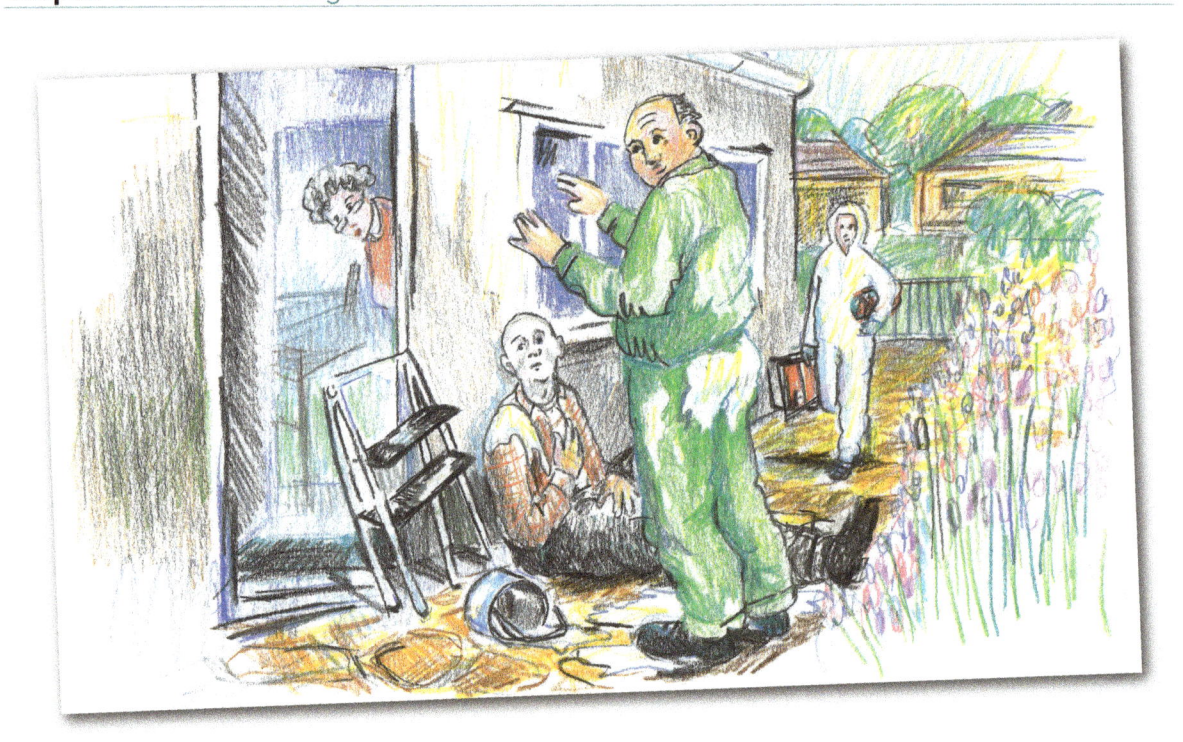

Pulmonary Embolism

You are on standby watching your colleague devour his McMammoth breakfast (its slogan is "It'll break you, fast!"). The fat oozing out of the generic meat burger is grossly mesmerising, but doesn't stop you suggesting that he cut out the middle man and just inject the fat straight into his artery. He smiles at you, losing some lettuce into his lap in the process. The MDT comes to the rescue, passing details of a 66-year-old man with difficulty breathing.

As you pull into a close lined with bungalows, you can see a worried looking woman waving frantically from one of the driveways. Your colleague rolls out of the cab and heads off to find the patient, while you turn the ambulance around. A quick glance up the side of the house reveals the patient and, even from a distance, he is looking rather grey. Well, his face is. The rest of him and the area surrounding him is covered in white paint. The tin was presumably resting on the small step ladder that is beside him.

You park up and put on your personal protective equipment, a Tyvek® coverall. It does make you look like a crime scene investigator, but you can't resist a smirk as you walk up the drive and spy your colleague who has already succumbed to the paint and is covered! However, the frivolity is short-lived as, up close, it is clear that your patient is a sick man.

The patient was painting the wall of the bungalow when he experienced a sudden

Pulmonary Embolism

onset of shortness of breath and dizziness, severe enough that he had to sit down, knocking the paint pot over in the process. He denies having chest pain or any respiratory symptoms in the past week. His medical history consists solely of ongoing treatment at a local oncology hospital for cancer of the prostate.

His observations are as follows:

General impression

Alert and orientated
Grey and sweaty

Airway

Patent

Breathing

Laboured
Respiratory rate: 32 breaths/min
SpO$_2$: 90% on air

Circulation

Palpable radial pulse
Heart rate: 140 beats/min
Blood pressure: 110/70 mmHg

> What are your likely differential diagnoses?

You consider the possible causes of breathlessness and come up with:[33]

- Asthma
- Chronic obstructive airways disease (COPD)
- Pulmonary oedema secondary to acute left ventricular failure
- Pneumonia
- Pneumothorax
- Pulmonary embolus
- Pleural effusion
- Metabolic acidosis
- Aspirin poisoning
- Renal failure.

You auscultate his chest and find it to be clear, which makes the most common causes of breathlessness (the first three items in the list above) unlikely. You persist, asking more questions and continuing with the clinical examination, and are rewarded with a new onset left calf swelling that the patient noticed on waking this morning. You lift up his trouser leg to find a swollen, red and tender calf, which looks suspiciously like a deep vein thrombosis (DVT). Putting the two together leads you to suspect a pulmonary embolism (PE) as the most likely cause.

You share your thoughts with your colleague, who dismisses your diagnosis. "He doesn't have any chest pain or he-mop-thingy," he protests. You turn to the patient who confirms that he has not been coughing up any sputum at all, let alone the pink, frothy stuff that is haemoptysis. He still denies having any chest pain.

> What are you going to do: **Listen to your colleague** (read on) or **Carry on with your diagnosis** (skip the next paragraph)?

Listen to your colleague

Your colleague has sown some seeds of doubt and you waver about your diagnosis. You whisk the patient away to hospital forgetting to make a pre-alert call as you scrabble about for another explanation for your patient's condition. Needless to say, the hospital staff are scathing at your failure to warn them about your arrival, particularly as the department is heaving and it takes some minutes to free up space in resus. After hearing your handover, the doctor concludes that the patient has a PE. "But he doesn't have chest pain or haemoptysis," you babble. The doctor sighs and turns back to the patient. You stand for a minute or two then slope off back to the ambulance.

Carry on with your diagnosis

Now is perhaps not the time to enlighten your colleague about a study you recently read that found the "classic" triad of dyspnoea, chest pain and haemoptysis only occurred in fewer than 13% of patients[34] and instead get busy applying oxygen before carefully wrapping the patient up in a blanket. You return to the ambulance and remove the patient's paint-covered clothes. After ensuring that your colleague has a towel to sit on for the drive to hospital, you record a 12-lead ECG (which shows a sinus tachycardia), request the phone and make a pre-alert call. This is fortunate, because the department is awash with patients, but the staff manage to make a space in resus.

After handing over the patient, the doctor agrees with your likely diagnosis and is reassured that you weren't fooled by the absence of chest pain and haemoptysis.

The scale of the problem

An embolus is a blood-borne substance (including air) that is transported from one part of the circulation to another, lodging in a vessel which is too small to allow the embolus to pass. When the embolus lodges in the pulmonary vessels, it is termed a pulmonary embolism (PE).[35] Deep vein thrombosis (DVT) and pulmonary embolism represent the spectrum of one disease known as venous thromboembolism (VTE).[36] Although an embolus can consist of air, fat or amniotic fluid, for example, the most common is a clot from a DVT.[37]

The exact incidence for PE is not known since accurate diagnosis is tricky. However, deaths from detected PE are declining, although 20% of patients die within 1 year of diagnosis. In Europe, PE accounts for 8–13 deaths per 1,000 women and 2–7 deaths per 1,000 men.[36]

Pathophysiology

Deep vein thrombosis (DVT) formation is often attributed to Virchow's triad of hypercoagulopathy, stasis and intimal (the innermost layer of an artery or vein) injury. However, Virchow actually described the consequences of thrombus formation, not the cause.[38] As with many processes in the human body, the exact mechanisms by which DVTs form are not fully understood, but appear related to the lower limb venous valve pockets (where most thrombi form) and altered (but not completely static) blood flow.[36]

The risk factors for developing a venous thromboembolism are well known and can be of assistance in identifying patients who may have a PE:[39]

- **High risk factors** (odds ratio greater than 10)
    - Fracture (hip or leg)
    - Major general surgery
    - Major trauma
    - Spinal cord injury
    - Previous VTE.
- **Moderate risk factors** (odds ratio 2–9)
    - Congestive heart or respiratory failure
    - Chemotherapy
    - Hormone replacement therapy
    - Cancer
    - Oral contraceptive therapy
    - Paralytic stroke
    - Postpartum
    - Previous VTE
    - Thrombophilia.
- **Low risk factors** (odds ratio less than 2)
    - Bed rest for more than 3 days
    - Immobility due to sitting (for example, prolonged car or air travel)

Pulmonary Embolism

- Increasing age
- Obesity
- Pregnancy
- Varicose veins.

Thrombi most often form in the deep veins of the calf (hence the name, deep vein thrombosis!) and can grow to lengths of 30–50cm.[40] The proximal end of the thrombus can extend into the popliteal vein, where the risk of embolisation is greater. Once the thrombus (or a portion) breaks off, it becomes an embolus, travelling up the femoral vein and into the iliac veins. From there it is free to ascend via the inferior vena cava to the heart (Figure 5.4). It continues into the right atrium, ventricle and finally into the lungs via the pulmonary trunk and left and right pulmonary arteries (the only arteries to carry deoxygenated blood), which divide and sub-divide until they form capillaries around the alveoli.

In healthy patients, an obstruction of up to 25% of the pulmonary arterial bed will only cause modest respiratory symptoms, most frequently a reduction in the partial pressure of oxygen. Once this increases to 30–50% there will also be cardiovascular compromise. Patients with pre-existing respiratory and/or cardiovascular disease will be symptomatic at much lower percentages.[39]

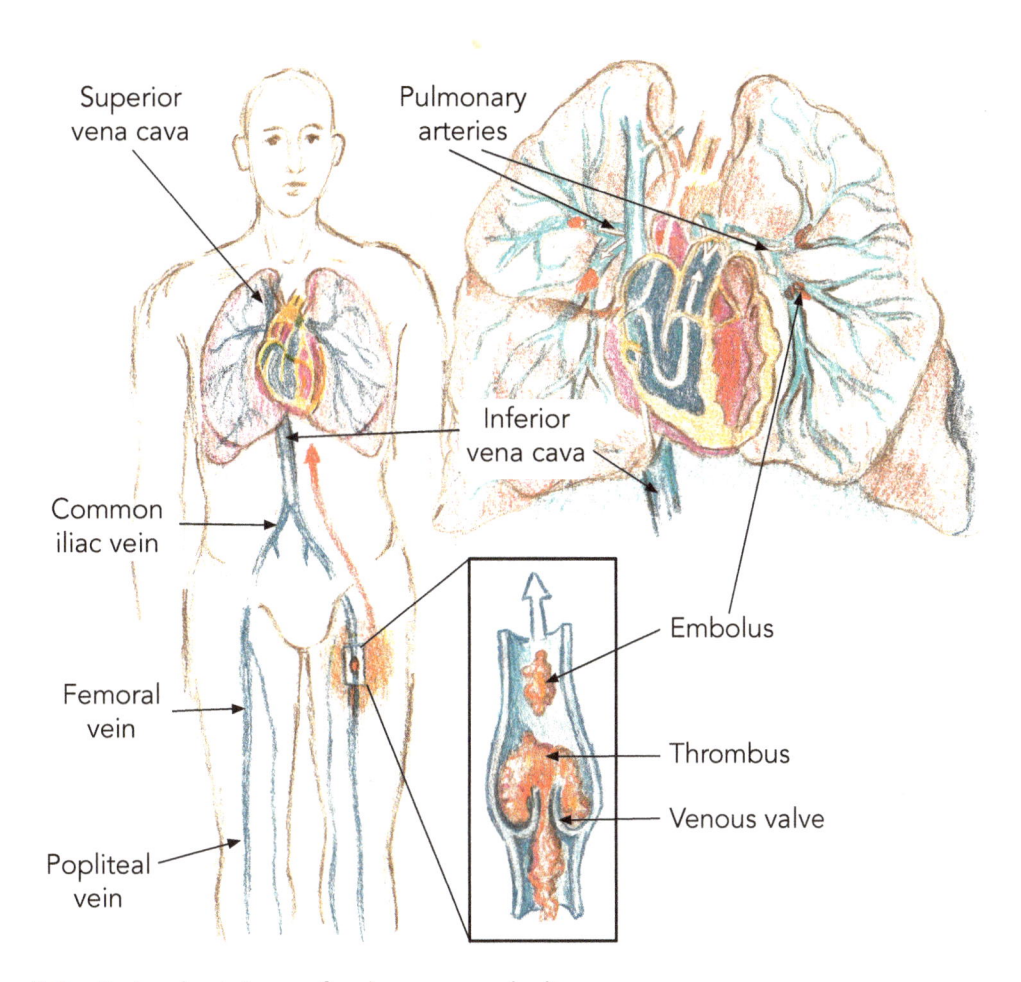

Figure 5.4 Pathophysiology of pulmonary embolism.

Chapter 5 Medical Emergencies

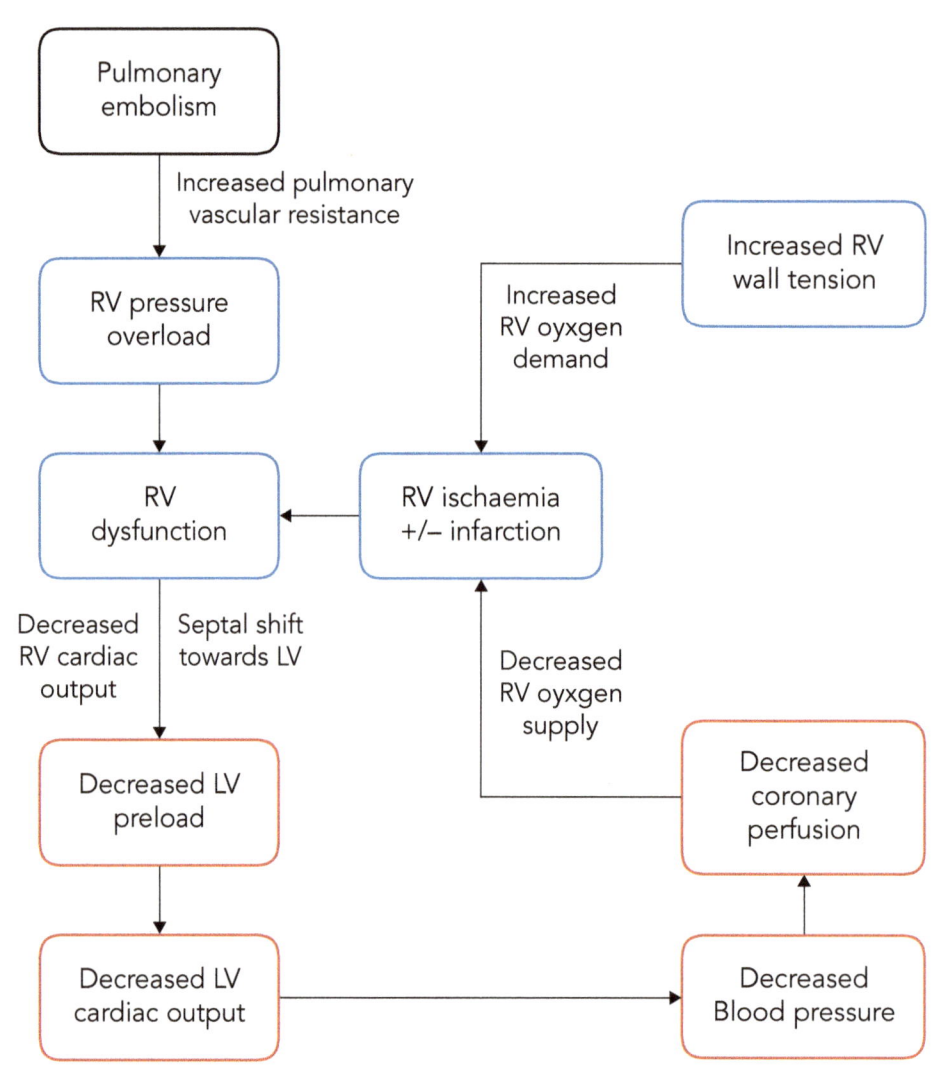

Figure 5.5 Right ventricular dysfunction due to acute pulmonary embolism.

Cardiovascular compromise is caused by increased pulmonary vascular resistance (Figure 5.5), which the right ventricle may not be able to overcome, resulting in sudden death.[39] In less severe cases(!), cardiogenic shock can result due to a combination of right ventricular pressure overload and dysfunction as the increase in wall tension increases oxygen demand while at the same time impeding supply. As the right ventricle enlarges, the intraventricular septum can deviate, which, coupled with a reduction in blood volume being pumped from the right side of the heart, results in a reduction in left ventricular cardiac output. Even with an increase in systemic vascular resistance, hypotension may follow, further reducing coronary artery perfusion and worsening ventricular ischaemia. Hypoxaemia can exacerbate this process further and is thought to be caused by a combination of processes including an increase is alveolar

Pulmonary Embolism

dead space, mismatched ventilation/perfusion (V/Q) and right-to-left shunting in patients who have a patent foramen ovale.[41,42]

Signs and symptoms

The patient's history and signs and symptoms cannot absolutely exclude or confirm the presence of a pulmonary embolism (PE), but there are tools which can help raise your index of suspicion. Two validated scores that do not require invasive tests and so lend themselves to pre-hospital use are the Wells score (Table 5.5) and Revised Geneva clinical prediction rule for PE (Table 5.6).[43–45] Most (80–90%) of patients will have at least one predisposing factor and so PE should be one of your differentials for any patient presenting with an acute onset of shortness of breath and/or chest pain.[43]

Common signs and symptoms of PE include difficulty breathing (dyspnoea) and rapid breathing (tachypnoea). Pleuritic chest pain is the most common symptom.[29]

Other signs and symptoms include:

- Signs:
    - respiratory rate greater than 20 breaths/minute
    - pulse rate greater than 100 beats/minute
    - pulse oximeter reading (SpO_2) less than 92% on air
    - signs of a DVT, which includes pain, swelling and/or tenderness on only one leg, often in the calf[36]

Table 5.5 Wells score (simplified).

Clinical feature	Points
Clinical signs and symptoms of DVT (minimum of leg swelling and pain with palpation of the deep veins)	3
An alternative diagnosis is less likely than PE	3
Heart rate more than 100 beats per minute	1.5
Immobilisation for more than 3 days or surgery in the previous 4 weeks	1.5
Previous DVT/PE	1.5
Haemoptysis	1
Malignancy (on treatment, treated in the last 6 months, or palliative)	1
Clinical probability simplified score	
PE likely	>4 points
PE unlikely	≤4 points

Source: Wells et al., 2000.

Table 5.6 Revised Geneva clinical prediction rule for PE (simplified version).

Indicator	Score
Over 65 years of age	1
Previous DVT or PE	1
Surgery or fracture in past month	1
Active cancer	1
Unilateral lower limb pain	1
Haemoptysis	1
Heart rate 75–94 beats per min	1
Heart rate over 94 beats per min	2
Pain on lower limb deep vein palpation and unilateral oedema	1
Clinical probability	
PE unlikely	0–2
PE likely	≥3

Source: Klok et al., 2008.

- Symptoms:
  - difficulty breathing (dyspnoea)
  - pleuritic chest pain
  - substernal chest pain
  - cough
  - haemoptysis (blood from the respiratory tract, usually coughed up)
  - syncope (faint).

The 12-lead ECG

Contrary to popular belief, the 'classic' S1Q3T3 pattern occurs in only 15% of patients with a PE. The most common change is sinus tachycardia, but right ventricular strain (the presence of one or more of right bundle branch block, S1Q3T3 and T wave inversion in the anterior leads) occurs in about 35% of patients.[46] The presence of right ventricular strain is an indicator of short-term adverse events (including death), so should not be ignored!

Management

The pre-hospital management for a pulmonary embolism (PE) is largely supportive of ABCs. Early recognition and prompt transport form the mainstay of treatment supplemented with oxygen and intravenous fluids, if required. If the patient is in cardiac arrest and pulmonary embolism is suspected, thrombolysis can be considered, although evidence for benefit is poor. If thrombolytic drugs are administered, CPR should be continued for 60–90 minutes.[47]

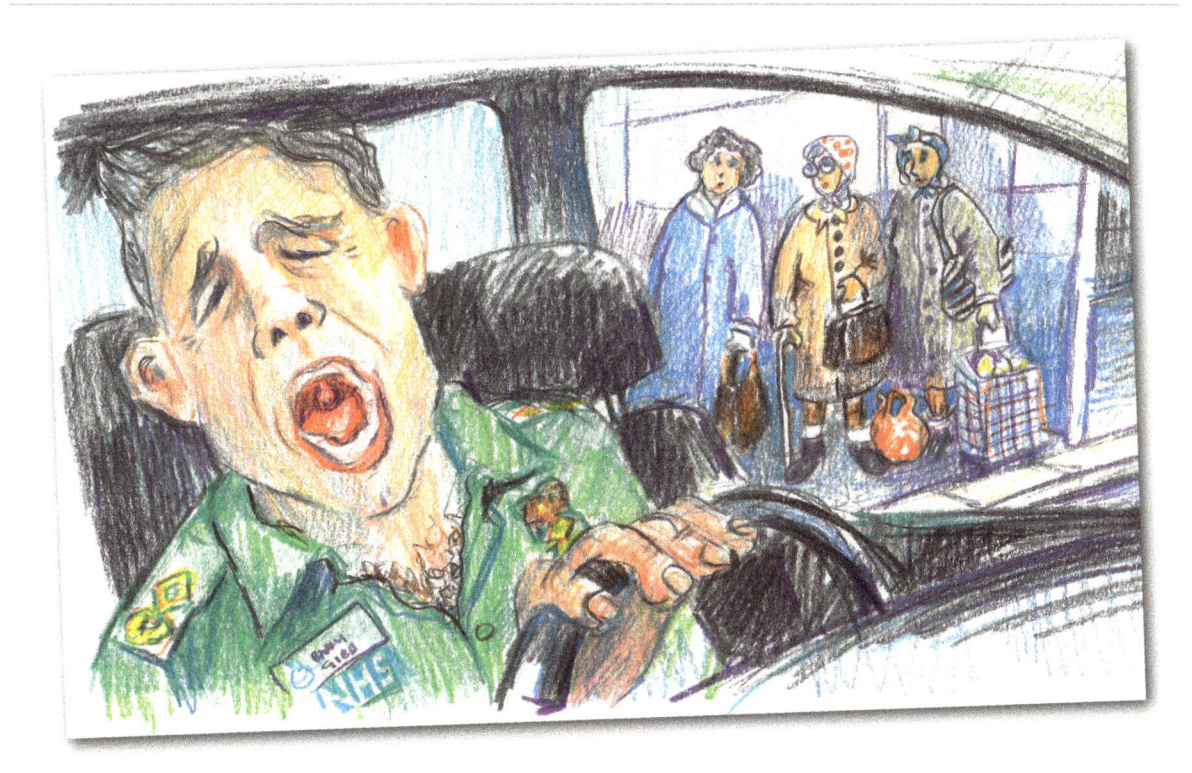

Addison's Disease

You are a single responder on standby contemplating your next job. Somewhere, approximately 8 minutes drive or so away, is a prospective patient about to call for an ambulance or have 999 called for them. Will it be an injury or illness? Perhaps they are just lonely, have toothache, can't find the remote for the TV…

In fact, over an hour ago, your next patient was descending a flight of stairs with two large cardboard boxes. Since she couldn't see the steps, she gingerly descended, wishing that her husband had moved them as he was asked to, before he nipped out for a round of golf. Without warning, she lost her balance and fell headfirst down the last few steps. The boxes and their contents did a good job of cushioning her head and torso, but one of her legs got caught in the balustrade of the stairs and there was a nasty cracking sound as her foot and lower leg rotated in opposite directions, fracturing her distal tibia and fibula. She let out a brief scream and then … nothing.

The patient wakes up over an hour later and is aware of a severe pain in her lower leg. With great effort, she crawls to the hall phone and dials 999. She manages to tell the call taker where she lives and that she has fallen and injured her leg. However, she is feeling drowsy and having trouble answering further questions. The call taker realises that this patient is not well at all as she is becoming unresponsive. The last thing she gets from the patient is 'add a son'.

Chapter 5 Medical Emergencies

They wonder if this relates to a child protection issue, having just completed an e-learning module on the very subject, and adds their concern to the patient's notes.

Seven minutes and 43 seconds drive away as it turns out, you catch yourself trying to hit the high notes of the Bee Gees hit, *Stayin' Alive*. You stop abruptly, but it is too late. You look up over the steering wheel to see a small collection of senior citizens, watching you from a nearby bus stop. Your wish for a job to escape the humiliation is fulfilled by the MDT, which passes details of a 53-year-old woman who has fallen with a leg injury. You note that she has become unresponsive and has a son who may be at risk. As you pass the bus stop, the ladies give you a cheery wave.

As you arrive on scene, you notice that there is a man on the drive pulling a set of golf clubs out of the boot of his car. You get out and introduce yourself and explain that you have received a call at this address. The smile disappears from his face and he scrabbles for the keys to open the front door. He ushers you in and as you enter the hallway, the patient comes into view. She is lying on her right side with her back to you. The old-fashioned Bakelite phone is lying on the floor and when you pick it up, the call taker is still on the other end. You replace the phone and turn to the patient. You notice that she looks rather thin. She is trying to say something to you, which sounds a bit like "add a son."

> What is she trying to draw your attention to: a **Child protection issue** (read on) or a **Life-threatening endocrine disease** (skip the next paragraph)?

Child protection issue

You turn to the husband, put on your concerned face and enquire about his son. He looks awkwardly at you and states that they have none, as Anisa (his wife) is unable to have children. You mumble an apology while wondering if your work boot will fit in your mouth. Perhaps the patient is making reference to a life-threatening endocrine disease…

Life-threatening endocrine disease

You can't quite make out what Anisa is saying, so you try to obtain a history from her husband. He starts on a long monologue about his trip to the golf club and a great shot on the 12th, and you have to drag him back to the present situation by asking him to fetch her medication. He returns with a mixture, but a couple of names jump out at you: hydrocortisone and fludrocortisone. You ask if Anisa has Addison's disease and the patient nods weakly. The husband is not so sure but does seem to recall her having some problem with her kidney glands.

The crew arrive and you pass on the story so far. They have no idea what you are talking about when you mention Addison's disease, but they do understand that a fall down the stairs, decreasing level of consciousness and distracting injury means treating the patient as if they have a spinal injury, and package her up efficiently while you record some baseline observations and gain intravenous access.

Her vital signs are as follows:

Airway

Patent

Breathing

Respiratory rate: 34 breaths/min with bilateral air entry
SpO$_2$: 94% on air

156

Circulation

  Rapid, thready pulse at a rate of 120 beats per minute
  Blood pressure: 80/45 mmHg

Disability

  GCS score: 13/15
  Blood sugar: 3.9 mmol/l

Exposure/Environment

  Temperature: 36.9°C

> What are you going to do first: **Administer hydrocortisone** (read on) or **Set up an intravenous infusion** (skip the next paragraph)?

Administer hydrocortisone

You give 100 mg hydrocortisone IV over the next couple of minutes. The crew are getting tetchy about time on scene, but you are concerned about how fast Anisa is deteriorating. Once this is done and the patient moved to the ambulance, you set up an intravenous infusion and en route to the emergency department, give repeated doses of normal saline, recheck her blood glucose and make a pre-alert call. By the time you arrive at hospital, 30 minutes later, Anisa's condition appears to be improving a little and after handing over to the hospital staff you say goodbye to her as she manages to mouth a 'thank you'. Not only that, but on your return to the ambulance, one of the crew has even made you a hot drink … and it's not even your birthday.

Set up an IV infusion

You elect to give fluids as the Anisa's blood pressure is so low. The crew are getting tetchy at the time spent on scene, but you insist on setting it up. However, you forget to lock off the tubing and pepper it with air bubbles. You curse, and start running fluid through to get rid of them. About 350 mls later, you finally get the giving set free of air, only to inadvertently rip the cannula out while trying to connect it up. With blood spilling on the hall carpet, the crew have had enough and take the patient from under your nose. By the time you have issued your apologies to the husband and cleared up the mess, the crew have already left scene. You find out later that she had a cardiac arrest en route and despite the best efforts of the crew and ED staff, she died. You can't believe how fast she went downhill and wonder if, had you administered hydrocortisone earlier, her death could have been prevented.

The scale of the problem

In 1855, Thomas Addison attributed "anaemia, general languor and debility, feebleness of the heart's action, irritability of the stomach and a peculiar change of colour of the skin" to a disease of the adrenal glands.[48] Today, Addison's disease falls under the umbrella term of primary adrenal insufficiency, which is a clinical syndrome caused by a number of diseases which all have decreased secretion of cortisol (the 'stress' hormone) and aldosterone by the adrenal glands in common.[49] Autoimmune Addison's disease (the most common type) affects around 1 in 10,000 people in the UK, typically affecting young and middle-aged people and is more common in women than men.[49,50]

Anatomy and physiology

The adrenal (or suprarenal) glands are situated in the retroperitoneum, within the renal fascia and on the superior and medical aspects on each kidney (that is, on top and towards the middle, Figure 5.6). They are shaped

Chapter 5 Medical Emergencies

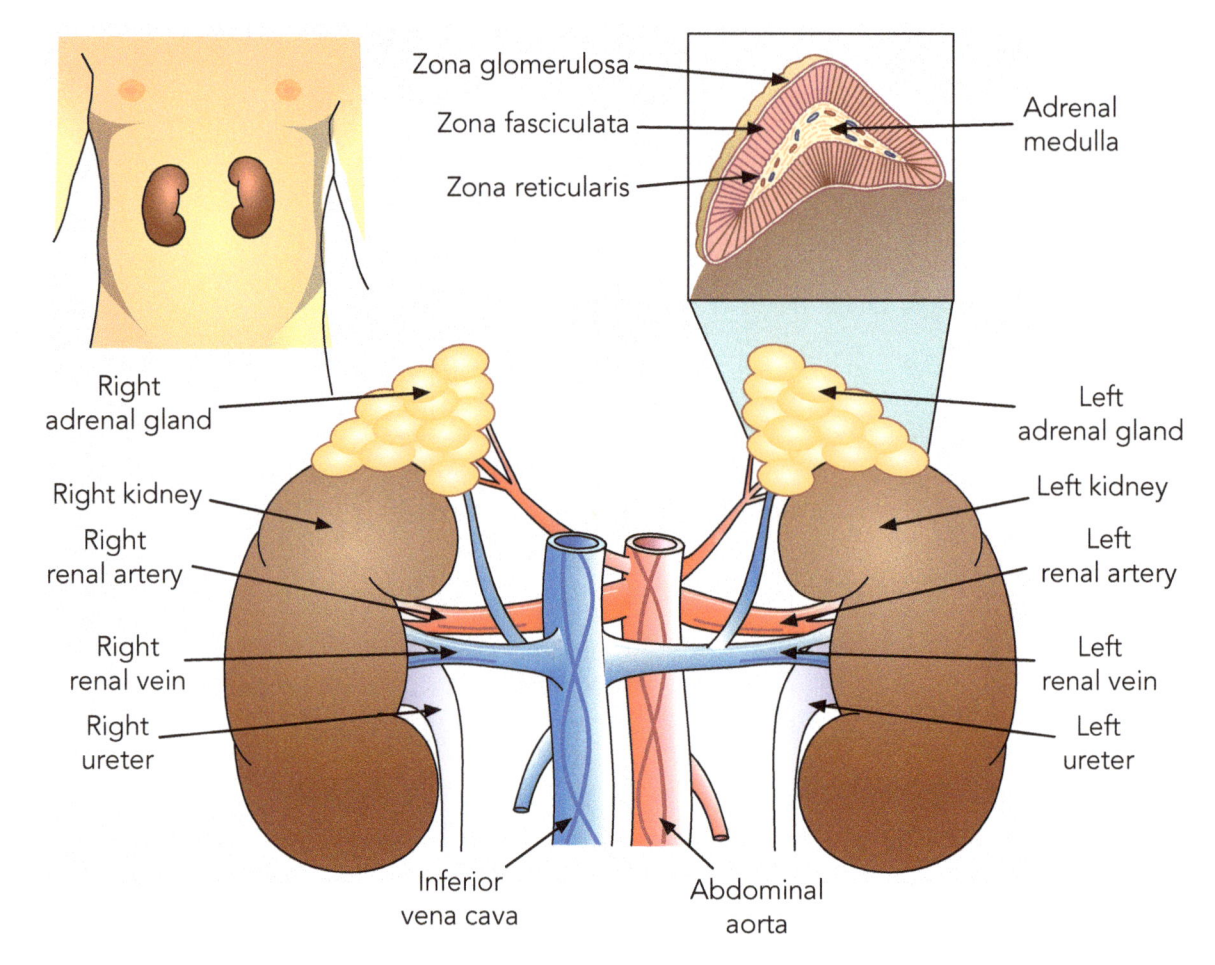

Figure 5.6 The kidneys and adrenal glands.

like a flattened pyramid, and in adults are around 3–5 cm tall, 2–3 cm wide and 1 cm deep.[18] When viewed in cross-section, it is clear that they are in fact two glands in one, with a smaller, inner medulla, responsible for secreting the catecholamines adrenaline and noradrenaline, and an outer cortex, which makes up over 80% of the gland.

The adrenal cortex is subdivided into three zones:

- An outer zona glomerulosa which secretes mineralocorticoids, the most important being aldosterone. This helps regulate levels of sodium (Na$^+$) and potassium (K$^+$), by increasing reabsorption of sodium from the distal tubules of the kidneys, the sweat glands and the gastrointestinal tract. It also increases excretion of potassium. Finally, aldosterone helps to regulate blood pressure as part of the renin-angiotensin-aldosterone pathway (more on that later).
- A middle zona fasciculata which secretes glucocorticoids, mainly cortisol (also known as hydrocortisone). Cortisol has a number of functions including glucose formation, the breakdown of proteins and triglycerides, reducing numbers of white blood cells involved in inflammatory processes and depressing the immune system response. It is also a permissive hormone, allowing other hormones to exert

their affects. For example, it is required for catecholamine synthesis and re-uptake into nerves.[51]

- An inner zona reticularis which secretes sex steroids such as oestrogen, progesterone and androgen. These are not crucial in acute emergencies, but can have a significant impact on the lifestyle of patients with Addison's disease.[52]

Sodium and potassium

Both these electrolytes are essential for life. Sodium is important in the excitability process of cell membranes, particularly in nerve and muscle tissue. It also plays a critical role in the regulation of plasma and extracellular volumes of water and regulation of blood pressure. Given its importance, there are a number of processes aimed at ensuring homeostasis of plasma sodium, one of which involves aldosterone.

Potassium is principally an intracellular electrolyte, but changes in extracellular potassium concentration affect the resting membrane potential of all body cells and thereby intracellular concentrations of potassium which is critical for cellular enzymes and protein synthesis. Abnormal rises in plasma potassium levels (hyperkalaemia) can affect cardiac and brain function, which in severe cases can be fatal.

Regulation of sodium and potassium

Raised plasma levels of potassium have a dramatic and rapid effect on the cells within the zona glomerulosa, resulting in release of aldosterone, which acts on the kidneys, increasing excretion of potassium in the urine until homeostasis is restored.

The mechanism by which falling levels of sodium stimulates aldosterone release is more involved and is linked to a mechanism responsible for control of blood pressure, namely the renin-angiotensin-aldosterone pathway (Figure 5.7).

Renin-angiotensin-aldosterone pathway

Aldosterone plays a key part in a multi-organ process that helps regulate plasma levels of sodium and blood pressure. It all starts with the juxtaglomerular apparatus situated between the afferent arteriole and distal tubule of nephrons in the kidneys. Either a drop in blood pressure or sodium results in the release of renin. Renin is a protein hormone, but acts like an enzyme, splitting angiotensinogen produced by the liver to form angiotensin I. This circulates to the lungs and is converted to angiotensin II by angiotensin converting enzyme (ACE, inhibitors of which are used to control blood pressure and generally end in –pril, for example, lisinopril and enalapril). Angiotensin II is a potent vasoconstrictor of arterioles, causing an increase in peripheral vascular resistance and blood pressure. It also acts on the cells of the zona glomerulosa, stimulating them to release aldosterone.

Compared with angiotensin II, aldosterone adopts a slow and steady approach, taking several hours to have an effect. It raises levels of plasma sodium by increasing reabsorption of sodium from the distal tubules and the salivary and sweat glands.

Glucocorticoids

In order to understand how cortisol (the chief glucocorticoid and 'stress' hormone) is secreted, it is necessary to turn your attention to a small area of the brain, located just under the thalamus – the hypothalamus. This area receives input from a number of different areas of the brain including the limbic system, cerebral cortex, thalamus, reticular activation system and external sensory signals from internal organs and even the retina. It forms the major interface between the nervous and endocrine systems.

In response to some form of stress, for example, cold, fasting/starvation, hypotension, haemorrhage, surgery, infection, pain from

Chapter 5 Medical Emergencies

wounds and fractures, severe exercise and even emotional trauma (such as when an audit letter arrives from the Heath and Care Professions Council), neurosecretory cells in the hypothalamus release-corticotropin releasing hormone (CRH). This hormone travels to the anterior pituitary gland where it is stimulated to release adrenocorticotrophic hormone (ACTH).

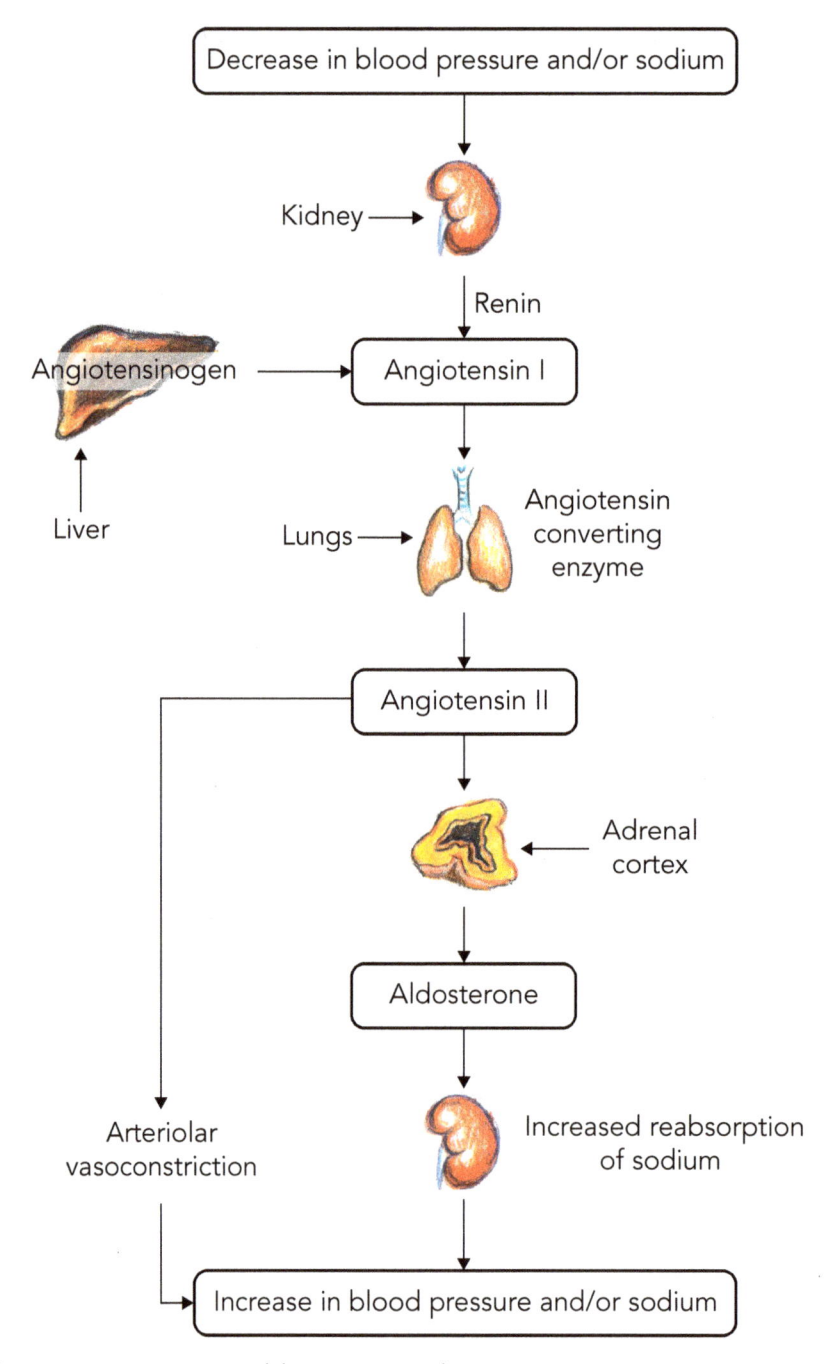

Figure 5.7 The renin-angiotensin-aldosterone pathway.

ACTH travels through the blood stream until it reaches the adrenal glands and stimulates the zona fasciculata to synthesise and release cortisol.[50]

Once blood levels of cortisol are high enough, levels of ACTH reduce thanks to a negative feedback mechanism acting on both the hypothalamus (inhibiting release of CRH) and the anterior pituitary.

Addison's disease

Causes of Addison's disease are summarised in Table 5.7. Pre-existing diseases are more commonly seen in patients with Addison's disease, particularly other autoimmune-related diseases such as Graves' disease, type 1 diabetes, premature ovarian failure and coeliac disease.[50,53,54]

The majority of patients with Addison's disease in developed countries, have the autoimmune form of the disease, whereby the adrenal cortex is progressively destroyed by the body's own immune system. Since the disease is slow to develop, patients are sometimes misdiagnosed with depression or anorexia until they present in crisis. Even then, up to a third of patients who present in crisis at a hospital will not have their condition identified.[55]

Adrenal crisis

A number of factors can lead to a patient with Addison's disease (and other causes of primary adrenal insufficiency) going into 'crisis'. The most common cause is vomiting and/or diarrhoea,[56] but other precipitating factors are given in Table 5.8. Around 8% of patients with Addison's disease will have at least one adrenal crisis requiring administration of hydrocortisone. The vast majority of these patients rely on a healthcare

Table 5.7 Causes of Addison's disease.

Cause	Notes
Autoimmunity	
Autoimmune polyendocrinopathy syndromes 1 and 2	Associated with other autoimmune diseases
Isolated autoimmune Addison's disease	
Infective	
Tuberculosis	A major cause worldwide in developing countries
Fungal	Often related to immunodeficiency
Genetic	Genetic mutations and other defects
Other	
Infiltration	Usually from malignant metastases or lymphoma
Haemorrhage	Bilateral bleeding in the adrenal glands is a rare cause, classically due to coagulation defects in meningococcal septicaemia (Waterhouse-Friderichsen syndrome)
Infarction	Associated with antiphospholipid syndrome
Iatrogenic	Bilateral adrenalectomy or drugs (for example, etomidate, ketoconazole)

Adapted from: Betterle et al., 2019.

Chapter 5 Medical Emergencies

Table 5.8 Common precipitating factors for adrenal crisis.

Cause	Incidence (%)
Vomiting	33
Diarrhoea	23
Flu-like illness	11
Major infection	6
Surgery	6
Blackout/LOC	6
Injury/severe pain	4
Shock	4
Other	3
Severe fatigue/inadequate medication	2
Unknown	1
Anxiety/psychological upset/stress	1

Adapted from: White & Arlt, 2010.

professional to administer a hydrocortisone injection. In one study, only 12% were able to administer it themselves, with a further 17% having the drug administered by a partner, relative or friend.[56]

Signs and symptoms

The most obvious signs of Addison's disease are cachexia and overpigmentation of the skin, which occurs due to loss of the negative feedback mechanism which controls melanocyte-stimulating hormone from the anterior pituitary gland.[57] The patient may look tanned, although this sign is sometimes subtle. Check for pigmentation of the palmar creases, and muddy brown patches in the mucous membranes of the lips and mouth. Enquire specifically about salt-craving, which can occur in hyponatraemia. Symptoms can be remembered by using the ADDISONS mnemonic:[55]

A	Always tired
D	Dizzy when standing
D	Drop in blood pressure on standing
I	Inexplicable weight loss
S	Skin colour changes
O	Only eating sparingly/anorexia
N	No strength in handgrip or limbs
S	Sick or nauseous

Patients in adrenal crisis typically present with severe hypotension or shock, acute abdominal pain, vomiting and pyrexia. As a result, there is a tendency for them to be misdiagnosed as an 'acute abdomen'. In children, hypoglycaemic convulsions are a common presentation.[58]

Other clues that may indicate your patient has Addison's disease include a MedicAlert bracelet and glucocorticoid and mineralocorticoid replacement medication, most commonly hydrocortisone and fludrocortisone.[59] In patients with type 1 diabetes, there may be a history of deteriorating blood sugar control, with recurrent hypoglycaemic episodes.[58]

Management of adrenal crisis

This is a life-threatening emergency. Patients are usually told to double or even treble their oral dose of hydrocortisone when unwell or injured, but they may not be able to manage medication orally if they are vomiting.[59] It is essential therefore that they receive intravenous (IV) hydrocortisone (or IM if IV access cannot be established) as soon as possible. The adult dose is 100 mg and the paediatric dose, 2–4 mg/kg.[60] Simplified regimens for children are found in the *JRCALC Clinical Guidelines*,[29] so follow local guidance and/or that of parents and carers. If you are in any doubt as to whether the patient has received an adequate dose of hydrocortisone, administer the drug.

In addition to administering hydrocortisone, you will need to correct hypotension and hypovolaemia with IV fluids, and hypoglycaemia with IV glucose. Frequently recheck blood glucose as these patients are at risk of recurring hypoglycaemia. Pre-alert the receiving hospital and make sure you pass on that the patient has Addison's disease to the staff, as the patient will require repeated doses of hydrocortisone.

Chapter 5 Medical Emergencies

References

1. Sampson HA, Muñoz-Furlong A, Campbell RL, Adkinson Jr NF, Allan Bock S, Branum A, et al. Second symposium on the definition and management of anaphylaxis: summary report – second National Institute of Allergy and Infectious Disease/Food Allergy and Anaphylaxis Network Symposium. *Annals of Emergency Medicine*, 2006 Apr;47(4):373–380.
2. Cardona V, Ansotegui IJ, Ebisawa M, El-Gamal Y, Fernandez Rivas M, Fineman S, et al. World Allergy Organization anaphylaxis guidance 2020. *World Allergy Organization Journal*, 2020 Oct;13(10):100472.
3. Panesar SS, Javad S, Silva D de, Nwaru BI, Hickstein L, Muraro A, et al. The epidemiology of anaphylaxis in Europe: a systematic review. *Allergy*, 2013 Nov 1;68(11):1353–1361.
4. Resuscitation Council UK. Emergency treatment of anaphylaxis [Internet]. 2021 Available from: https://www.resus.org.uk/media/337/download
5. Turner PJ, Gowland MH, Sharma V, Ierodiakonou D, Harper N, Garcez T, et al. Increase in anaphylaxis-related hospitalizations but no increase in fatalities: an analysis of United Kingdom national anaphylaxis data, 1992–2012. *Journal of Allergy and Clinical Immunology*, 2015 Apr 1;135(4):956–963.e1.
6. Conrado AB, Ierodiakonou D, Gowland MH, Boyle RJ, Turner PJ. Food anaphylaxis in the United Kingdom: analysis of national data, 1998–2018. *British Medical Journal*, 2021 Feb 17;372:n251.
7. Pumphrey RS. Lessons for management of anaphylaxis from a study of fatal reactions. *Clinical & Experimental Allergy*, 2000 Aug;30(8):1144–1150.
8. Simons FER. Anaphylaxis: recent advances in assessment and treatment. *Journal of Allergy and Clinical Immunology*, 2009 Oct;124(4):625–636.
9. Paiva M, Piedade S, Gaspar Â. Toothpaste-induced anaphylaxis caused by mint (Mentha) allergy. *Allergy*, 2010 Sep 1;65(9):1201–1202.
10. Simons FER. 9. Anaphylaxis. *Journal of Allergy and Clinical Immunology*, 2008 Feb;121(2, Supplement 2):S402–S407.
11. Marieb E, Hoehn K. *Human anatomy & physiology*, 11th edition. Pearson; 2019.
12. Prussin C, Metcalfe DD. 5. IgE, mast cells, basophils, and eosinophils. *Journal of Allergy and Clinical Immunology*, 2006 Feb;117(2, Supplement 2):S450–S456.
13. Lee JK, Vadas P. Anaphylaxis: mechanisms and management. *Clinical & Experimental Allergy*, 2011 Jul 1;41(7):923–938.
14. Simons FER, Frew AJ, Ansotegui IJ, Bochner BS, Golden DBK, Finkelman FD, et al. Risk assessment in anaphylaxis: Current and future approaches. *Journal of Allergy and Clinical Immunology*, 2007 Jul;120(1, Supplement):S2–24.
15. Simons FER, Gu X, Simons KJ. Epinephrine absorption in adults: Intramuscular versus subcutaneous injection. *Journal of Allergy and Clinical Immunology*, 2001 Nov;108(5):871–873.
16. Diabetes UK. Diabetes: Facts and stats [Internet]. 2016 Available from: https://www.diabetes.org.uk/professionals/position-statements-reports/statistics/diabetes-prevalence-2016#:~:text=There%20are%20almost%203.6%20million,with%20diabetes%20in%20the%20UK.
17. Alwafi H, Alsharif AA, Wei L, Langan D, Naser AY, Mongkhon P, et al. Incidence and prevalence of hypoglycaemia in type 1 and type 2 diabetes individuals: a systematic review and meta-analysis. *Diabetes Research and Clinical Practice*, 2020 Dec;170:108522.
18. Drake RL, Vogl W, Mitchell AWM, Gray H. *Gray's anatomy for students*, 3rd edition. Philadelphia: Churchill Livingstone/Elsevier; 2015.
19. Jolles S. Paul Langerhans. *Journal of Clinical Pathology*, 2002 Apr;55(4):243–243.
20. Rang HP, Dale MM, Ritter JM, Flower RJ, Henderson G. *Rang & Dale's pharmacology*, 7th edition. London: Churchill Livingstone; 2011.
21. Murphy KG, Bloom SR. Gut hormones and the regulation of energy homeostasis. *Nature*, 2006 Dec 14;444(7121):854–859.
22. Cryer PE. The barrier of hypoglycemia in diabetes. *Diabetes*, 2008 Dec;57(12):3169–3176.
23. Briscoe VJ, Davis SN. Hypoglycemia in type 1 and type 2 diabetes: physiology, pathophysiology, and management. *Clinical Diabetes*, 2006 Jul 1;24(3):115–121.
24. Quesada I, Tudurí E, Ripoll C, Nadal Á. Physiology of the pancreatic α-cell and glucagon secretion: role in glucose

homeostasis and diabetes. *Journal of Endocrinology*, 2008 Oct 1;199(1):5–19.
25. Graveling AJ, Frier BM. Hypoglycaemia: an overview. Primary Care Diabetes, 2009 Aug;3(3):131–139.
26. Elliott J, Heller S. Hypoglycaemia unawareness. *Practical Diabetes International*, 2011 Jun 1;28(5):227–232.
27. Deary IJ, Hepburn DA, MacLeod KM, Frier BM. Partitioning the symptoms of hypoglycaemia using multi-sample confirmatory factor analysis. *Diabetologia*, 1993 Aug;36(8):771–777.
28. Bailey CJ, Day C. Hypoglycaemia: a limiting factor. British Journal of Diabetes & Vascular Disease, 2010;10(1):2–4.
29. Joint Royal Colleges Ambulance Liaison Committee, Association of Ambulance Chief Executives. JRCALC Clinical Guidelines. Cited from JRCALC Plus (Version 1.2.13) [Mobile application software]. Bridgwater: Class Publishing Ltd; 2021.
30. Moore C, Woollard M. Dextrose 10% or 50% in the treatment of hypoglycaemia out of hospital? A randomised controlled trial. Emergency Medicine Journal, 2005 Jul 1;22(7):512–515.
31. Walker A, James C, Bannister M, Jobes E. Evaluation of a diabetes referral pathway for the management of hypoglycaemia following emergency contact with the ambulance service to a diabetes specialist nurse team. Emergency Medicine Journal, 2006 Jun 1;23(6):449–451.
32. Roberts K, Smith A. Outcome of diabetic patients treated in the prehospital arena after a hypoglycaemic episode, and an exploration of treat and release protocols: a review of the literature. Emergency Medicine Journal, 2003 May 1;20(3):274–276.
33. Woollard M. 4 Shortness of breath. Emergency Medicine Journal, 2004 May 1;21(3):341–350.
34. Stein PD, Terrin ML, Hales CA, Palevsky HI, Saltzman HA, Thompson BT, et al. Clinical, laboratory, roentgenographic, and electrocardiographic findings in patients with acute pulmonary embolism and no pre-existing cardiac or pulmonary disease. Chest, 1991;100(3):598–603.
35. Lawrence H, Moore T, LLM STDBsMM, *MRCP PXMMBc*. Crash course respiratory medicine, 5th edition. FRCP OUMPF, editor. Elsevier; 2018.
36. Khan F, Tritschler T, Kahn SR, Rodger MA. Venous thromboembolism. *The Lancet* [Internet]. 2021 May 10; Available from: https://www.sciencedirect.com/science/article/pii/S0140673620326581
37. Giordano NJ, Jansson PS, Young MN, Hagan KA, Kabrhel C. Epidemiology, pathophysiology, stratification, and natural history of pulmonary embolism. Vascular and Interventional Radiology, 2017 Sep 1;20(3):135–140.
38. Bagot CN, Arya R. Virchow and his triad: a question of attribution. *British Journal of Haematology*, 2008 Oct 1;143(2):180–190.
39. Konstantinides SV, Meyer G, Becattini C, Bueno H, Geersing G-J, Harjola V-P, et al. 2019 ESC Guidelines for the diagnosis and management of acute pulmonary embolism developed in collaboration with the European Respiratory Society (ERS): The Task Force for the diagnosis and management of acute pulmonary embolism of the European Society of Cardiology (ESC). *European Heart Journal*, 2020 Jan 21;41(4):543–603.
40. Tapson VF. Acute pulmonary embolism. *New England Journal of Medicine*, 2008 Mar 6;358(10):1037–1052.
41. Wood KE. Major pulmonary embolism. Chest, 2002 Mar 1;121(3):877–905.
42. Kasper W, Geibel A. Patent foramen ovale in patients with haemodynamically significant pulmonary embolism. *The Lancet*, 1992;340(8819):561.
43. Le Gal G, Righini M, Roy P-M, Sanchez O, Aujesky D, Bounameaux H, et al. Prediction of pulmonary embolism in the emergency department: the revised Geneva score. *Annals of Internal Medicine*, 2006 Feb 7;144(3):165–W29.
44. Klok FA, Mos ICM, Nijkeuter M, Righini M, Perrier A, Le Gal G, et al. Simplification of the revised Geneva score for assessing clinical probability of pulmonary embolism. Archives of Internal Medicine, 2008 Oct 27;168(19):2131–2136.

45. Wells PS, Anderson DR, Rodger M, Ginsberg JS, Kearon C, Gent M, et al. Derivation of a simple clinical model to categorize patients probability of pulmonary embolism: increasing the models utility with the SimpliRED D-dimer. Thrombosis and Haemostasis, 2000 Mar;83(3):416–420.
46. Vanni S, Polidori G, Vergara R, Pepe G, Nazerian P, Moroni F, et al. Prognostic value of ECG among patients with acute pulmonary embolism and normal blood pressure. American Journal of Medicine, 2009 Mar;122(3):257–264.
47. Lott C, Truhlář A, Alfonzo A, Barelli A, González-Salvado V, Hinkelbein J, et al. European Resuscitation Council Guidelines 2021: cardiac arrest in special circumstances. *Resuscitation*, 2021 Apr 1;161:152–219.
48. Addison T, Wilks SS, Daldy TM. *A collection of the published writings of the late Thomas Addison*, M.D. London: New Sydenham Society; 1868. 324 p.
49. Husebye E, Løvås K. Pathogenesis of primary adrenal insufficiency. Best Practice & Research Clinical Endocrinology & Metabolism, 2009 Apr;23(2):147–157.
50. Betterle C, Presotto F, Furmaniak J. Epidemiology, pathogenesis, and diagnosis of Addison's disease in adults. *Journal of Endocrinological Investigation*, 2019 Dec;42(12):1407–1433.
51. Greenstein B, Wood D. *The endocrine system at a glance*, 3rd edition. Chichester: Wiley-Blackwell; 2011. 144 p.
52. Arlt W. Quality of life in Addison's disease – the case for DHEA replacement. *Clinical Endocrinology*, 2002 May 1;56(5):573–574.
53. Myhre AG, Aarsetøy H, Undlien DE, Hovdenak N, Aksnes L, Husebye ES. High frequency of coeliac disease among patients with autoimmune adrenocortical failure. *Scandinavian Journal of Gastroenterology*, 2003 May;38(5):511–515.
54. Falorni A, Laureti S, De Bellis A, Zanchetta R, Tiberti C, Arnaldi G, et al. Italian addison network study: update of diagnostic criteria for the etiological classification of primary adrenal insufficiency. *Journal of Clinical Endocrinology and Metabolism*, 2004 Apr;89(4):1598–1604.
55. Addison's Disease Self Help Group. Diagnosing Addison's Disease: A Guide For GPs [Internet]. Addison's Disease Self-Help Group. 2020. Available from: https://www.addisonsdisease.org.uk/diagnosing-addisons-disease-a-guide-for-gps
56. White K, Arlt W. Adrenal crisis in treated Addison's disease: a predictable but under-managed event. *European Journal of Endocrinology*, 2010 Jan 1;162(1):115–120.
57. Innes JA, Dover AR, Fairhurst K, Britton R, Danielson E. *Macleod's clinical examination*, 14th edition. Edinburgh: Elsevier; 2018.
58. Arlt W, Allolio B. Adrenal insufficiency. *The Lancet*, 2003;361(9372):1881–1893.
59. Baker SJK, Wass JAH. Addison's disease. *British Medical Journal*, 2009 Jul 2;339(jul02 1):b2384–b2384.
60. National Institute for Health and Care Excellence. Hydrocortisone [Internet]. NICE; 2021. Available from: https://bnfc.nice.org.uk/drug/hydrocortisone.html#indicationsAndDoses

6   Trauma

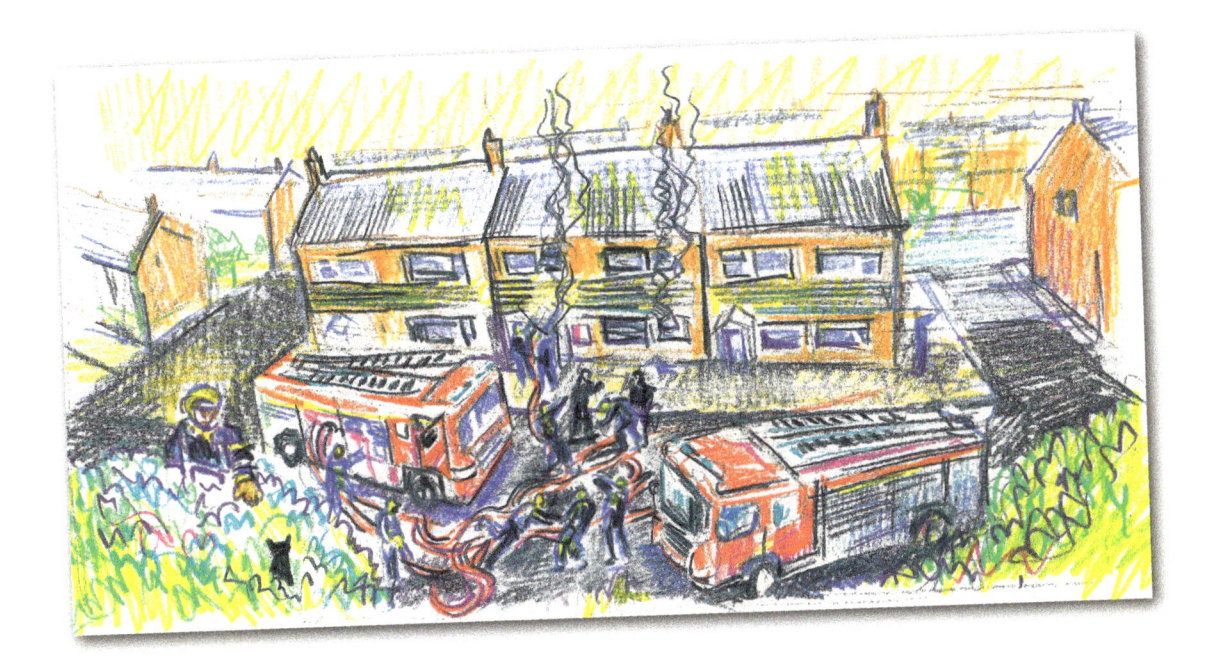

Thermal Burns

You are on standby on the coldest day of the year. Thanks to your vehicle being left outside overnight, you spend 10 minutes scraping the ice off the windscreen and trying to get the vehicle warmed up. This has done nothing for your mood, although your colleague does generate a bit of cheer when he attempts to pole dance using one of the yard's lampposts.

It all goes really well until he ends the routine with an erotic lick of the metal pole and gets his tongue stuck to the metal. Once everyone on station has had a look and their photo taken, you donate the last of your (tepid) cup of tea in freeing him by carefully pouring it over his tongue.

However, out on standby, and despite the heater being on full blast, you are starting to lose the feeling in your feet. "What we need is a good fire," sighs your colleague. No sooner have the words been uttered, when the MDT flashes up your next job. It's a request from the fire service to attend a house fire … with persons reported.

As you turn into the street a few minutes later, you spot the address thanks to two fire tenders

Chapter 6 Trauma

and a sea of firefighters already on scene. Smoke is streaming out of the windows, which have all been opened. You park up and find the incident commander who confirms that there is one female inside, close to the origin of the fire. This has now been extinguished and with the smoke clearing, he deems it safe for you to enter. You walk into the property and are directed by a firefighter in breathing apparatus to the living room. Your patient is lying on a sofa, naked except for a few charred remains of her clothes. It looks like she has extensive burns from her head to her knees.

> **?** Assuming her burns are circumferential, what percentage of total body surface area (TBSA) is this?

There is no getting away from the fact that this is a serious burn. Her eyes are opaque from having been burnt, but you are more concerned about the sooting around her mouth and nose. Your colleague turns up with a carry chair and sheet. The patient is awake and trying to speak, although she is difficult to understand with her husky voice. You discover that she is 50 years old, she has difficulty breathing and she is in pain.

> **?** What are you going to do now: **Cool the burn** (read on) or **Administer oxygen** (skip the next paragraph)?

Cool the burn

You set about trying to find some way of getting water from the kitchen to the living room. After a few minutes of messing about, ice-cold water arrives in a dirty washing up bowl one of the firefighters found outside. The patient's skin feels cool to touch and you do not want that dirty water anywhere near your patient, so you elect to place the patient on high-flow oxygen, wrap her in the sheet and set off for the ambulance.

Administer oxygen

Although the patient has only been briefly cooled with water (when the firefighters extinguished the flames), the low ambient temperature, the absence of clothes and the coolness of the patient's skin leads you to suspect that she is at greater risk of hypothermia. You apply high-flow oxygen via a non-rebreathing mask and lift the patient onto the waiting carry chair.

Once on the ambulance, your colleague sets about trying to obtain some baseline observations, while you auscultate her chest. Collectively, you obtain the following:

Airway

Patent, hoarse voice, soot in mouth and nose, nasal hair singed

Breathing

Shallow, around 36 breaths/min
Widespread coarse crackles with bilaterally reduced air entry
Pulse oximeter cannot obtain a reading

Circulation

You cannot locate radial or brachial pulses due to the severe burns
Pedal pulse is palpable
Cannot obtain a blood pressure

Disability

Patient is alert but disorientated

Exposure/Environment

Full thickness burns front and back from head to knees, about 80% TBSA

> **?** What are you going to do next: **Get IV access** (read on) or **Get going** (skip the next paragraph)?

168

Get IV access

You know that administering intravenous fluids and analgesia is important, so you set about trying to find a vein. Her arms are severely burnt and your eyes keep drifting towards her fingertips, which are blackened and gnarled. This, coupled with the smoky, burnt flesh smell is proving to be a distraction. You hunt in vain for a vein in her feet before your colleague suggests using the intraosseous kit, but you can't find that either. Minutes have gone by and even the fire service are wondering why you are still on scene.

Get going

The major trauma centre (MTC) is not far away so you elect to set off. En route, you continue reassessing your patient's airway while bobbing back down to her feet in a futile attempt to find a vein. On a particularly violent right-hand turn, the intraosseous kit slides out from its hiding place and you are able to finally gain vascular access. The patient settles a little with some morphine, but you arrive at hospital having only just set up an intraosseous infusion.

Thanks to your pre-alert call, a large team has assembled, including the burns team and you leave to the sound of the consultant loudly stating that since mortality is percentage TBSA plus the patient's age, she has a 130% chance of dying.[1]

The scale of the problem

There are around 130,000 visits to an emergency department (ED) in England each year for burns and scalds.[2] In England and Wales, serious burn injury (defined as requiring at least a 72-hour stay in hospital) is responsible for 5.4% of all serious trauma.[3]

Burn injury most commonly occurs in the home (over 30%) with the kitchen being the favoured location. The most common sources of injury are:[4]

- Cup of tea in children
- Petrol ignition in adults
- Bathing, kettle spills and central heating radiators in the elderly.

Anatomy and physiology

The skin is the largest body organ, both in terms of surface area and weight. In adults, skin has a surface area of 2 m^2 and weighs 5 kg.[5] It is comprised of two main layers, the epidermis and dermis. Under the skin, is a supportive subcutaneous layer, known as the hypodermis or superficial fascia (Figure 6.1).[6]

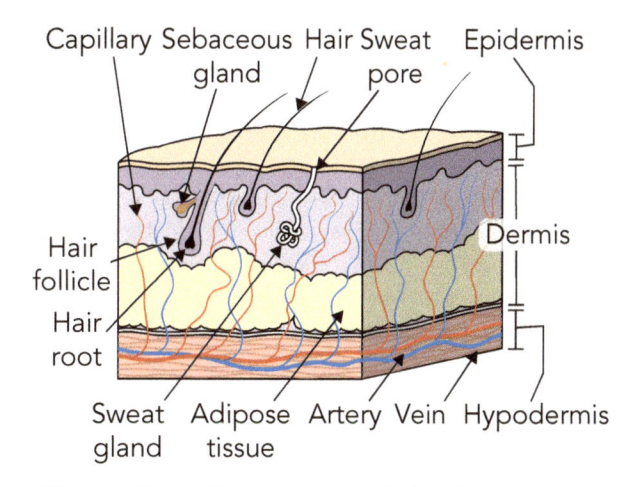

Figure 6.1 Cross-section of the skin.

Epidermis

This is the outermost layer and consists of five sublayers. Most of the cells (90%) are keratinocytes, which produce a tough, fibrous protein (keratin). This helps protect the skin and tissues from heat and microbes. Keratinocytes also produce lamellar granules which decrease water entry and loss, and prevent entry of foreign material. Around 8% of the cells are melanocytes, which produce melanin. This is taken up by keratinocytes, protecting the cell's nucleus from the harmful effects of ultraviolet (UV) light. Keratin is either a yellow-red or brown-black pigment and contributes to skin colour. The remaining cells consist of Langerhans cells, which help in the body's immune response and Merkel cells, which are involved in touch perception. It takes around 2–3 weeks for a cell, starting at the lowest layer of the epidermis, to become a keratinocyte and migrate up to the top layer (stratum corneum) and slough off.[5]

Dermis

This deeper layer of skin mostly consists of connective tissue, elastin and an extracellular matrix, which provides strength and pliability. However, it also contains blood and lymphatic vessels, nerve fibres, hair follicles and sebaceous and sweat glands. The dermis is divided into two regions, the papillary and reticular. The papillary region consists of connective tissue that anchors the epidermis and a dense network of capillaries and small blood vessels, in nipple-like projections called dermal papillae. These play an important part in temperature regulation. In addition, the dermal papillae also contain free nerve endings, which act as pain receptors, and fine touch receptors (Meissner corpuscles).[5]

The reticular region makes up 80% of the dermis and consists of dense, irregular connective tissue. Interlocking collagen fibres run in various planes, forming 'lines of cleavage'. Surgeons try to make incisions parallel to these lines, since the skin does not gape as much, resulting in less scarring.[7]

Hypodermis

Also known as the superficial fascia, this layer contains subcutaneous fat, connective tissue, sweat glands, muscle and bone. It helps to insulate the body, absorb shocks to the skeletal system and enables the skin to move easily over underlying structures.

Physiology

The skin provides a range of functions, which any damage can impair:[5,7]

- Protects by forming a physical barrier to microbes and foreign material, helping to prevent infection.
- Sensory perception of pain, pressure, heat and cold.
- Thermoregulation using nerves, blood vessels and sweat glands to control body temperature.
- Excretion of trace amounts of water and body waste, while helping to prevent dehydration.
- Maintains mineralisation of bones and teeth and synthesises vitamin D.
- Absorption of lipid-soluble substances such as fat-soluble vitamins and drugs through the skin.

Burns classification

Although crucial for subsequent burns management and decisions about surgery, the depth of a burn is hard to determine and does not affect pre-hospital treatment, although may give an indication as to cause (Table 6.1).[8]

Pathophysiology of burns

Thermal burns include flame, scalds and contact burns. Flame burns are more common in adults and are often associated with smoke inhalation and other traumatic injuries. These are more likely to result in deep dermal or full-thickness burns (Table 6.1).

Scalds are the most common cause of burn in children, usually due to spillages of hot drinks or immersion in hot bath water.[9] They generally cause epidermal or superficial dermal, burn injury.

Table 6.1 Burns classification.

Classification	Other names	Example causes	Appearance	Sensation	Healing time
Epidermal	Superficial, 1st degree	UV light	Dry and red, blanches with pressure, no blisters	May be painful	Less than 7 days
Superficial dermal	Superficial partial thickness, 2nd degree	Scald (spill or splash)	Pale pink, fine blisters, blanches with pressure	Very painful	Less than 14 days
Mid-dermal	Superficial partial thickness, 2nd degree	Scald (spill), flame	Dark pink with large blisters, delayed capillary refill	May be painful	14–21 days
Deep dermal	Deep partial thickness, 2nd degree	Scald (spill), flame	Blotchy red, may blister, no capillary refill Children: dark lobster red with mottling	No sensation	Over 21 days
Full thickness	3rd degree	Scald (immersion), flame, steam, high-volt electricity	White, waxy or charred. No blisters or capillary refill Children: dark lobster red with mottling	No sensation	Does not heal without grafting

Source: New Zealand Guidelines Group, 2007.

Direct contact burns are caused by brief contact with a very hot object, or (more commonly), prolonged contact with a cooler object. Typical patient groups include epileptics and those who misuse alcohol or drugs.

Irreversible damage to the epidermis can be caused by exposure to 44°C heat for six hours, or 65°C for one second.[10] Burns injuries are characterised by a local response and, if the total body surface area (TBSA) burned is greater than 20%, a systemic response.[9]

Local response

At skin level, burns form three zones of injury:[11]

- Zone of coagulation: the point of maximal injury, with irreversible damage to tissue due to protein coagulation.
- Zone of stasis: surrounding the zone of coagulation and characterised by reduced tissue perfusion. Potentially salvageable with adequate resuscitation.
- Zone of hyperaemia: surrounds the zone of stasis and is characterised by increased tissue perfusion. Usually recovers.

Chapter 6   Trauma

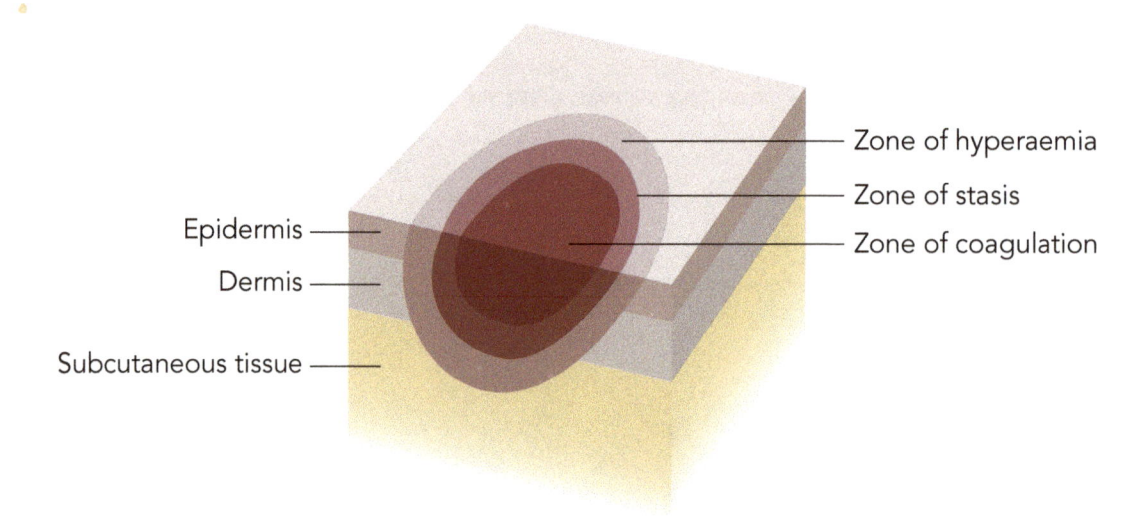

Figure 6.2   Zone of burn injury.

The zones spread out from the point of injury in three dimensions, including deeper into dermal tissue (Figure 6.2).

Systemic response

The level of inflammatory response is related to the %TBSA that is burned. Once the burn covers more than 20% TBSA, the inflammatory response can exert systemic effects.[11] Capillary permeability increases, leading to loss of intravascular proteins and fluid into interstitial space. Peripheral and splanchnic vasoconstriction occur and myocardial contractility decreases. Combined with fluid loss from the burn, this results in hypotension and end-organ hypoperfusion. In the lungs, there can be bronchoconstriction and the development of acute respiratory distress syndrome in any severe burns. Initially, there is a reduction in metabolic rate ('ebb phase'), but this can double in the days following burn injury ('flow phase').[12]

Acute smoke inhalation injury

Smoke inhalation is a killer. Around 60% of fire-related fatalities are attributed to smoke inhalation and it has a greater contribution to overall mortality and morbidity of burn injuries than either %TBSA or age.[13]

Naso-oropharygeal and mucosal burns are common,[14] but thermal injury below the vocal cords is rare since heat is effectively exchanged in upper airway passages.[15] When air, steam and/or smoke are at sufficiently high temperatures to cause thermal injury to the lower airways, rapid oedema of the glottis develops resulting in fatal airway obstruction.

Systemic toxins are the products of incomplete combustion and include carbon monoxide (CO) and hydrogen cyanide. CO is an odourless, colourless gas that binds to haemoglobin with 250 times the affinity of oxygen. This results in a shift of the oxygen-dissociation curve to the left, decreasing the oxygen carrying capacity of the blood. Cyanide adversely affects internal respiration by preventing aerobic production of adenosine triphosphate (ATP).[14]

Particulates and irritants have the greatest effect on the pathophysiological processes that occur due to smoke inhalation. Soot impregnated with toxins can reach the alveoli suspended in air. The types of chemicals vary, depending on what has been burning, but they trigger a cascade of events, resulting in pulmonary oedema and ventilation/perfusion (V/Q) mismatch.[16] Water-soluble gases such as ammonia and hydrogen chloride react with the mucous membranes, producing strong alkalis and acids leading to intense and prolonged inflammatory reactions. Lipid-soluble irritants act more slowly as they dissolve into cellular membranes.

History

Identify the mechanism, including the cause of the burn, how it came into contact with the patient and any first aid undertaken. Note when the injury occurred, how long the patient was exposed to the source and the duration of any cooling. Don't forget to be alert for signs of non-accidental injury.

Assessment

Pre-hospital estimation of TBSA of burn injury is poor, with the 'rule of nines' (Figure 6.3) underestimating burns of less than 20%, overestimating burns over 40% and is not accurate in children under 14 years of age.[11,17]

The whole hand (palm and adducted fingers) represents about 0.82% TBSA in adults and 0.77% in children, making accurate calculations tricky. However, the palm alone is 0.5% TBSA[18] and is suitable for burns less than 15% or greater than 85% TBSA. Note that these methods will generally underestimate %TBSA in obese patients.[19]

Lund and Browder charts are more accurate, but these are cumbersome to complete in the back of an ambulance. However, it is only necessary to determine an approximate value for TBSA to determine the need for direct admission to a MTC and/or intravenous fluids.[17] Remember that erythema (reddening) should not be included when calculating

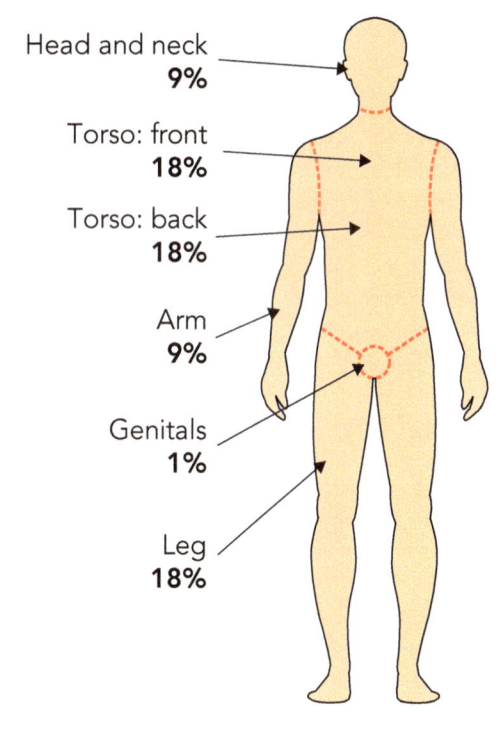

Head and neck **9%**
Torso: front **18%**
Torso: back **18%**
Arm **9%**
Genitals **1%**
Leg **18%**

Figure 6.3 Rule of nines.

TBSA of burn injury but consideration of obesity and large breast should factor in your estimation.[17,20]

Management

Safety

Don't get burnt yourself. Let the nice people in fire retardant clothing bring your patient to you.

Stopping the burning process

The patient needs to be removed from the source of the burn if it is safe to do so. Clothing should be removed unless it is sticking to the patient as should jewellery, which may become constrictive as tissues swell.

Cooling

Burns should be cooled for 20 minutes preferably with running water (between 8 and 15°C).[17,21] There is little evidence that ice causes damage to underlying tissues, but runs the risk of making the patient hypothermic so is not recommended.[22,23] Cooling should commence immediately after the burn has occurred, but there is limited evidence to suggest cooling up to three hours after the burn has occurred is still beneficial.[21] If running water is not available or practicable, then gel-based body blankets can be used without causing hypothermia.[21]

Covering/dressing

Patients with burns lose heat from non-epithelialised areas of skin due to evaporation. With the thermoregulatory function of the skin disrupted, patients are at risk of hypothermia, even on a warm day. Hypothermia is part of the lethal triad in trauma and for each 1°C reduction in body temperature, the mortality rates increases significantly,[24] and there is weak evidence that patients admitted to hospital with burns who are hypothermic, have an increased mortality.[25] Once cooling has been completed, cover the burn with a clean sheet or Clingfilm, but take care not to apply it circumferentially as it can become constrictive as oedema develops.[17]

Assessment of <C>ABC

Follow the <C>ABC approach for burns as you would any traumatic injury. However, inhalation injury is a particular concern and occurs in around 22% of all burns, 60% if facial burns are present.[14] Signs of inhalation injury include:[11]

- Full thickness or deep dermal burns to face, neck or upper torso
- Singed nasal hair
- Soot in sputum or oropharynx
- Dyspnoea, hoarseness, cough or stridor
- Cyanosis
- Altered level of consciousness.

Administer high-flow oxygen and consider beta$_2$ agonist for bronchospasm. Consider early the need for tracheal intubation if the airway is at risk.[21] High-flow oxygen is beneficial in carbon monoxide (CO) poisoning and can reduce the half-life of carboxyhaemoglobin considerably. Cyanide poisoning can be treated with hydroxocabalimin (vitamin B$_{12}$), which actively binds to cyanide allowing it to be excreted in the urine, although this is not routinely used by UK ambulance services.[21]

Fluids

Fluid loss in burns is not due to open burn wounds, but intravascular fluid loss via capillary leakage into the interstitial tissues.[18] Any signs of shock in the first hour after injury likely due to another cause. Burns with a TBSA of >10% in children or 15% in adults may require fluid depending on TBSA and journey time to the hospital.[17]

Analgesia

Cooling and covering burns can provide temporary pain relief but this should be supplemented with intravenous analgesia as soon as practicable.

Transport

Patients should be transported to the most appropriate hospital. Follow local guidance, particularly if you have a regional burns unit nearby.

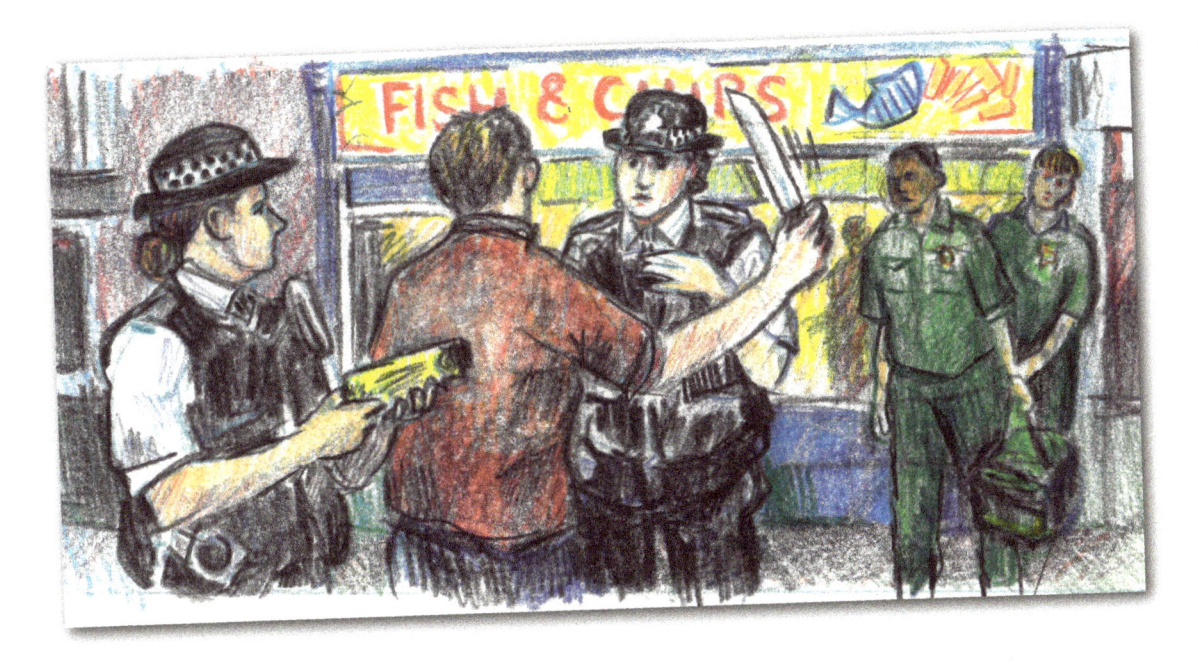

Conducted Electrical Devices

You are on standby and it's hot. The sun is setting, but the concrete and tarmac are still radiating warmth, which is rather pleasant until you have to leave the air-conditioned cab and carry someone down a flight of stairs. However, sweaty armpits are not your main concern – it's the number of people in beer gardens. Everywhere you have been so far, you can count the people without a drink in their hand in single figures. The significance of this statistic is not lost on your colleague either. "It's going to be a busy night," he murmurs. "Lots of people fighting, mark my words." No sooner have the words left his lips than the MDT is bleeping into life with details of a man in his 30s brandishing a knife outside a fish and chip shop. Your colleague immediately contacts the emergency operations centre (EOC) to determine whether the police are on scene. The response is that the call has come from police and they are 'on their way'. "In that case, we'll be standing off until they arrive on scene," replies your colleague.

As you approach the scene and contemplate where you are going to park up without getting accosted by inebriated members of the public, you see two police cars speeding towards the location of the fish and chip shop. One officer waves at you as they pass, but the second slows and winds down their window. "Going to 'A Salt N Battered' for a chap with a knife?" the officer asks. "Just waiting for you to arrive," your colleague replies. The officer smiles, before saying, "We're here!" and drives off to support their colleague. You set off in pursuit of the police

Chapter 6   Trauma

vehicle, although it has already disappeared around the corner. You arrive on scene a minute later to find the two police officers already on scene and out of the vehicles. The officer who stopped to speak to you has circled around to the back of the assailant and drawn her Taser. Her colleague is facing the man holding the knife and clearly trying to engage in conversation with him. You park up on the other side of the road, open the side door of the ambulance and glove up before grabbing the response bag.

Despite the efforts of the officer facing the assailant, he continues to get agitated. Then, a number of things happen in quick succession. You have one of those moments where everything seems to happen in slow motion, as you can already picture the sequence of events that is about to unfold. The assailant raises the knife and takes a step towards the officer facing him, just as a member of the gathering crowd shouts to the man warning him that there is a copper behind him with a Taser. The man makes to turn around to spot the new threat, but he is too slow. The police officer with the Taser discharges the weapon. You see a blur of metal wires leaving the cartridge on the front of the Taser, followed almost immediately with a scream from the assailant as the officer who has fired the Taser yells the word "Taser" several times. The man goes rigid … and falls flat on his face. The officers run forward and subdue the man and within 30 seconds he is handcuffed. The officer with the Taser looks at you and asks if you can remove the barbs.

> What are you going to do: **Suggest removal at hospital** (read on) or **Remove the barbs** (skip the next paragraph)?

Suggest removal at hospital

You aren't too keen on pulling the barbs out of the man's back, so you sheepishly suggest taking the patient to hospital. The officer gives you a 'you're kidding, right?' look before asking if you have a pair of gloves handy. You give her a pair from your pocket and she promptly removes the cartridge from the end of the Taser, gathers up the wire and pulls out the barbs, inserting them barb first into the cartridge. A police van arrives just as the officers are assisting the man to his feet, and within 5 minutes he is packed into the van and on his way to the local police station.

Remove the barbs

You ask whether the barbs need to be kept for evidential purposes and the officer shakes her head. "Have you got one of those yellow bins?" she asks. You nod and your colleague opens the response bag to retrieve it. The officer removes the cartridge from the Taser and shows it to you. "No shocks, I promise," she says, winking. You explain to the patient what you are intending to do and he grunts in response. You stretch the skin slightly around the barb before pulling sharply and firmly on it. It doesn't come out as easily as you expect, so you pull more firmly on the second. A quick wipe with an alcohol wipe and, two plasters later, your work is done. You manage to get a set of clinical observations, which don't suggest anything alarming, before the police van is on scene and the patient is bundled off to the local police station.

Scale of the problem

The Taser is a conducted electrical device (CED, although sometimes referred to as a conducted electrical weapon, CEW), a hand-held, single-shot device designed to temporarily incapacitate a person by causing a temporary, but painful, muscle contraction. In the UK, the Taser X26 has been approved for use by trained police officers (Figure 6.4).[26] Taser is actually an acronym for Thomas A. Swift Electronic Rifle, which was coined by

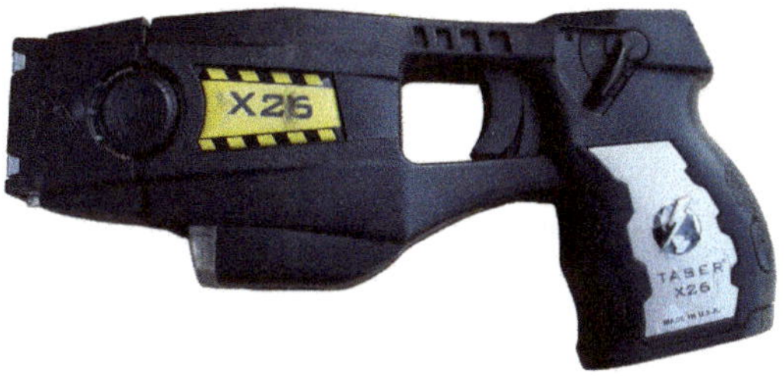

Conducted Electrical Devices

Figure 6.4 Taser X26.
Source: Junglecat (Own work) [CC BY-SA 3.0 or GFDL], via Wikimedia Commons.

its inventor, Jack Cover, and named after his favourite childhood book character.[27]

UK police officers 'use' a Taser about 32,000 times a year. However, it is important to understand that 'use' covers a number of actions and the vast majority of 'uses' do not involve discharge of a Taser (Table 6.2).[28]

Taser: mechanism of action

When a Taser is fired, two barbed darts are propelled from the replaceable cartridge by the release of compressed nitrogen.[29] The maximum range of the device is 6.4 m, although the distance at which the barbs will attach themselves to a person is likely to be much less.[26] Even if the dart does not penetrate the skin (for example, if it only attaches to the patient's clothing), the electrical impulse can still be transmitted. A standard discharge is a 5-second burst producing an initial arcing voltage of 50,000 V, although the voltage received by the subject is around 1,200 V, with a current of 2.1 mA.[27]

Firing the Taser or using the angled drive stun technique can result in incapacitation of the subject.

Table 6.2 Taser types of use definitions.

Level of use	Type of use	Definition
Highest level	Fired	The Taser is fired with a live cartridge installed. When the trigger is pulled, the probes are fired towards the subject with the intention of completing an electrical circuit and delivering an incapacitating effect.
	Angled drive stun	The officer fires the weapon with a live cartridge installed. One or both probes may attach to the subject. The officer then holds the Taser against the subject's body in a different area to the probe(s), in order to complete the electrical circuit and deliver an incapacitating effect.
	Drive stun	The Taser is held against the subject's body and the trigger is pulled with no probes being fired. Contact with the subject completes the electrical circuit which causes pain but does not deliver an incapacitating effect.
Non-discharges	Red dot	The weapon is not fired. Instead, the Taser is deliberately aimed and then partially activated so that a laser red dot is placed onto the subject.
	Arcing	Sparking of the Taser without aiming it or firing it (Figure 6.5).
	Aimed	Deliberate aiming of the Taser at a targeted subject.
Lowest level	Drawn	Drawing of the Taser in circumstances where any person could reasonably perceive the action to be a use of force.

Adapted from: UK Government, 2020.

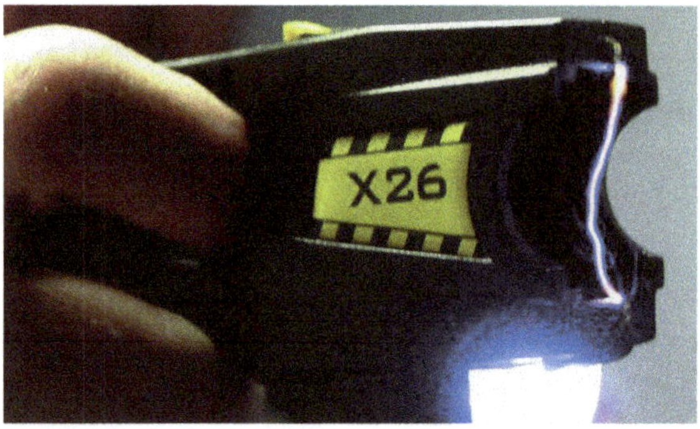

Chapter 6 Trauma

Figure 6.5 A Taser being 'arced'. Note that there is no cartridge installed on the device. *Source*: jasonesbain (Taser) [CC BY 2.0], via Wikimedia Commons.

Although the mechanism is not completely understood, the delivery by the device of approximately 100 microcoulombs of electrical charge over 100 microseconds at a rate of about 20 pulses per second inhibits alpha-motor neurons.[30]

Alpha-motor neurons are important as they innervate the majority of your skeletal muscle fibres (called extrafusal muscle fibres). The nuclei of these nerves are located in the anterior grey horn of the spinal cord and the brain stem (which only innervate the muscles located on the head). Their response to muscle spindle-mediated proprioception helps maintain muscle tone and keep you upright. The Taser interrupts this process by causing uncontrollable skeletal muscle contraction while being discharged. Since voluntary movement is inhibited, as well as the ability to respond to proprioceptive messages from muscle spindles, subjects tend to fall over if they are standing.[5] However, this process ceases as soon as the electrical discharge stops, which is why you tend to see officers acting swiftly to subdue a subject once the Taser has been fired.[31]

Myocardial capture

Myocardial capture (that is, obtaining an electrical response from the heart's conducting system) has been demonstrated in a swine model when Taser barbs straddle the heart, even during a 5 second burst. However, ventricular fibrillation/tachycardia (VF/VT) could not be induced unless prolonged shocks (10–40 seconds) were applied, and even then, this was not consistent.[32]

Electrical current and its effect on the heart rhythm are well studied and form the basis of cardiac pacing and defibrillation. Cardiovascular implanted electronic devices (CIEDs) are known to be vulnerable to electromagnetic interference (EMI).[33] The most common complication of EMI is oversensing, leading to bradycardia mode inhibition or the pacemaker reverting to noise-aversion pacing (that is, it reverts to asynchronous pacing, providing a constant pacing rate irrespective of underlying electrical heart activity).[34] However, determining whether CEDs present a risk to patients with CIEDs is difficult to determine due to a lack of evidence.

Ironically, although a theoretical model of the human heart has shown risk of VF/VT in the event that Taser barbs strike a subject and straddle their heart,[35] it appears that unless the subject has a CIED fitted, myocardial capture does not occur. However, given that the average age of a subject Tasered is 30 years of age (±10 years) and the average age of a patient having a CIED fitted is 75 years (±11 years), this is not a common scenario.[33] However, despite this, the Defence Scientific Advisory Council Sub-Committee on the Medical Implications of Less-Lethal Weapons (DOMILL) has recommended that officers avoid the frontal chest overlying the heart (where tactically possible).[36]

One final concern relates to patients who have an internal cardio-defibrillator (ICD) and the risk of the device shocking its owner inappropriately following exposure to a Taser discharge. This is possible, although with discharges of 5 seconds, ICDs will not have time to charge the capacitor before the Taser-induced electrical interference comes to an end.[37] However, prolonged discharge can lead to inappropriate defibrillation (at least in the animal model).[27]

Pathophysiology

Serious injury and death from CED exposure is rare, with most injuries occurring secondary to a fall or fume ignition.[38] Table 6.3 lists a number of reported injuries following CED exposure.[27] The main concern relates to whether the deaths that have occurred following CED exposure are due to the device itself, although there is no evidence to suggest that this is the case, with the exception, arguably of fume ignition.[38] However, it is apparent that the groups of subjects most at risk of adverse outcomes following exposure to a CED are those most likely to be 'Tasered'.[39]

Table 6.3 Reported injuries following CED exposure.

Barb injuries	Injuries from falls
Superficial puncture wounds	Contusions, abrasions
Osseous penetration of fingers and the skull	Lacerations, haematomas
Intracerebral perforation	Fractures
Ophthalmological injuries	Intracranial bleeding
Pharyngeal perforation	Facial fractures
Pneumothorax	Chipped tooth
Testicular torsion	Miscarriage
Electrical injuries	Ingestion of the barb
Vertebral compression fractures	
Burns	

Adapted from: Pasquier et al., 2011.

A review by DOMILL identified the following medical implications of Taser use:[40]

- The physiological burden as a result of Taser-induced muscle contraction and pain, accompanied with the likely stress of the situation, could adversely affect subjects who are elderly, who have pre-existing medical conditions, such as heart disease or asthma
- Although a Taser discharge has not been shown to cause uterine contraction, falls during pregnancy lead to higher probability of Caesarean section and lower birth weight
- Certain subject groups are at increased risk of injury during a fall, such as those with osteoporosis or clotting disorders and patients taking anti-coagulants
- A Taser discharge probably does not induce epileptic convulsions. It is more likely that emotional stress and physical exertion are the culprits
- There is potential for a Taser to be used because of behaviour that has been induced by an underlying medical or mental health condition, such as epilepsy (post-ictal), diabetes (hypoglycaemia) and learning difficulties, or because of communication problems due to language barriers and/or hearing/visual impairments
- Although CIEDs are unlikely to be damaged by a Taser (they have to be able to resist the much higher energy of defibrillation), the effect on vagal nerve stimulators and cochlear implants is unknown.

Management

Incidents involving a Taser require you to be situationally aware and to carry out a dynamic risk assessment as you do not want to get hit by a Taser barb or get in between the police and the assailant.

Ensure you are well out of the way and only come forward when invited to by officers. The only exception to this might be when they are managing a person with acute behavioural disturbance (ABD) and you suspect that the airway has been compromised.

Most people who have been incapacitated with a Taser will not require a trip to the emergency department (ED). However, they still need a prompt medical assessment to determine the presence of:[17]

- Neck and back injuries
- Secondary injuries, for example, that occur as a result of falling
- Cardiac symptoms such as chest pain and arrhythmias
- ABD
- Taser barbs embedded in the skin.

If you are asked to remove the Taser barbs, ensure that they are detached from the Taser first. Either ask the officer to remove the cartridge from the Taser or cut the wires with a pair of scissors. Before removing the barbs, ask the officer whether they wish to keep the barbs for evidential purposes. If so, ensure there is an appropriate receptacle for them to be placed in, as they are essentially a biohazardous sharp. Alternatively, ensure they are placed in a sharps bin.

To remove a Taser barb:[17]

1. Stretch the skin around the barb
2. Pull sharply and firmly to remove the barb
3. Clean the area with an alcohol/antiseptic wipe
4. Cover the site with a dressing
5. Enquire about tetanus status and advise tetanus booster within 72 hours, if appropriate.

NOTE: You should not remove barbs that are attached to:

- Skin where blood vessels are close to the skin surface, for example, neck and groin
- One or both eyes
- The face
- The genitalia
- The mouth, or have been swallowed
- The scalp
- Joints, for example, finger.

Also, broken barbs should be left in situ. In all of these cases, cut the wire close to the barb, leaving approximately 4 cm of wire, and transfer to the local ED. Patients fitted with CIEDs, vagal nerve stimulators and other implanted devices need transfer to the ED, as do patients with evidence of ABD. In addition, patients with pre-existing medical conditions, that you deem to be at increased risk of harm following a Taser incapacitation, should be transferred.[26] Ensure you record a 12-lead ECG on any patient complaining of chest pain, or who has cardiac symptoms, a significant cardiac history or CIEDs.[17]

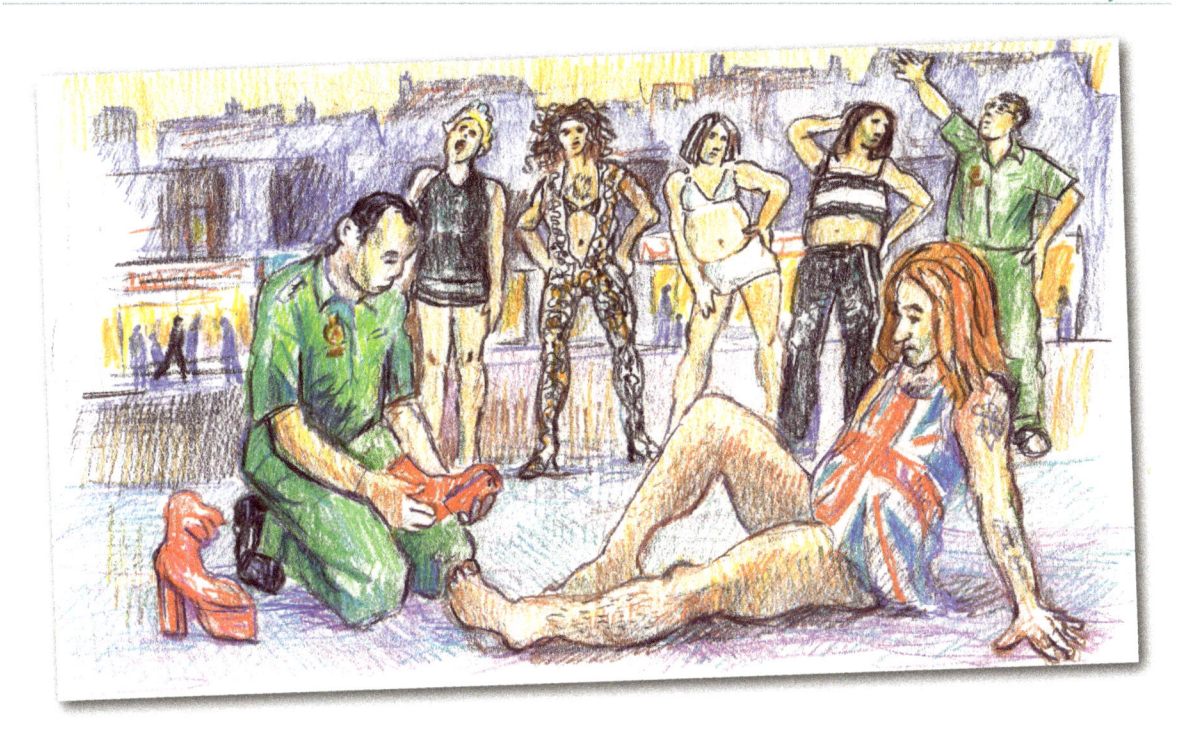

Ankle Injuries

You are on standby in town as dusk settles on another Saturday afternoon, with your colleague and a student who is on their first placement. As you reflect on the shift, you are quietly impressed with the student's composure thus far. They have seen their first death and handled the condolences with dignity and respect, managed an impressive sleight of hand to avoid eating a chocolate proffered by a confused woman with suspicious looking dark matter under her fingernails, and is now buried in an article about ankles and a city in Canada. You mull the last one over and are just about to enquire about it when you spot your next patient.

A gaggle of women are tottering your way. The flame-haired beauty in the middle of them is wearing a Union Jack dress and holding her shoes, one of which is missing a heel. "Blimey, it's the Spice Girls!" exclaims your colleague and, as you take stock of the five women, it does indeed appear that they are wearing appropriate attire for the group. "Your next patient is Ginger Spice," you call back to the student, "open up the back doors and drop the step will you?"

To avoid getting another job, your colleague contacts the emergency operations centre (EOC) to pass you a running call and you both exit the cab to greet the patient.

As you approach, the patient gives you a queasy smile and says "Hello boys!" in a very deep voice. You invite the patient to hop up into the ambulance and take a seat on the trolley. You introduce yourself and ask them their name. "Rob," he replies, "except at weekends when I'm Mandy." "Mandy it is

Chapter 6 Trauma

then," you reply, although explain that for the purposes of your paperwork, you will need to use his real name. The patient nods in agreement while you absent-mindedly lift up the jaw of your student, which has almost hit the floor at the situation unfolding in front of them.

With your student temporarily incapacitated, you decide to obtain a history. The patient explains that he has been out with his friends in his new 6" high heels, when he caught his left heel in a broken paving slab, breaking it off the shoe and inverting his ankle. He was helped to his feet and has managed to weight bear, but states that his ankle throbs and you can see swelling over his lateral malleolus.

Your student seems to have recovered as they are now fidgeting in their seat as if wanting to say something.

> What should you do now: **Apply a box splint and go to the ED** (read on) or **Listen to your student** (skip the next paragraph)?

Apply a box splint and go to the ED

Although he has a distal pulse and sensation, there could be a fracture lurking under that swelling and, ignoring your student, you decide to play it safe. You apply a box splint to the patient, although he grumbles at the pressure being applied to his lateral malleolus. Still, some Entonox soon puts a stop to that, although his maniacal laughter at the sound of his voice after inhaling the gas is rather unnerving.

You trundle across town to the ED, which is busy with patients and crews waiting to hand over. After a long wait for triage, the nurse examines his ankle, removes the box splint and asks the patient to take some steps. He does so, and is able to weight bear, although it looks painful. She directs him to the waiting room and turns her attention to the next crew, leaving you to slope off back to the ambulance with your trolley, the box splint and Entonox wondering what went wrong. Your student subsequently writes a critical reflection on the incident (using a published model of reflection no doubt) entitled 'The mentor who would not listen'.

Listen to your student

Your student has adopted an uncanny resemblance to a young child desperate for a wee, but you correctly interpret this as a desire to become involved and so invite them to speak up. "We could use the Ottawa ankle rules," they blurt out, passing you the article they were reading. You nod your assent, and they review the history, confirming that the patient could walk immediately after the incident, and examine the patient's foot and ankle for bony tenderness in a number of locations.

At the end of the examination, they triumphantly exclaim that the patient does not have any bony tenderness and thinks their ankle is not likely to be broken. If this is true, it opens up the possibility of using the local walk-in centre, which can see minor injuries, although you know from past experience that they don't like broken limbs.

> What should you do now: **Apply a box splint and go to the ED** (go back five paragraphs) or **Visit the local walk-in centre** (read on)?

Visit the local walk-in centre

You explain to the patient about the possibility of going to the walk-in centre instead of travelling across town to the ED, which pleases them no end since they

Ankle Injuries

live nearby. You call ahead and are given the usual grilling from a staff member who enquires about potential social problems and asks whether you think it is broken. "No," you reply "he's been assessed using the Ottawa ankle rules and everything checks out fine." There is a pause on the line while the nurse processes what you have just said, giving you time to wink at your student. It seems there is no room to wriggle out of accepting the patient now you have played your 'Ottawa ankle rule' trump card, and they ask when you will be arriving.

On arrival at the walk-in centre, you ask the patient to weight bear and walk out of the ambulance, which he manages, although it is painful. Still, your colleague finds a wheelchair near the entrance and the patient drops gratefully into it. You book him in and park him up next to the most prudish-looking couple you can find. You walk out of the centre with Mandy blowing you kisses and telling anyone who will listen what a fantastic ambulance crew you are.

The scale of the problem

It is not possible to say exactly how many ankle sprains occur each year in the UK, or indeed accurately determine how many attend an emergency department (ED). However, the best guesstimate for the general population visiting the ED with an ankle sprain is 302,000 new cases per year, with around 42,000 of those considered severe (defined as being unable to weight bear on arrival in the department, with lateral ankle tenderness but no fracture on X-ray).[41]

Patients who sustain a sprain tend to be younger and male, until the age of 35 years of age, when women sprain their ankle more often. Common causes include tripping, sports injury and walking.[42]

Anatomy and physiology

The foot is a mobile structure and functions to support bodyweight and transmit power for walking, running etc. It is shaped like an arch, with the heel and metatarsal heads making contact with the ground.[43] This helps to absorb and distribute downward forces from the body when standing and moving across various terrain.[44] There are 26 bones in the foot (28 if you count the two sesamoid bones on the dorsal surface of the 1st metatarsal) and they are shown in Figure 6.6.

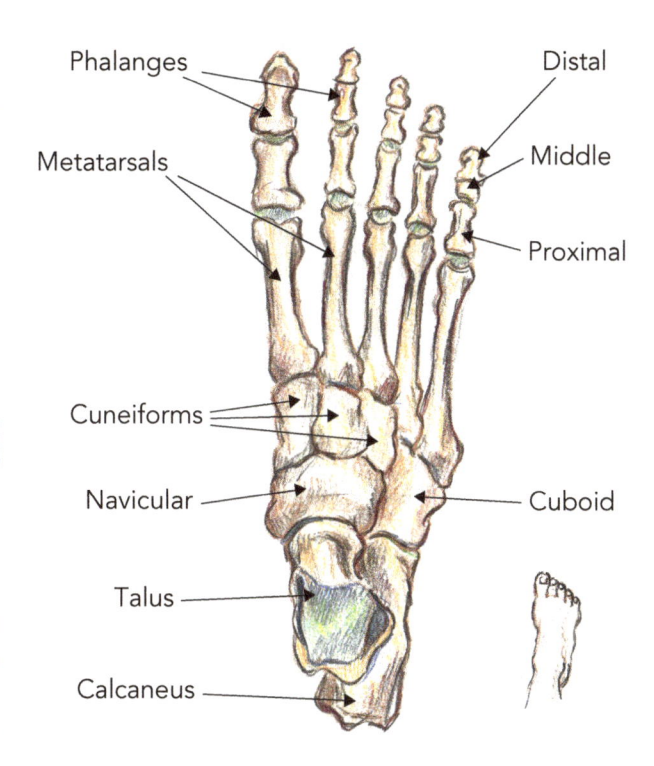

Figure 6.6 The bones of the foot.

The ankle is a synovial joint consisting of the talus in the foot and the tibia and fibula of the leg. It is mostly a hinge-joint, allowing for dorsi- and plantarflexion, although some inversion and eversion of

Chapter 6 Trauma

the foot is possible when the ankle joint is plantarflexed (Figure 6.7).[45]

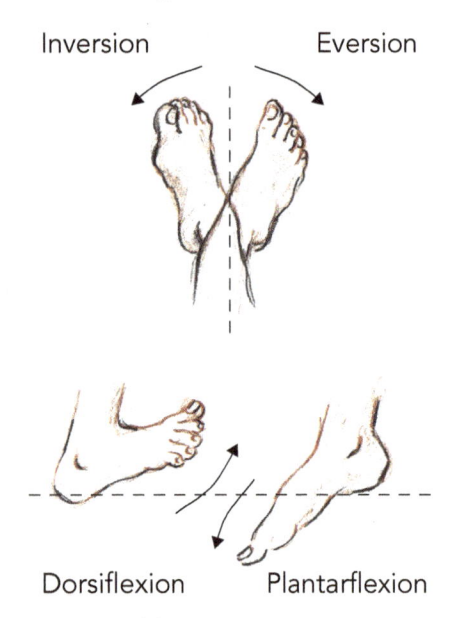

Figure 6.7 Ankle joint movements.

The stability of the ankle joint is maintained in part by a three-sided mortise consisting of the medial and lateral malleoli and the tibial plafond (the underside of the distal tibia, which articulates with the talus).[46] In addition, muscle power and a number of ligaments all contribute to ankle stability (Figure 6.8 and 6.9).

The ankle ligaments are organised into three complexes (a complex is a collection of three or more ligaments that are related in function):[46]

- **Syndesmotic ligamentous complex**
  Anterior and posterior tibiofibular, transverse tibiofibular and interosseous ligaments. Located between the distal tibia and fibula and resists forces that might affect the structural integrity of the mortise.
- **Deltoid (or medial) ligamentous complex**
  Tibionavicular, tibiocalcaneal and superficial and deep tibiotalar ligaments. Provides medial stability of the talus and prevents lateral displacement.
- **Lateral ligamentous complex**
  This consists of the anterior and posterior talofibular and calcaneofibular ligaments and provides lateral support, although is not as strong as the deltoid complex.

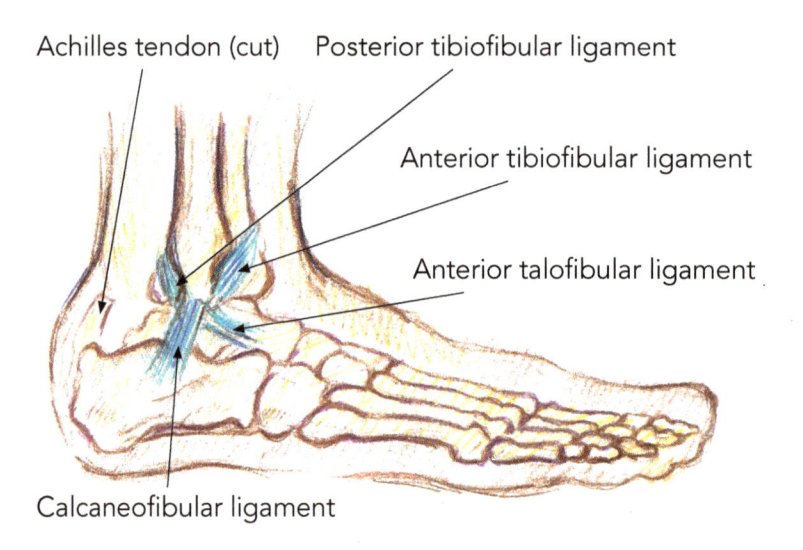

Figure 6.8 Lateral view of the ankle joint.

Ankle Injuries

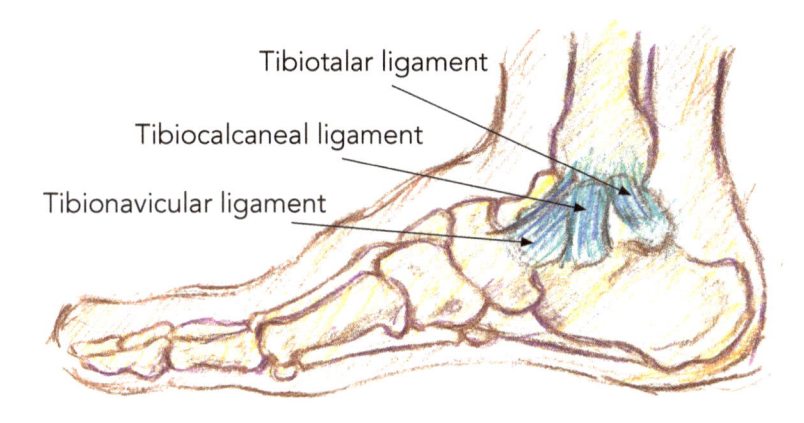

Figure 6.9 Medial view of the ankle joint.

Pathophysiology

The most common ankle injury is a partial tear of the anterior talofibular ligament due to ankle inversion with plantarflexion.[47] The medial ligaments are less commonly injured, but tend to lead to prolonged disability if they are.[43] High ankle (syndesmotic) sprains are caused by dorsiflexion and eversion of the ankle with internal rotation of the tibia. This can lead to anterior and posterior tibiofibular ligamentous injury

Sprains are graded on a scale of 1–3 based on severity:[48]

- **Grade 1** – Few fibres of part of the ligament are torn.
- **Grade 2** – Complete rupture of part of the ligament complex (most commonly rupture of the anterior talofibular ligament of the lateral ligamentous complex).
- **Grade 3** – Complete disruption of the ligament complex with associated instability.

History

The classic presentation is the patient 'going over on' or 'twisting', their ankle. These vague terms encompass everything from a mild, self-limiting grade 1 sprain, to a significant ligamentous complex rupture with associated fracture. It is vital therefore that you determine the exact mechanism of injury. A good way to do this is to produce a mental image of the direction, magnitude and duration of the force that was applied to the ankle. It can be useful for the patient to show you the position of the ankle at the time of injury (although do get them to use the uninjured ankle to do this!).[43] Check whether the patient could weight bear immediately after injury occurred and be alert for any repeated 'giving way' of the joint and past injuries, which could indicate a weakened joint.

Examination

Assuming there is no obvious deformity, you can move onto examination of the injury. It is important to conduct a systematic examination, so you don't miss any important signs. A common approach consists of examining the joint above, looking, feeling and moving the joint before checking function and nerves and vessels:[48]

Joint above

Expose both legs above the knee joint and palpate around the knee to ensure that this has not been injured. This is important as it helps establish a rapport (since this should not be painful), but forces are often transmitted up the limb and it will ensure you do not miss an injured knee or proximal humeral head fracture.

Look

Compare limbs and look for ecchymosis (bruising) and swelling, which will be present with a ligamentous injury or fracture.

Feel

Starting just distal to knee, palpate the fibular head and then work your way down the tibia and around to the medial malleolus and ligament. Check the Achilles tendon to ensure it is still intact, by asking the patient to kneel on a chair and squeezing their calf. The foot should plantarflex if the tendon is intact (Simmons test). Also note any bilateral swelling between the tendon and the malleoli as this indicates the presence of an effusion within the ankle joint. Next, examine the foot, paying particular attention to the tarsometatarsal joints and the base of the 5th metatarsal, which is vulnerable to avulsion fractures. Finally, examine the lateral malleolus and ligaments.

Move

Active (the patient moves the joint) and passive (you do the manipulating) movements often reveal a classic limitation in plantar flexion and virtually absent dorsiflexion. Resisted movements usually demonstrate normal power, although resisted eversion can be painful in calf muscle tears and avulsion fractures of the base of the 5th metatarsal. Stress testing of the joint is tricky just after injury and requires adequate analgesia, but the anterior draw test is helpful to confirm a complete rupture of the anterior talofibular ligament.[47] You do this by asking the patient to support their lower leg at the thigh and then you push backwards with one hand on the tibia while the other pulls forward on the heel.

Function

If the patient can manage it, observe them walking and, in the case of chronic ankle problems, you can have lots of fun making them stand on one leg (to check proprioception and muscle balance, not for enjoyment). If they can do this, get them to try it with their eyes closed, although do hold onto them as if they fall over and damage something else, it won't look good.

Nerves and vessels

Don't forget to check for equal sensation and distal pulses (usually the dorsalis pedis).

Ottawa ankle rules

In addition to ligamentous injury, you will need to identify underlying fractures, if present. The most reliable way of doing this is to utilise the Ottawa ankle and foot rules (Figure 6.10). These rules were originally conceived to prevent unnecessary X-rays of ankles and feet,[49] but have now been validated in a wide range of settings and are very good at excluding fractures in adults of all ages and in children over 5 years of age.[50,51]

Management

Assuming you do not suspect a fracture or a grade 3 sprain (identified by an unstable ankle joint and inability to weight bear), and there is no history of repeated 'giving way' of the joint, you will need to consider whether the patient will manage at home with their injury. This is particularly important for the elderly and determining their social situation should be part of the history.[52]

Initial management of ankle sprains is based on the mnemonic PRICE: protect, rest, ice, compression and elevation, and avoiding HARM: heat, alcohol, running, massage. There is no consistent advice on management, but a common regimen might consist of:[53,54]

Ankle Injuries

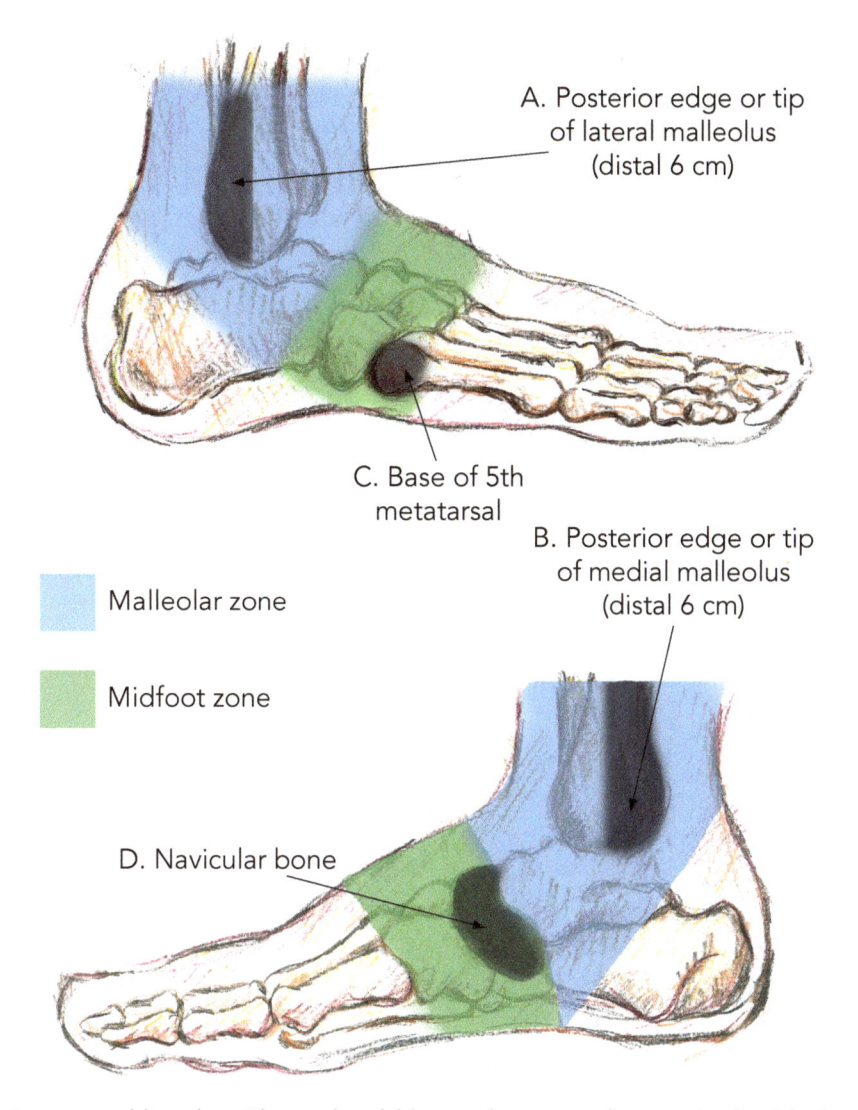

Figure 6.10 Ottawa ankle rules. There should be no bony tenderness in the black zones.

A. Posterior edge or tip of lateral malleolus (distal 6 cm)
B. Posterior edge or tip of medial malleolus (distal 6 cm)
C. Base of 5th metatarsal
D. Navicular bone

Malleolar zone
Midfoot zone

First 48–72 hours:

- Protect from further injury
- Rest injured ankle
- Apply an ice pack for up to 10–30 minutes every 2 to 3 hours
- Use an elasticated bandage to compress the joint. Discontinue after 48 hours or if distal tissue become cyanosed or painful
- Elevate the limb above heart level
- Pain can be managed with paracetamol or other non-steroidal anti-imflammatory drugs.

After 72 hours:

- Heat – This should be avoided in the first 72 hours, as it exacerbates inflammation. However, after this time, it can be soothing
- Alcohol – Can increase bleeding and swelling
- Running – Increases the risk of further injury
- Massage – As with heat, after 72 hours this may be symptomatically beneficial.

Chapter 6   Trauma

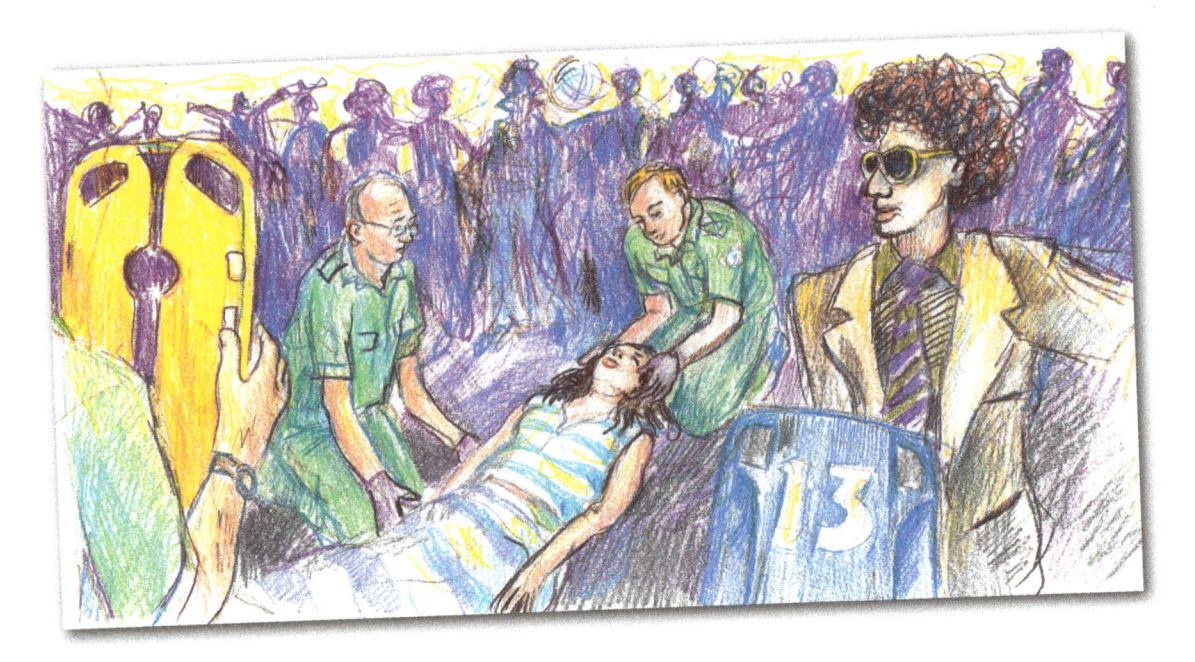

Pelvic Trauma

You are sat on standby with the oldest member of the ambulance service. Rumours are rife that he is over 70 years of age, but this is clearly an exaggeration, probably. Having never worked with him before, your colleagues have been embellishing his reputation for the past week, ever since the orders listing your pairing, were published. "Don't get him started on the 101 uses for blankets," you are warned by one colleague. "If you ask for oxygen to be administered, don't be surprised if he just opens a window," another sagely advises.

Actually, the shift does not turn out to be quite as bad as you feared, mainly because he is engrossed in his new smartphone, which despite having to squint and frequently lift his half-moon glasses up and down to read the screen, he seems to have got the hang of. Following a particularly tricky extrication at the last job, he is perusing search results about spinal immobilisation. "Ha, just as I thought," he exclaims triumphantly, "we used to walk patients to the ambulance and get them to lie on the spinal board. I knew it would come back into fashion." He thrusts his phone under your nose and you spot a research article that concluded applying a collar and asking the patients to get out of the vehicle themselves resulted in the least amount of neck motion.[55] You also note that they used healthy volunteers and none were elderly. Further discussion is prevented by the MDT, which is passing you details about a 19-year-old female who has fallen from height. The major trauma co-ordinator rings before you have pulled away from the standby point asking for an update. You politely tell them that you will update them once on scene.

The address is about 10 minutes away, and by the time you arrive, an RRV paramedic and one of the bronze officers is already on scene. Quite a party is taking place at the house and, given that it is mid-week and past midnight, you imagine that the neighbours must be thrilled. Guessing by the attire, it is a 70s themed party, which has probably helped sales in the local charity shops. The RRV paramedic quickly updates you about the patient, who is currently looking quite perky and grinning broadly, clearly bemused at having her head held by the bronze officer.

It turns out that the patient was leaning out of an attic window (about 25 feet from the ground) to chat to some friends hanging out of the window on the floor below. She lost her balance, sliding down the roof and falling onto the ground floor bay window, before rolling off onto a wheelie bin and then onto the pavement. After a rapid trauma assessment, the RRV paramedic can only elicit low back pain and significant swelling and bruising to the patient's right hip and thigh.

A particularly inebriated student has been creeping closer and closer to the patient, and is staring intently at her. After loitering for 5 minutes, he pipes up with "She needs a CT scan, her." You thank him for his medical advice and ask him to step back as he is starting to get in the way. However, he fails to comply despite several more requests. Your colleague approaches the student and, for a brief moment, you think he is going to hit him. Instead, he whispers something into the student's ear and you can see the colour draining from the young lad's face before your eyes. He slinks off and is not seen again. "Tetley doctors, eh?" your colleague grins, "he'll not be bothering us again." The RRV paramedic looks at you quizzically. "As in Tetley's, the bitter," you explain.

Despite the fall, the patient appears stable, but given the mechanism and possible back and hip injury, and the fact that the patient, by her own admission, is under the influence of alcohol and MDMA (ecstasy), you elect to fully immobilise her.

> **?** What do you want to use: a **Longboard** (read on) or **Orthopaedic (scoop) stretcher** (skip the next paragraph)?

Longboard

You turn to your colleague and ask for the longboard. He looks over his half-moon glasses at you with his stern teacher face. "Given the swelling around her hip, do you not think that log rolling the girl is a bad idea?" You realise he's right. She does appear well, but you are going to have a hard time excluding a pelvic fracture on the street. You need a scoop stretcher.

Orthopaedic (scoop) stretcher

Concerned about the possibility of a fractured pelvis, you opt for the scoop. Your colleague nods in approval and starts to chat about the merits of the new yellow scoops over the silver ones you used to have. "Of course, the old scoops could fold up and practically fit in your pocket, although they did tend to bend rather. There was this one time, when old Moggy and me were in the . . ." You politely drag him back from his nostalgic road trip to the present, and he trots off to get the scoop and trolley, collaring a couple of students to help him. The bronze officer and RRV paramedic are ready to lift the patient, to enable you to insert the pelvic binder. Just a vertical lift of a couple of centimetres is enough to get it in place.

> **?** What landmark did you use to position the pelvic binder: **Iliac crests** (read on) or **Greater trochanters** (skip the next paragraph)?

Chapter 6 Trauma

Iliac crests

You palpate the hips and find the iliac crests, such an easy landmark to find. However, your colleague is looking down at you over his half-moon glasses with his stern teacher face. "Do you not think that you've placed that binder a little high on this missy, and placing the binder over the top of her femurs would be a better idea?" You realise he is right and sulkily slide the binder down to the correct level.

Greater trochanters

You palpate the patient's proximal femurs and find the greater trochanters, making sure the binder is centred over this point. It looks like it is too low, but you are confident with your placement. After applying a blanket between her legs, they are strapped together, and she is placed on the scoop. You ask her boyfriend, who is accompanying you to hospital, to take a photo of the house to show the MTC staff how far she has fallen. Once en route, you make a pre-alert call, but can tell the doctor on the phone is unmoved with the patient's impressively normal observations, and tells you to go through triage. On arrival at the MTC, you ask the boyfriend to show the doctor the photo of the house and he revises his decision, electing to place the patient in resus. You find out later that the swelling to the hip was just soft-tissue trauma and that otherwise, she had a very lucky escape.

Scale of the problem

Fractures of the pelvic ring are relatively uncommon, occurring in around 7% of major trauma cases. As with other significant trauma, older patients falling from standing are becoming an increasingly frequent mechanism of injury. In one MTC, falls from standing represented 38% of all pelvic ring fractures; the same as road traffic collisions (RTCs).[56]

Anatomy

The pelvis is an area of the body surrounded by the pelvic bones and lower part of the vertebral column. The pelvic ring is made up of two pelvic (also called innominate or hip) bones, which themselves are comprised of three fused bones (ilium, ischium and pubis), and the sacrum (Figure 6.11).[57] The pelvic bones articulate anteriorly at the pubic symphysis joint, and posteriorly at the sacroiliac joints. Pelvic ring stability is dependent on the rigidity of the bones and the ligamentous connections. Posteriorly, this is provided by the sacroiliac and iliolumbar ligaments, which resist rotational and vertical shear forces. Anterior stability is provided by the symphysis pubis ligament.[58]

Mechanism of injury

Figure 6.12 shows three main types of pelvic ring fracture and the direction of forces required to cause them. The Young-Burgess system of classifying pelvic ring fractures includes a fourth type (combined mechanical), which is actually a combination of the other three:[59]

Lateral compression (LC) fractures: These are the most common type of pelvic ring fracture[56] and are caused by internal rotation of the pelvic ring due to a direct force applied to the iliac crests, or indirectly via the femoral head.[60] These forces typically result in pubic rami fractures on one or both sides anteriorly, and places severe strain on the sacroiliac joints. If these become displaced, the pelvis will be unstable. The typical mechanism of injury is a side-impact RTC or fall.[58]

Anterior-posterior compression (APC) fractures: These are typically caused by a frontal collision between a pedestrian and a vehicle, front-seat passengers in a frontal RTC and crush injury.[60] With these mechanisms, either the pubic rami are fractured, or the symphysis pubis is disrupted, resulting in the

Pelvic Trauma

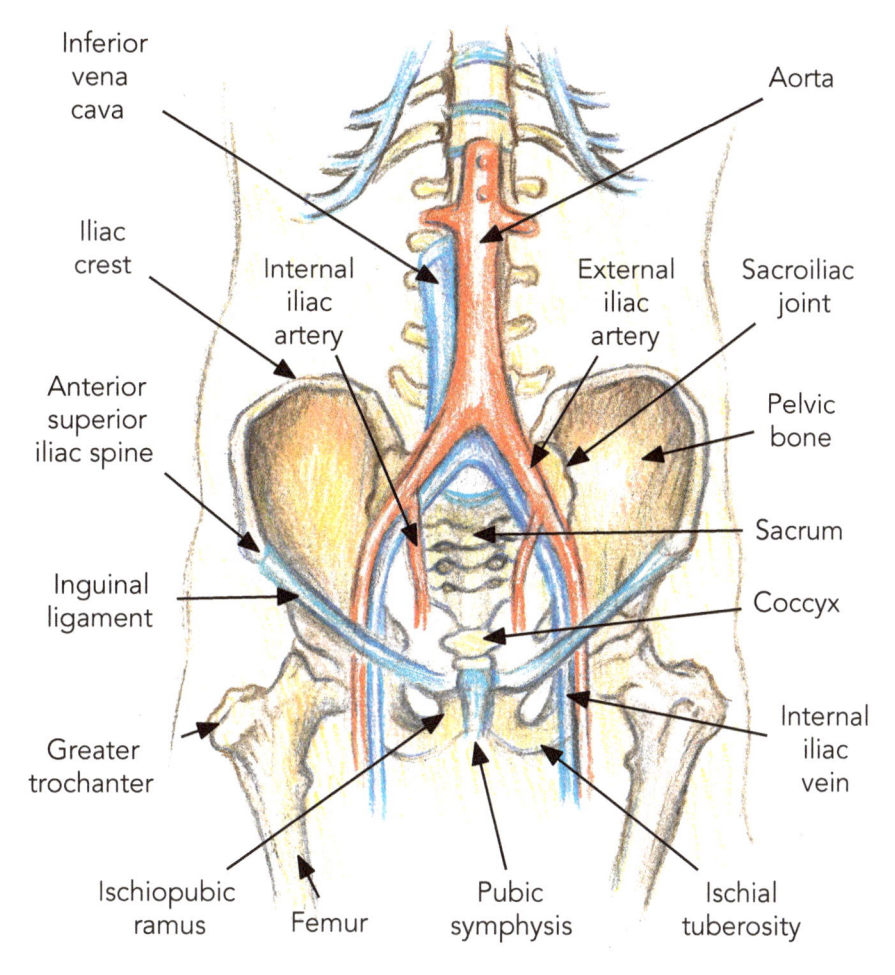

Figure 6.11 The pelvis.

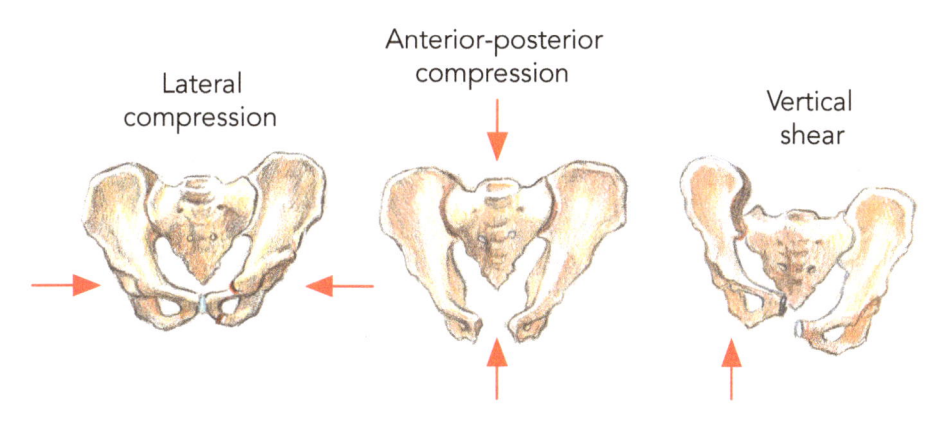

Figure 6.12 Types of pelvic ring fractures.

pelvic bones springing apart and externally rotating. This is often called an 'open book' injury. Posteriorly, the sacroiliac ligaments can be torn and/or the posterior aspect of the pelvic bones fractured.

Vertical shear (VS) fractures: These are the least common type of injury but are the most likely to kill your patient.[61] These fractures occur when one of the pelvic bones is displaced vertically, leading to a fracture of the pubic rami and disruption of the sacroiliac joint on the same side. These are typically caused by falls from height, with the patient landing on one leg first. Because of this, blood vessels are often torn, leading to severe retroperitoneal haemorrhage (which can easily accommodate the body's entire blood volume) and severe damage to soft tissues.[62]

Combined mechanical (CM) fractures: These are really a combination of other types of fractures and are typically caused by a multitude of forces applied in different directions, for example, during a rollover RTC.

Tile's classification

One of the other classification systems in common use, is Tile's classification, which is based on pelvic disruption and degree of stability (Table 6.4).[63] It is worth knowing the basic sub-classifications, since these are often mentioned in the literature about pelvic trauma.

Table 6.4 Tile's classification of pelvic trauma.

Type	Description
A	**Stable**
A1	Pelvic fracture not involving the pelvic ring
A2	Stable, minimally displaced pelvic ring fractures
B	**Rotationally unstable**
B1	Open book
B2	Lateral, ipsilateral (same-side as impact) compression
B3	Lateral, contralateral (opposite-side to impact) compression. Called a bucket-handle as the affected pelvic bone rotates anteriorly and superiorly like the handle of a bucket
C	**Rotational and vertically unstable**
C1	Unilateral
C2	Bilateral
C3	Associated with an acetabular fracture

Source: Tile, 1988.

Haemorrhage

All pelvic fractures cause some bleeding, although the source can vary. Bleeding from cancellous bone that has been fractured is common, but bleeding can also occur from lacerations to retroperitoneal veins and the internal iliac arteries. Arterial bleeding accounts for up to 25% of haemodynamically unstable pelvic ring fractures,[58] but most bleeding is actually low-pressure bleeding (that is, not arterial) and usually responds well to appropriate stabilisation (such as with a pelvic binder or external fixator) and tamponade.[64] Reducing the pelvic volume is an important step in controlling bleeding, as just a 3 cm gap at the symphysis pubis can lead to an increase in pelvic volume of 1.5 litres.[65]

Compared with adults, pelvic ring fractures are rare in children, due to the higher proportion of cartilage, which makes the pelvic ring more ductile (able to deform), and so is less likely to result in haemodynamic instability.[66] However, the intra-pelvic visceral organs are vulnerable, and significant damage can occur even in the absence of a pelvic fracture.

Associated abdominal injuries

As well as the potential vascular damage that pelvic ring fractures can cause, the soft-tissues are also vulnerable, and injuries to the anorectum, vagina, urethra and nerves can occur. The most common is bladder injury, typically caused by a fractured pelvic rami being compressed into the bladder, or a Tile type C fracture causing tearing of the bladder wall.[62]

Urethral and anorectal injuries are more common with straddle injuries, for example, when a motorcyclist straddles the fuel tank during an RTC, resulting in the separation of the two pelvic bones and severe tearing of the pelvic floor.[62]

Recognition

As with any trauma patient, you should consider the MOI to provide an indication as to possible underlying injuries. Pelvic ring fractures usually require high forces, so it is no surprise that the most common cause are RTCs. Front-seat passengers in head on collisions, and those on the side of impact in T-bone type collisions in cars, are most common. These are closely followed by motorcyclists, pedestrians and falls from heights.[67,68] However, as mentioned earlier, a significant sub-group are the elderly, who will typically fall from standing and may have osteoporosis.[60]

In the alert and orientated patient (that is, with a Glasgow coma score of 15/15) with no distracting injury, enquire about pain in the pelvic area, including lower back, groin and hips. The presence of any of these should lead to immobilisation. Clearly, if the patient is unresponsive, or under the influence of alcohol or other drugs, and the mechanism is suggestive of pelvic ring fracture, assume there is a fracture and immobilise appropriately.[17]

A clinical examination should include looking for deformity, bruising and swelling over bony prominences, pubis, perineum and scrotum. If one leg is shorter than the other, deformed and/or rotated, and there is no fracture in that leg, then this could indicate a pelvic fracture.[69] Wounds over the pelvis, or bleeding from the patient's urethra, vagina (in ladies, obviously) and/or rectum could be a sign of open pelvic fracture.[60]

Springing the pelvis is not recommended, because it is an unreliable test, only detecting the most serious pelvic disruption, and could dislodge blood clots leading to further blood loss.[17]

Management

As with all trauma patient management, adopt a <C>ABCDE approach. Any pelvic fracture may cause life-threatening haemorrhage, so in cases where the patient is obviously haemodynamically compromised (that is, has signs of shock), or has suffered a traumatic cardiac arrest where a pelvic fracture is suspected, apply a pelvic binder. In open pelvic fractures, consider packing the wound with gauze or haemostatic dressings. Don't forget to consider other causes of bleeding (remember blood on the floor, plus four more).[70]

Unless you are supremely confident that the patient does not have a pelvic fracture, immobilise their pelvis. Do not log roll the patient, utilise a small vertical lift instead, to insert a pelvic binder, and use an orthopaedic stretcher to immobilise and transport the patient (unless you have a vacuum mattress).

Practise permissive hypotension (that is, only administer intravenous fluids to patients with a systolic blood pressure of less than 90 mmHg, and in 250 ml boluses). Don't forget to administer tranexamic acid once you have obtained intravenous access and transport the patient to a MTC where possible.[17]

Chapter 6 Trauma

Pelvic binders

Commercial pelvic binders have been shown to reduce Tile type A, B1 and C fractures adequately, with no important displacement of fractures, irrespective of device.[71] Concerns have been expressed with their use in lateral compression fractures (Type B2 and B3), but there is no good evidence that their use is detrimental to the patient with these fractures.[72]

Given the high energy forces that typically cause pelvic ring fractures, the patient may have femur fractures too. These should generally be reduced by the use of a traction splint (such as the Kendrick Traction Device) that does not have a manufacturer's contraindication of pelvic fractures. However, if the patient is severely haemodynamically compromised, it is acceptable to pull the legs out to length, apply a commercial pelvic binder (that is, not a DIY binding technique) and then keep the legs together using a figure of eight bandage of straps.[73]

Positioning

The correct placement of pelvic binders is very important. Pelvic binders should be centred over the greater trochanters (Figure 6.11), but are commonly placed too high, such as over the iliac crests, which can actually compound pelvic fractures.[74] Where possible, pelvic binders should be placed directly against the patient's skin.[73]

References

1. Sheppard NN, Hemington-Gorse S, Shelley OP, Philp B, Dziewulski P. Prognostic scoring systems in burns: a review. *Burns*, 2011 Dec;37(8):1288–1295.
2. NHS Digital. Hospital Accident & Emergency Activity 2019–2020 [Internet]. NHS Digital. 2020. Available from: https://digital.nhs.uk/data-and-information/publications/statistical/hospital-accident–emergency-activity/2019-20
3. Kalson NS, Jenks T, Woodford M, Lecky FE, Dunn KW. Burns represent a significant proportion of the total serious trauma workload in England and Wales. Journal of the International Society for Burn Injuries, 2012 May;38(3):330–339.
4. National Burn Care Group. UK Burn Injury Data 1986–2007. UK: UK National Burn Care Group; 2008.
5. Marieb E, Hoehn K. *Human anatomy & physiology*, 11th edition. Pearson; 2019.
6. Hall S, Stephens J, LLM STDBsMM, MRCP PXMMBc. *Crash course anatomy and physiology*, 5th edition. Smith CF, editor. Elsevier; 2018.
7. Thompson G, Sciarra J, editors. *Wound care made incredibly visual*. Ambler: Lippincott Williams & Wilkins; 2008.
8. New Zealand Guidelines Group. *Management of burns and scalds in primary care*. Wellington: Accident Compensation Corporation; 2007.
9. Greaves I, Porter K, Wright C, editors. *Trauma care pre-hospital manual*, 1st edition. Boca Raton: CRC Press; 2018.
10. Moritz AR, Henriques FC. Studies of thermal injury. Am J Pathol. 1947 Sep;23(5):695–720.
11. Hettiaratchy S, Dziewulski P. Pathophysiology and types of burns. *British Medical Journal*, 2004 Jun 12;328(7453):1427–1429.
12. Sheridan R. *Burns: a practical approach to immediate treatment and long-term care*. London: Manson Publishing; 2012.
13. Giebułtowicz J, Rużycka M, Wroczyński P, Purser DA, Stec AA. Analysis of fire deaths in Poland and influence of smoke toxicity. *Forensic Science International*, 2017 Aug;277:77–87.
14. Toon MH, Maybauer MO, Greenwood JE, Maybauer DM, Fraser JF. Management of acute smoke inhalation injury. Critical Care and Resuscitation, 2010 Mar;12(1):53–61.
15. Prien T, Traber DL. Toxic smoke compounds and inhalation injury – a review. *Burns Including Thermal Injury*, Dec;14(6):451–460.
16. Murakami K, Traber DL. Pathophysiological basis of smoke inhalation injury. *Physiology*, 2003 Jun 1;18(3):125–129.
17. Joint Royal Colleges Ambulance Liaison Committee, Association of Ambulance Chief Executives. JRCALC Clinical Guidelines. Cited from JRCALC Plus (Version 1.2.13) [Mobile application software]. Bridgwater: Class Publishing Ltd; 2021.
18. Muehlberger T, Ottomann C, Toman N, Daigeler A, Lehnhardt M. Emergency pre-hospital care of burn patients. *The Surgeon*, 2010 Apr;8(2):101–104.
19. Butz DR, Collier Z, O'Connor A, Magdziak M, Gottlieb LJ. Is palmar surface area a reliable tool to estimate burn surface areas in obese patients? Journal of Burn Care & Research, 2015 Jan 1;36(1):87–91.
20. Enoch S, Roshan A, Shah M. Emergency and early management of burns and scalds. *British Medical Journal*, 2009 Apr;338(apr08 1):b1037–b1037.
21. Battaloglu E, Greasley L, Leon-Villapalos J, Young A, Porter K. Expert Consensus Meeting: Management of Burns in Pre-Hospital Trauma Care [Internet]. 2020. Available from: https://fphc.rcsed.ac.uk/media/2957/2020-09-20-burns-consensus.pdf
22. Cuttle L, Pearn J, McMillan JR, Kimble RM. A review of first aid treatments for burn injuries. *Burns*, 2009 Sep;35(6):768–775.
23. Cuttle L, Kempf M, Kravchuk O, Phillips GE, Mill J, Wang X-Q, et al. The optimal temperature of first aid treatment for partial thickness burn injuries. *Wound Repair & Regeneration*, 2008 Oct;16(5):626–634.
24. Lonnecker S, Schoder V. Hypothermia after burn injury – influence of pre-hospital management. *Der Chirug*, 2001 Feb 12; 72(2):164–167.
25. Hostler D, Weaver MD, Ziembicki JA, Kowger HL, McEntire SJ, Rittenberger JC,

et al. Admission temperature and survival in patients admitted to burn centers. *Journal of Burn Care & Research*, 2013 Oct;34(5):498–506.
26. College of Policing. Conducted energy devices (Taser) [Internet]. 2020. Available from: https://www.app.college.police.uk/app-content/armed-policing/conducted-energy-devices-taser/
27. Pasquier M, Carron P-N, Vallotton L, Yersin B. electronic control device exposure: a review of morbidity and mortality. *Annals of Emergency Medicine*, 2011 Aug;58(2):178–188.
28. UK Government. Police use of force statistics [Internet]. GOV.UK. 2020. Available from: https://www.gov.uk/government/collections/police-use-of-force-statistics
29. Taser International. Taser X26E ECD User Manual [Internet]. 2011. Available from: https://prismic-io.s3.amazonaws.com/tasr%2F9324bd84-e504-4062-a53e-a607e353c0e1_x26-user-manual.pdf
30. Ho JD, Miner JR, Lakireddy DR, Bultman LL, Heegaard WG. Cardiovascular and physiologic effects of conducted electrical weapon discharge in resting adults. *Academic Emergency Medicine*, 2006 Jun;13(6):589–595.
31. Jauchem JR. TASER® conducted electrical weapons: misconceptions in the scientific/medical and other literature. Forensic Science, Medicine and Pathology, 2015 Mar;11(1):53–64.
32. Zipes DP. TASER Electronic control devices can cause cardiac arrest in humans. *Circulation*, 2014 Jul 1;129(1):101–111.
33. Vanga SR, Bommana S, Kroll MW, Swerdlow C, Lakkireddy D. TASER conducted electrical weapons and implanted pacemakers and defibrillators. 2009 Annual International Conference of the IEEE Engineering in Medicine and Biology Society, 2009 Sep;3199–3204.
34. Olshausen G von, Rondak I-C, Lennerz C, Semmler V, Grebmer C, Reents T, et al. Electromagnetic interference in implantable cardioverter defibrillators: present but rare. *Clinical Research in Cardiology*, 2016 Jan 29;1–9.
35. Leitgeb N, Niedermayr F, Loos G, Neubauer R. Cardiac fibrillation risk of TASER X-26 dart mode application. Wiener Medizinische Wochenschrift, 2011 Dec;161(23–24):571–577.
36. Defence Scientific Advisory Council Sub-Committee on the Medical Implications of Less-lethal weapons. Statement on the Medical Implication of Use of the Taser X26 and M26 Less-lethal Systems on Children and Vulnerable Adults [Internet]. 2012. Available from: http://data.parliament.uk/DepositedPapers/Files/DEP2012-0729/96605%20Library%20Deposit.pdf
37. Wenzel BJ, George S, Lakkireddy D, Vanga S, Bommana S, Gussak I, et al. Algorithm for quantitative 3 dimensional analysis of ECG signals improves myocardial diagnosis over cardiologists in diabetic patients. *Annual International Conference of the IEEE Engineering in Medicine and Biology Society*, 2011;2011:965–968.
38. Kroll MW, Brave MA, Pratt HMO, Witte KK, Kunz SN, Luceri RM. Benefits, risks, and myths of TASER® handheld electrical weapons. Human Factors and Mechanical Engineering for Defense and Safety, 2019 Dec;3(1):7.
39. O'Brien AJ, Thom K. Police use of TASER devices in mental health emergencies: a review. *International Journal of Law and Psychiatry*, 2014 Jul;37(4):420–426.
40. Ministry of Defence, Scientific Advisory Committe on the Medical Implications of Less-Lethal Weapons. Scientific Advisory Committee on the Medical Implications of Less-Lethal weapons triennial review [Internet]. 2014. Available from: https://www.gov.uk/government/publications/scientific-advisory-committee-on-the-medical-implications-of-less-lethal-weapons-triennial-review
41. Bridgman SA, Clement D, Downing A, Walley G, Phair I, Maffulli N. Population based epidemiology of ankle sprains attending accident and emergency units in the West Midlands of England, and a survey of UK practice for severe ankle sprains. Emergency Medicine Journal, 2003 Nov 1;20(6):508–510.
42. Al Bimani SA, Gates LS, Warner M, Ewings S, Crouch R, Bowen C. Characteristics of patients with ankle sprain presenting to an emergency department in the south of England (UK): a seven-month review. *International Emergency Nursing*, 2018 Nov 1;41:38–44.

43. Wardrope J, English B. *Musculo-skeletal problems in emergency medicine*, Oxford: Oxford University Press; 1998. 348 p.
44. Drake RL, Vogl W, Mitchell AWM, Gray H. *Gray's anatomy for students*, 3rd edition. Philadelphia: Churchill Livingstone/Elsevier; 2015.
45. Innes JA, Dover AR, Fairhurst K, Britton R, Danielson E. *Macleod's clinical examination*, 14th edition. Edinburgh: Elsevier; 2018.
46. Koval KJ, Zuckerman JD. *Rockwood's handbook of fractures*, 2nd revised edition. London: Lippincott Williams and Wilkins; 2001.
47. Tiemstra JD. Update on acute ankle sprains. *American Family Physician*, 2012 Jun 15;85(12):1170–1176.
48. Wardrope J, Driscoll P, Laird C, Woolard M, editors. *Community emergency medicine*, Edinburgh: Churchill Livingstone Elsevier; 2008. 305 p.
49. Stiell IG, Greenberg GH, McKnight RD, Nair RC, McDowell I, Worthington JR. A study to develop clinical decision rules for the use of radiography in acute ankle injuries. *Annals of Emergency Medicine*, 1992 Apr;21(4):384–390.
50. Bachmann LM. Accuracy of Ottawa ankle rules to exclude fractures of the ankle and mid-foot: systematic review. *British Medical Journal*, 2003 Feb 22;326(7386):417–417.
51. Jonckheer P, Willems T, De Ridder R, Paulus D, Holdt Henningsen K, San Miguel L, et al. Evaluating fracture risk in acute ankle sprains: Any news since the Ottawa Ankle Rules? A systematic review. *European Journal of General Practice*, 2016 Jan 2;22(1):31–41.
52. Purcell D. *Minor injuries: a clinical guide*, 3rd edition. Edinburgh; New York: Churchill Livingstone; 2016.
53. Chelsea and Westminster Hospital NHS Foundation Trust. Care of your ankle injury [Internet]. 2021. Available from: https://www.chelwest.nhs.uk/your-visit/patient-leaflets/medicine-services/care-of-your-ankle-injury
54. Oxford University Hospitals NHS Trust. Ankle sprain advice [Internet]. 2015. Available from: https://www.ouh.nhs.uk/patient-guide/leaflets/files/12384Pankle.pdf
55. Gabrieli A, Nardello F, Geronazzo M, Marchetti P, Liberto A, Arcozzi D, et al. Cervical spine motion during vehicle extrication of healthy volunteers. *Prehospital Emergency Care*, 2020 Sep 2;24(5):712–720.
56. Leach SET, Skiadas V, Lord CE, Purohit N. Pelvic fractures: experience of pelvic ring fractures at a major trauma centre. *Clinical Radiology*, 2019 Aug 1;74(8):649.e19–649.e26.
57. Drake R, Vogl AW, Mitchell AWM. *Gray's anatomy for students*, 4th edition. Philadelphia: Elsevier; 2019.
58. McCormack R, Strauss EJ, Alwattar BJ, Tejwani NC. Diagnosis and management of pelvic fractures. *Bulletin of the NYU Hospital for Joint Diseases*, 2010;68(4):281.
59. Burgess AR, Eastridge BJ, Young JW, Ellison TS, Ellison PS Jr, Poka A, et al. Pelvic ring disruptions: effective classification system and treatment protocols. *Journal of Trauma*, 1990 Jul;30(7):848–856.
60. Garlapati AK, Ashwood N. An overview of pelvic ring disruption. *Trauma*, 2012 Apr 1;14(2):169–178.
61. White MA, Logterman S, Mauffrey C. Pelvic vertical shear injuries and sacroiliac joint disruptions. In: Giannoudis PV, editor. Fracture reduction and fixation techniques: spine-pelvis and lower extremity [Internet]. Cham: Springer International Publishing; 2020, pp. 77–90. Available from: https://doi.org/10.1007/978-3-030-24608-2_6
62. Leenen L. Pelvic fractures: soft tissue trauma. *European Journal of Trauma and Emergency Surgery*, 2010 Apr 1;36(2):117–123.
63. Tile M. Pelvic ring fractures: should they be fixed. *Journal of Bone and Joint Surgery*, 1988;70(1):1–12.
64. Abrassart S, Stern R, Peter R. Unstable pelvic ring injury with hemodynamic instability: what seems the best procedure choice and sequence in the initial management? *Orthopaedics & Traumatology: Surgery & Research*, 2013 Apr;99(2):175–182.
65. Mears DC. *Pelvic and acetabular fractures*. Thorofare Slack; 1986. 534 p.
66. Tuovinen H, Söderlund T, Lindahl J, Laine T, Åström P, Handolin L. Severe pelvic fracture-related bleeding in pediatric patients: does it occur? *European Journal of Trauma and Emergency Surgery*, 2012 Apr 1;38(2):163–169.

Chapter 6 Trauma

67. Gabbe BJ, de Steiger R, Esser M, Bucknill A, Russ MK, Cameron PA. Predictors of mortality following severe pelvic ring fracture: results of a population-based study. *Injury*, 2011 Oct;42(10):985–991.
68. Papadopoulos IN, Kanakaris N, Bonovas S, Triantafillidis A, Garnavos C, Voros D, et al. Auditing 655 fatalities with pelvic fractures by autopsy as a basis to evaluate trauma care. *Journal of the American College of Surgeons*, 2006 Jul;203(1):30–43.
69. Lee C, Porter K. The prehospital management of pelvic fractures. Emergency Medicine Journal, 2007 Feb 1;24(2):130–133.
70. Greaves I, Porter K, Ryan J, Garner J. *Trauma care manual*, 2nd edition. London: Hodder Arnold; 2008. 336 p.
71. Knops SP. Comparison of three different pelvic circumferential compression devices: a biomechanical cadaver study. *Journal of Bone & Joint Surgery*, 2011 Feb 2;93(3):230.
72. Toth L, King KL, McGrath B, Balogh ZJ. Efficacy and safety of emergency non-invasive pelvic ring stabilisation. *Injury*, 2012 Aug;43(8):1330–1334.
73. Scott I, Porter K, Laird C, Greaves I, Bloch M. The prehospital management of pelvic fractures: initial consensus statement. Emergency Medicine Journal, 2013 Jan 12;30(12):1070–1072.
74. Henning S, Norris R, Hill CE. Pelvic binder placement in a regional trauma centre. *Journal of Paramedic Practice*, 2018;10(11):5.

7 Obstetrics and Gynaecology
Aimee Yarrington

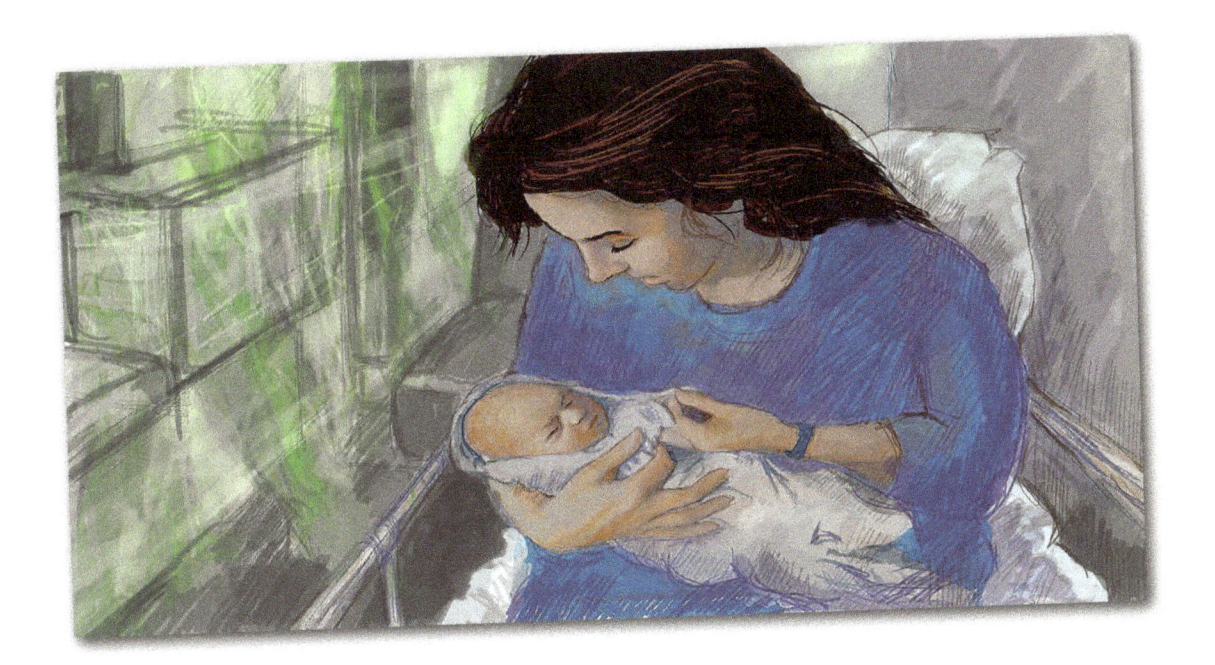

Care of the Newborn

You are on standby at one of your favourite people-watching spots. Spring should be in the air but the weather has suddenly turned very cold and grey; perhaps working over the bank holiday is the better option, you think. It's the height of the shopping rush hour and you are just finishing off the remains of your second hot cross bun when there is a group call over your radio: "Any available crew able to deal, outstanding red call, birth imminent, control standing by." Your over-excited colleague pleads "ohhhhhh please can we see if we are close? I love babies!" You begrudgingly agree, thinking a hot chocolate would be nicer, but then you think back: it's been a while since you caught a baby, and so you agree to call up. You are surprised that they send you, but indeed you are very close – only 4 minutes away. There is an update on the MDT that flashes "Mother stating urge to push" as your colleague squeals with delight.

The trip takes you longer than you thought, as you were diverted for the 'Easter Bunny Hop' event in the square, and you arrive at the location 8 minutes later. You were given a road name and told to look for a green car; as you pull up you see a man frantically jumping up and down on the spot and waving at you.

Chapter 7 Obstetrics and Gynaecology

"Over here, it's coming, and on my new car seat too, it's already made a heck of a mess!"

As you approach the front seat of the car you see a woman who is quite clearly in the second stage of labour and bearing down with a contraction. "Can you get the heat on?" you shout at the very anxious father-to-be. "What do I call you?" you add in quickly to the mother-to-be. "Jayne," she answers after the contraction subsides. "It's coming," she adds, "I can feel it!" Sure enough it is: as she pulls away the blanket that was protecting her modesty you see the distinct, almost crowning, fetal head. You quickly reassure Jayne: "it's okay, just breathe through it, it will all be over shortly," you say, thinking to yourself you'd rather have had that hot chocolate!

> You now have to decide quickly: risk trying to **Move the patient to the ambulance** (read on) or **Stay put** and catch the baby in the car (skip the next paragraph)?

Move the patient to the ambulance

You shout to your colleague to bring the stretcher and ask Jayne to swing her legs round so she is facing you. However, it dawns on you that not only is this baby coming a lot faster than you thought, but you are now directly in the line of Jayne's waters breaking! Suddenly she shouts "here comes another one!" and at that she bears down, her waters break and the baby's head is born, covering your shirt in warm amniotic fluid. Your crew mate, who is now standing next to you, can't move for the laughter and hands you a towel. As you bring it to your shirt to mop up, some of the warm fluid manages to seep through to the band of your trousers. Jayne bears down again and you realise as the baby falls into your arms that the towel your colleague kindly passed you was for the baby, not your now-soaking shirt!

Stay put

You can see that moving Jayne to the ambulance now would not be a wise move: the amniotic sac is still intact so there will be all that fluid to deal with and you have only just mopped the back out after the last patient. You grab the towel and an incontinence pad from the stretcher your colleague has brought round and put the blanket that was covering Jayne onto the floor of the car with the pad on top. You shut her door and run round to jump in the driver's seat. You shut the door and turn up the heating to maximum; it's a little too warm for comfort and, as the dad jumps into the back seat, small beads of sweat break out on his forehead. Jayne has the urge to push again, and with the next contraction her waters break and hit the dash with some force. Jayne breathes the baby's head out beautifully, and with the next contraction she puts her hands down and you help bring her beautiful baby girl up towards her. You rub the infant down with the towel you had put on the heater to warm and the baby girl begins to cry and pink up.

You rub the baby until she is dry, and at 1 minute you calculate her APGAR score to be 9, and with all the crying, she soon starts to pink up further. With the baby placed skin-to-skin on her mother she calms from her initial cry, opens her large dark eyes and looks up at you – what a moment! The baby's 5-minute APGAR score is now 10 and you start to relax slightly as the baby is reacting normally and making that transition to extra-uterine life as normal.

Jayne starts to complain of increasing abdominal pain and you notice a small gush of blood, no more than 200 ml, onto the incontinence pad on the car floor. It quickly stops; you feel down and look at the baby's cord, which is flat, white and opaque and

Care of the Newborn

no longer has a pulse in it. You deduce that the placenta has separated and that it is no longer of use. You decide to separate mum and baby now before you try to manoeuvre them out of the car, as it would be difficult for them if they were still attached. Opening the maternity pack, you locate the two clamps and scissors and, after fixing the clamps in place and cutting between them, free the newborn from the safety of her mother. You shout to your colleague through the window and tell him you are ready to move. Jayne wraps the baby snugly in another blanket she had in a bag in the back of the car and she then suddenly has an overwhelming urge to push. As she does so the placenta plops down onto the blanket underneath her. You manage to get her underwear and trousers back on, grabbing the maternity pad from the pack for her, returning Jayne to a dressed state to maintain her dignity when removing her from the car.

Your colleague is ready with the stretcher outside the door, so you pass the baby to dad and ask him to follow in a few minutes. Jayne jumps up with surprising speed and is out of the door and on the stretcher before you have a chance to run round the car. You retrieve the placenta and bag it up, then assist your colleague with moving Jayne into the ambulance. Your colleague has done a good job of getting the ambulance warm and it remains warm despite having the doors open for a short time to get Jayne in and settled. You ask dad for a nappy and a hat from Jayne's hospital bag and put both on the baby. Your colleague takes the baby for a cheeky cuddle then places her skin-to-skin with Jayne with two blankets over the top to ensure she stays warm.

A wise colleague once told you to always ensure that babies arrive at the maternity ward warm. You call through, inform the midwives that you will be arriving shortly and make your way to the local maternity ward, where you are greeted at the door by a cheerful midwife who congratulates you on knowing to keep the baby warm.

Physiology of transition

The fetal circulation is very different to that of the neonate, primarily because the source of oxygen is the placenta and not the lungs. Oxygen from the uterine artery enters the maternal side of the placenta and follows its concentration gradient into vessels within the villi on the fetal side of the placenta. The villi contain capillaries that merge and form the umbilical vein, which contains blood with the highest oxygen saturation within the fetal circulation (approximately 70–80%). The umbilical vein enters the fetus and branches at the level of the liver to provide some hepatic blood flow. However, the majority of the blood enters the inferior vena cava (IVC) via the ductus venosus (Figure 7.1).

Blood flow preferentially serves the heart and brain, so even though blood from the ductus venosus and IVC merge near the heart, the more well oxygenated blood from the ductus venosus is preferentially shunted to the left atrium via the foramen ovale.[1] The poorly oxygenated blood from the IVC enters the right atrium and merges with blood from the superior vena cava (SVC) and enters the right ventricle. Due to high pulmonary vascular resistance caused by the lung being filled with fluid, much of the blood in the pulmonary arteries is shunted to the descending aorta via the ductus arteriosus, which then oxygenates the abdominal organs and lower extremities before returning to the placenta via the two umbilical arteries. This is possible because of the placenta's low resistance to flow, making the right side of the heart have a higher pressure than the left; the opposite of neonatal circulatory pressures.

As previously mentioned, the more oxygenated blood from the ductus arteriosus

Chapter 7 Obstetrics and Gynaecology

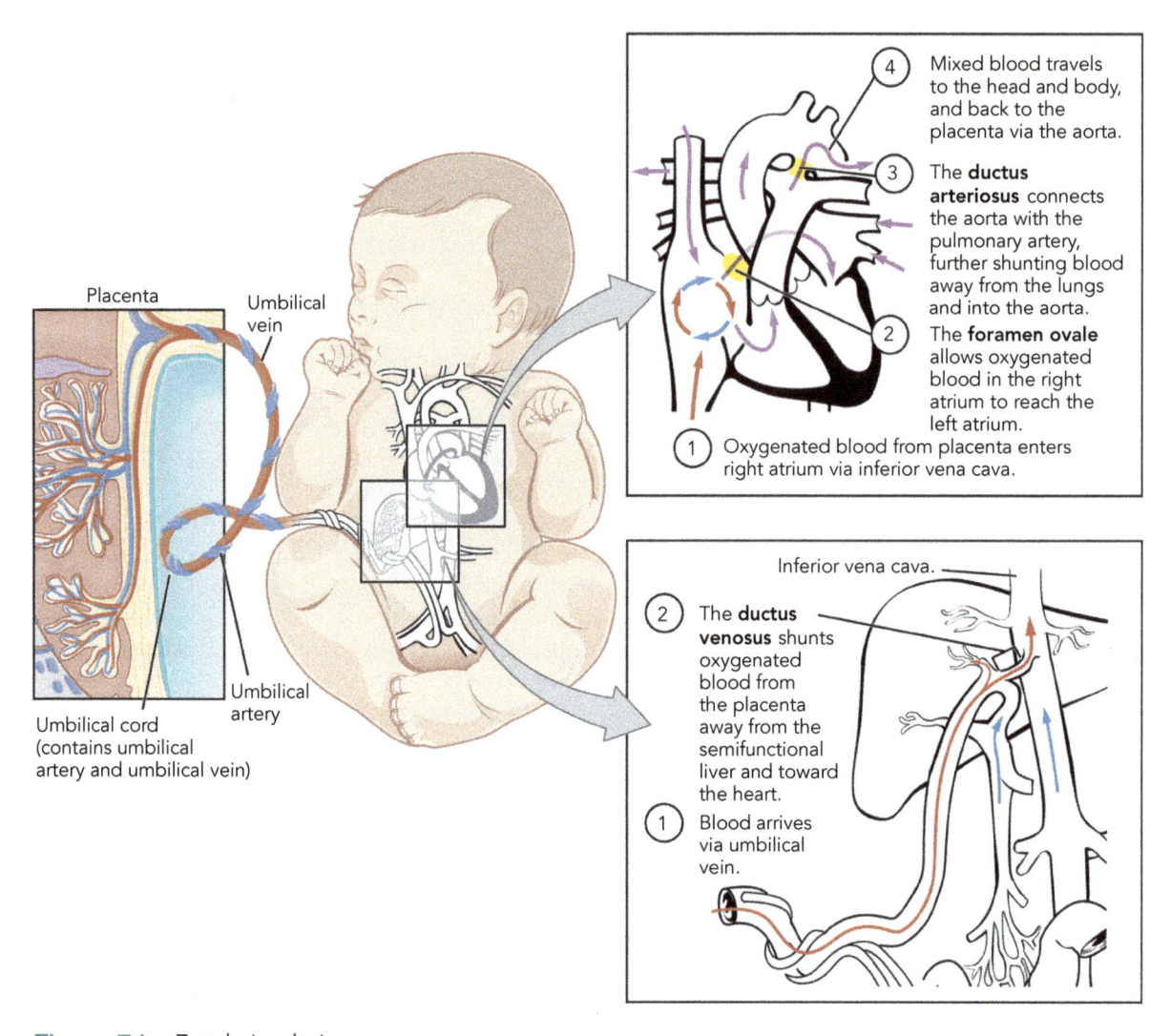

Figure 7.1 Fetal circulation.
Source: OpenStax College [CC BY 3.0 (https://creativecommons.org/licenses/by/3.0)], via Wikimedia Commons.

is preferentially directed to the left atria via the foramen ovale; a shunt that is responsible for around 25% of cardiac output. This blood is mixed with a small amount of blood returning from the pulmonary veins before leaving the heart via the ascending aorta and supplying the coronary and carotid arteries with blood. Therefore the oxygen saturations of blood supplying the heart and brain, have a slightly higher oxygen saturation (approximately 65%) compared with the post-ductal aorta (around 60%).[2]

Transition

In the first 60 seconds of the baby's life after birth, the newborn circulation changes significantly (Figure 7.2). The newborn's first breaths are crucial in starting this transition but may not occur immediately after birth; you

202

Care of the Newborn

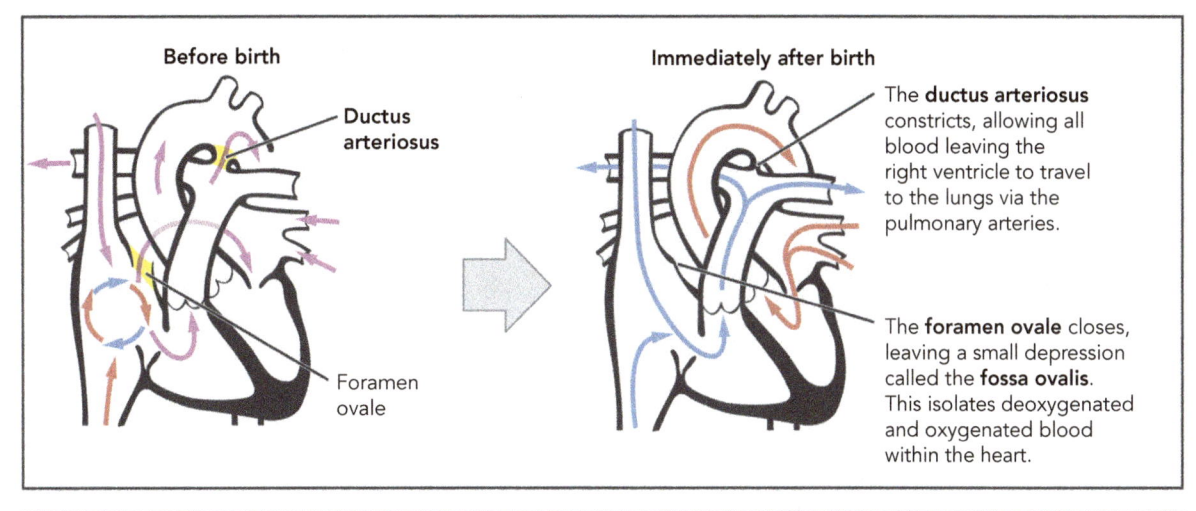

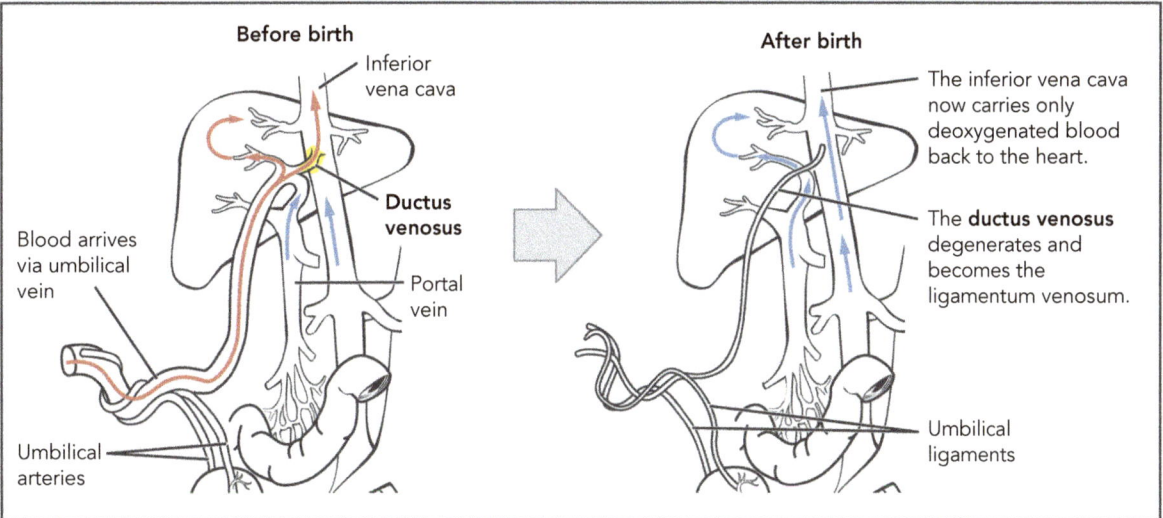

Figure 7.2 Changes that occur during fetal transition.
Source: OpenStax College [CC BY 3.0 (https://creativecommons.org/licenses/by/3.0)], via Wikimedia Commons.

literally have to wait for the baby to 'catch its breath'. This is not always a huge cry out after the birth and the onset of regular respirations needs to be determined. It can be quite an anxious period, but remember that while the cord is still pulsating the baby is still receiving an oxygenated supply of blood from the placenta and its mother.

Clearance of the lung fluid and aeration of the lungs leads to a decrease in pulmonary vascular resistance. In addition, the low resistance placental bed is disconnected as (for example, by cord clamping) increasing systemic vascular resistance. This increases pressure in the left atrium, effectively closing the foramen ovale as pressure on the left side of the heart increases and becomes higher than the right.

Blood flow across the ductus arteriosus is reversed immediately after birth, although as blood oxygen levels increase, the vessel becomes increasingly constricted causing functional closure.

Chapter 7   Obstetrics and Gynaecology

Assessment of the newborn

Calculating the APGAR score

Due to the transition physiology, the APGAR score is not calculated at birth, but instead delayed for 1 minute following birth, and then repeated after 5 minutes. It is primarily a tool to determine the need for resuscitation; a score of 7 or less at 1 minute indicates a baby in need of resuscitation whereas a baby scoring more than 7 should not.[3]

The component parts of the APGAR test can be difficult to remember so don't be afraid to use an aide memoire to remember the components of the score (Table 7.1). If you find it hard to remember each of the component parts, you may find it easier to remember the mantra: colour, tone, breathing, heart rate. This gives all the elements needed to help work out the score, apart from the grimace, which in most basic terms refers to how the baby is responding to extra-uterine life – whether they are pulling away, sneezing or crying appropriately. Note that if you are not in attendance for the birth then the APGAR score must not be retrospectively completed, but it is always worth documenting a score when you first arrival on scene in these cases.

Observations

As with all patients, physiological observations should be performed on the newborn and documented accordingly.

Oxygen saturations

Newborn oxygen saturation probes should be placed on the right hand of the baby in order to capture the pre-ductal (that is, oxygen saturation before blood mixed with shunted blood from the ductus arteriosus) (Figure 7.3). Pulse oximetry levels are initially lower than the standard expected is because birth is a hypoxic event (Table 7.2).[4] Most healthy babies tolerate this level of hypoxia well and are not affected by the low blood oxygen levels.[4] It is when the infant is already compromised (for example, they are premature or they are growth-restricted) that the low oxygen levels cause increased difficulties within the transitional period. It is these infants that may need additional support in the transition.

Respiratory and heart rates

Respiratory and heart rates need to be determined with a stethoscope to avoid errors in calculation; normal values for a newborn are a heart rate of 110–160 bpm and a respiratory rate of 30–40 per minute.[3]

Table 7.1   AGPAR score.

Score	0	1	2
Appearance	Blue or pale all over	Blue at extremities, body pink	Body and extremities pink
Pulse rate	Absent	<100	≥100
Grimace or response to stimulation	No response to stimulation	Grimace/feeble cry when stimulated	Cry or pull away when stimulated
Activity or muscle tone	None	Some flexion	Flexed arms and legs that resist extension
Respiration	Absent	Weak, irregular gasping	Strong, lusty cry

Source: JRCALC, 2021.

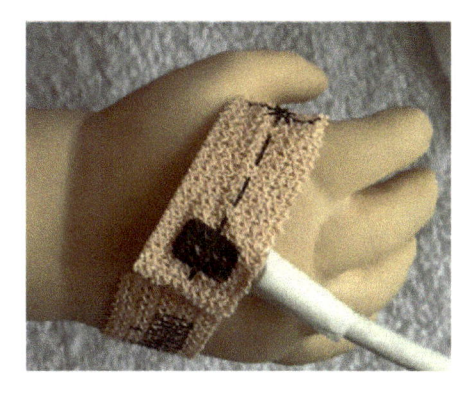

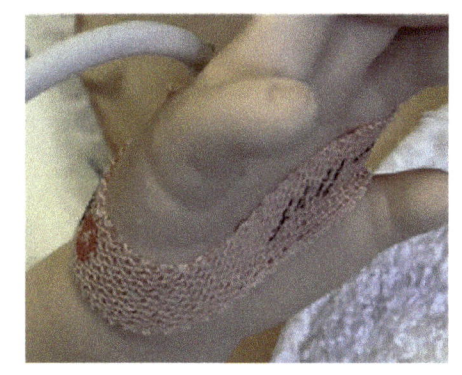

Figure 7.3 Correct placement of the oxygen saturation probe on a newborn.

Table 7.2 Acceptable pre-ductal SpO_2 values.

Time after Birth	Expected SpO_2
2 minutes	65%
5 minutes	85%
10 minutes	90%

Source: Madar et al, 2021.

Ideally, these values should be checked when the newborn is at rest and not crying.[5] During resuscitation, you can also determine the heart rate using the ECG.[4]

Blood glucose

Newborns have a naturally low blood glucose level, and therefore do not routinely need a capillary blood glucose test. A newborn usually has sufficient glucose stores to provide them with a supply until breastfeeding is established, which is normally on day 3. A newborn blood glucose at the age of 1–2 hours will be just under 2 mmol/l.[6] However, if newborn resuscitation is required, then blood glucose should be measured to rule out other potential causes of the requirement for resuscitation.

Care of the newborn

As soon as the baby is born it must be dried thoroughly since newborns lose heat very quickly, and placing them skin-to-skin with their mothers once dry, will not only keep them warm but will also help to regulate the newborn's vital signs and assist in their transition to extra-uterine life. Skin-to-skin contact is recommended for infants following birth and ideally, separation in the first hour of life should be avoided.[7] This promotes a positive bond between mother and baby and may even reduce the risk of postnatal depression.[8] In addition to keeping them warm, skin-to-skin contact also helps to regulate the infant's heart rate, breathing rate and blood glucose level. An added benefit for the mother is the rise in oxytocin levels, which will increase further if she breastfeeds. Raising the level of oxytocin should increase the likelihood of the placenta being delivered (part of third stage management). It is important to remember when assisting with skin-to-skin contact, that the baby needs to be covered. Ideally the baby should have a hat and a nappy to prevent heat loss; the nappy will prevent further cooling if the baby urinates and becomes wet again. Once the baby is on the skin, cover them with two towels or blankets to ensure they are kept warm.

Cutting the cord

It is very important that the cord is not clamped and cut immediately at birth, since up to a third (around 150 ml) of the baby's circulating blood volume is either within the cord or placenta. Most newborns quickly make the transition to using their lungs for oxygenation instead of the placenta, and the blood in the cord and placenta will fully return to the newborn within 10–20 minutes. You will know when this is complete because the cord will stop pulsating and will go from being full of blood to being flat, white and opaque (Figure 7.4). While the cord is still pulsating, do not raise the baby higher than the breast, in order to maximise the blood transfused. Even in cases where a newborn requires chest compressions, delay cord clamping until you reach the requirement for chest compressions (typically around the 3 minutes after birth).

Resuscitation

Around 85% of babies born at term will spontaneously initiate breathing within 10 to 30 seconds of birth, with most babies pinking up and crying or establishing regular respirations within 90 seconds. Another 10% of babies will respond through drying and stimulation with a further 5% responding to positive-pressure ventilations; fewer than 0.3% will require chest compressions.[4]

In the event that resuscitation is required, aeration of the lungs is key, as without this no further progress can be made. If possible, perform the initial inflation breaths with the cord intact. This will allow for the oxygenated blood to feed the newborn while they are not breathing for themselves. The cord should only be cut once chest compressions are commenced when possible. If practicalities dictate that the cord needs to be cut, then this should not be undertaken until at least 1 minute after birth regardless of gestation.[10]

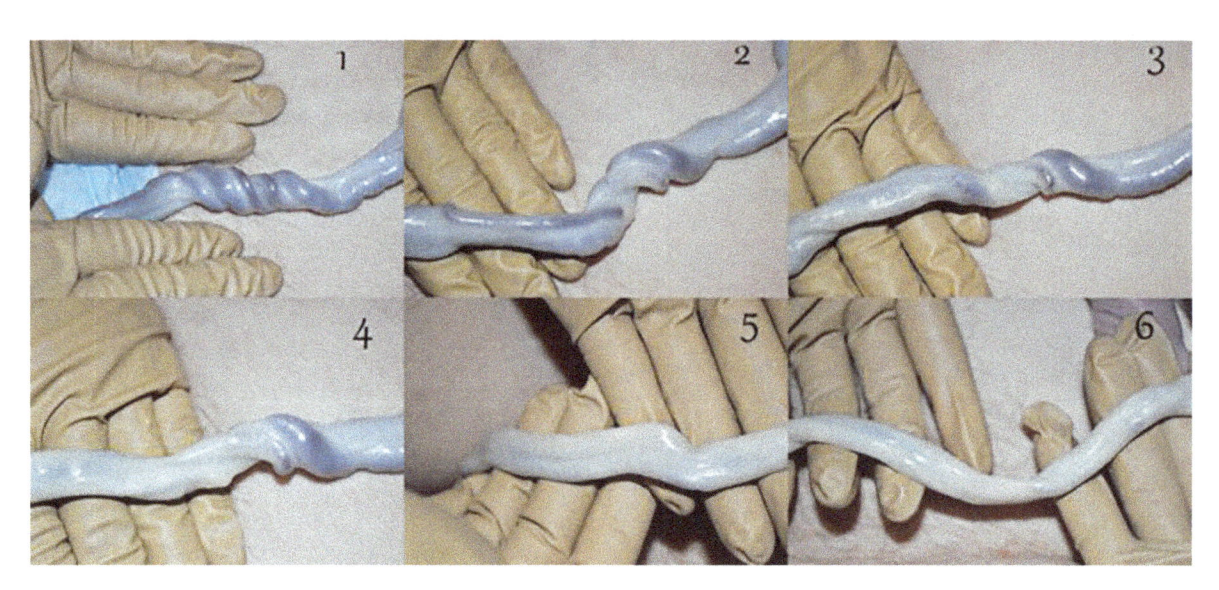

Figure 7.4 Unclamped cord over the course of 15 minutes.
Reproduced with the kind permission of Lyndsay King (nurturingheartsbirthservices.com).

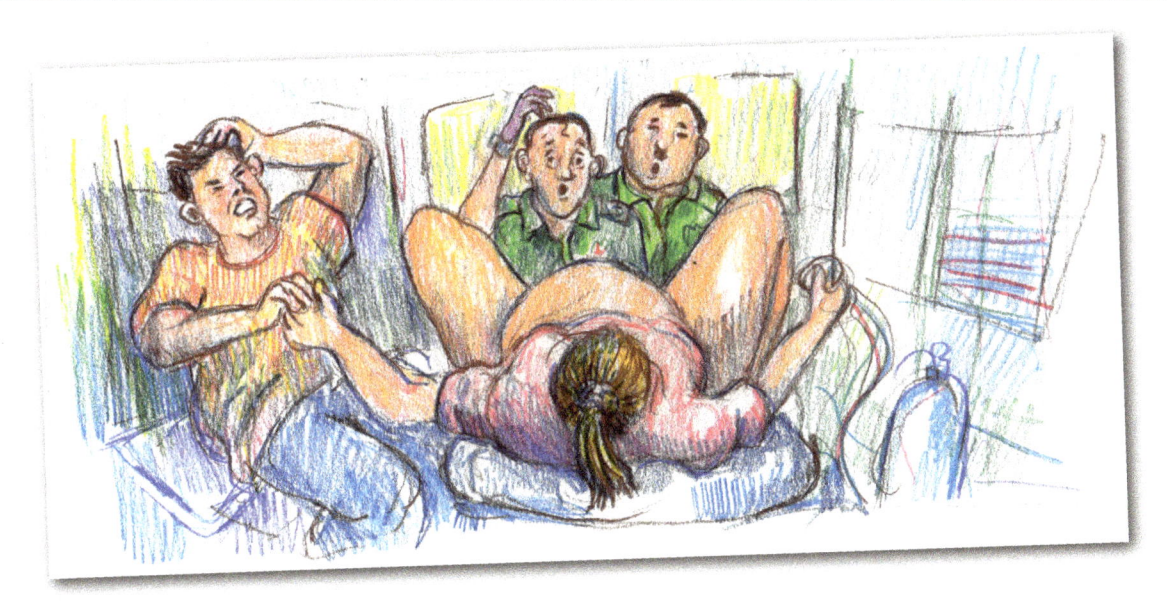

Childbirth Complications

You are on standby with the most vulgar staff member on your station. He is just getting started with his latest bedroom exploits, when you are saved by the MDT passing you brief details of a maternity call. "Another job for the maternataxi," sighs your colleague as you start the ambulance and head for the address. It is not far away and you receive no further details relating to the incident before you arrive at the address a few minutes later.

Your colleague rolls out of the ambulance and saunters up the drive to the house. A maternity pack seems like a good idea, so you grab one before heading to the house. The patient's father is outside, chain-smoking and looking rather pale. He nods towards the front door and you smile in acknowledgement.

Having ascended the steep stairs with a tight quarter-turn near the top, you look straight up into the bathroom to quite a sight. The patient is lying semi-recumbent on the bathroom floor, naked below the waist. The floor looks wet, probably due to the patient's waters breaking. The dad-to-be looks relieved at your presence, but winces as his partner crushes his hand in response to a strong contraction. However, your heart stops as you spot a 10–15 cm loop of umbilical cord that has emerged from the patient's vagina. The patient explains that she had been experiencing strong, but infrequent contractions for a couple of hours when her waters had broken. At this point she had noticed the cord and instructed her husband to phone for an ambulance.

> What are you going to do: **Leave the cord** (read on) or **Replace it into the vagina** (skip the next paragraph)?

Chapter 7   Obstetrics and Gynaecology

Leave the cord

You recall that minimal handling of the cord is a good idea, but know you need to do something with it. You elect to place a dry pad in the patient underwear and contemplate how you are going to get her out of the bathroom and into the ambulance.

Replace it into the vagina

"We need to replace the cord," you say to your colleague, "use two fingers to replace the cord gently into the vagina." Your colleague looks aghast, "What!?" Given the lewd one-sided conversation just prior to the call, you are surprised at his sudden coyness so step in and complete the manoeuvre. With the cord safely inside the vagina, you use a dry dressing in the patient's underwear and plan your next move.

Her contractions are not frequent and you are confident that birth is not imminent. You turn to your colleague and suggest that now would be a good time to head for the nearest consultant-led maternity unit. He looks immensely pleased at this suggestion and with an impressive sleight of hand, pick-pockets the ambulance keys from you and heads off downstairs stating that he will fetch the carry chair. Having already ascended the stairs, you know that this is going to be a tricky carry.

> What are you going to do: **Wait for the carry chair** (read on) or **See if the patient can walk** (skip the next paragraph)?

Wait for the carry chair

Your colleague does not emerge straight away and you are wondering if he is sharing a cigarette with the father downstairs. He emerges from the stairs several minutes later, puffing away. You assist the patient onto the chair and set off down the stairs. Your colleague is profusely perspiring as you struggle round the quarter-turn of the stairs and keeps having to adjust his grip on the bottom of the carry chair. Without warning, the patient yells out as she is struck with a particularly strong contraction and grabs the banister. At the same time, she splays her legs, knocking the greasy hands of your colleague from the chair. He stumbles forward into her lap and the chair starts to descend down the stairs. Only your quick actions prevent you all from negotiating the rest of the stairs at high speed. No one is hurt, but this clearly is not going to work. After untangling everyone from the chair, you all descend the stairs with the patient gingerly walking down the remaining steps (read on).

See if the patient can walk

The patient experiences a particularly strong contraction, but it eases off quickly. She agrees to try the stairs and between you and the husband, she safely makes it down to the ground floor and out of the front door to the ambulance. Your colleague has only just got the carry chair from the ambulance and looks rather miffed that he has to put it back again.

Having made it to the ambulance you assist the patient up the stairs and she reaches the trolley. She eases herself onto the trolley and flops onto her back, clearly exhausted by the whole ordeal. You reach for the Entonox to minimise the effects of the contractions and overhear your colleague chatting to the husband about cava. You set about obtaining some baseline observations and getting the husband aboard and so don't notice straight away that the patient is looking rather pale. It takes a glance at the monitor and a systolic blood pressure

Childbirth Complications

of 85 mmHg to turn your attention back to the patient. You ask her how she is feeling and she complains about feeling dizzy.

> What are you going to do: **Wet the baby's head** (read on) or **Change the mother's position** (skip the next paragraph)?

Wet the baby's head

Your colleague has his eyes on the husband's bottle of cava sticking out of a hastily packed bag. Given that your colleague's driving is bad enough already, without being under the influence of alcohol, this is not a good idea and you suggest that he gets ready to go. Your mind turns to cava … caval … caval occlusion! She needs to be moved off her back and into another position (Read on).

Change the mother's position

Mum lying on her back with a full-term fetus compressing her great vessels is not a good idea and is probably responsible for her dropping blood pressure, so you elect to change her position. You recall that a expectant mothers over 20 weeks should be placed in a left lateral position. On the other hand, an all-fours position with the patient's head down and bottom in the air is good for cord prolapse, but will make it difficult to strap her onto the trolley.

> What position are you going to use: **All-fours** (read on) or **On her side** (skip the next paragraph)?

All-fours

You can only manage to get a seatbelt around the back of the patient's thighs and with your colleague driving the ambulance like he has stolen it, you come unstuck on the first right-hand corner. You lose your balance and the patient rolls over the sidebar, but is saved injury by landing on you. Placing the patient on their side is going to be the safer option.

On her side

All-fours is great, but is not going to work in the ambulance, so you elect to place the patient on her side. However, placing her left lateral will mean she will face the wall and make it harder to continue to support and monitor her en route. Instead, you ask her to roll onto her right side and place a wedge under her hips to raise her pelvis upward releasing the pressure of the baby's head on the cord. With the patient safely strapped in, you are ready to go.

Just before you set off, there is a knock at the door. The view that greets you on opening the door lifts your spirits … it's a community midwife. She steps in and you briefly explain the events so far. "Great, I'll pop a urinary catheter in and we can get off." Your colleague has stuck his head through the bulkhead window and looks rather incredulous. "Can't she have a wee when she gets to hospital?" he asks. He has a point, things seem rather time-critical for a wee. The midwife patiently explains why a catheter is necessary, and sets about inserting it. Once the catheter is in place, she fills the patient's bladder with saline and then clamps the catheter off. That done, you set off for the local maternity hospital and the midwife makes a pre-alert call. The patient is whisked away to theatre for an emergency Caesarean section. Your colleague appears to have recovered as he is chatting up an unimpressed receptionist, leaving you to clean up the vehicle. Just as you are preparing to leave, you are tapped on the shoulder by the midwife. "Mum and baby are doing fine," she beams "and they want to name the baby after you."

Chapter 7 Obstetrics and Gynaecology

The scale of the problem

In 2019, there were over 640,000 births in England and Wales, most of which went without a hitch and resulted in a healthy boy or girl.[9]

Three complications that can occur during childbirth and will be covered in this section include:

- Cord prolapse, which has an annual incidence of 0.1–0.6% (about 4,800 births), although this increases to 1% in breech births.[10]
- Shoulder dystocia, which has an annual incidence of 0.58–0.70% (about 5,600 births).[11]
- Breech presentation, which has an incidence of 20% at 28 weeks, gestation, reducing to 3–4% at term (about 32,000 births).[12]

Stages of labour

Normal labour follows a sequence of progressively painful uterine contractions which cause effacement and dilation of the cervix, descent of the fetus though the maternal pelvis, leading to spontaneous vaginal birth of the baby. Subsequently, the placenta and membranes are expelled.[13] Typical time frames are shown in Table 7.3.

Table 7.3 Typical time frames in labour.

Stage of labour	First pregnancy	Subsequent pregnancies
First	12–14 hours	6–10 hours
Second	60 mins	Up to 30 mins
Third	20–30 mins	20–30 mins

Source: MacDonald & Johnson, 2017.

First stage

This stage commences with the onset of regular contractions, which cause cervical dilation from 0 to 10 cm. Established labour is signified by regular contractions (about 3–4 in 10 minutes) lasting around 1 minute. By 8 cm dilated, women typically become vocal, requesting epidurals and demanding that the baby is born, for example.[14] However, examination of the cervix is only undertaken by a midwife and not a pre-hospital clinician, so other signs of labour must be addressed to make a full assessment.

Second stage

This stage starts once the cervix is fully dilated and ends with the birth of the baby. Women may have a strong urge to push, which can feel similar to the sensation of wanting to open their bowels … which might also happen, so be prepared!

Third stage

After the birth of the baby, the third stage commences, ending with the expulsion of the placenta. If this stage lasts more than 60 minutes, the placenta is classed as being retained, which is why if it is not expelled by 30 minutes out-of-hospital, you must transport the mother to a maternity unit. In addition, if the placenta partially separates, life-threatening haemorrhage can ensue (postpartum haemorrhage).[14]

Cord prolapse

If the umbilical cord descends below the presenting part, it is said to be prolapsed. Note that the presenting part does not actually have to be visible from the introitus (the entrance to the vagina). If this happens, the cord can become occluded by pressure from the presenting part, resulting in serious fetal morbidity or death. It comes in three presentations:[13]

- Cord presentation – Loops of cord below the presenting part, but the membranes remain intact

Childbirth Complications

- Cord prolapse – The membranes rupture and the cord descends below the presenting part
- Occult (hidden) presentation – A loop of cord lies beside the presenting part. This cannot be felt by a vaginal examination.

In the absence of a midwife, you will only know that the cord has prolapsed if you check the introitus, which is why it is vital to perform a visual check if the mother's waters have broken (that is, the membranes have ruptured). Remember NO internal or cervical examinations are permitted in pre-hospital practice.

Management

This is a time-critical emergency. If the mother has been on the phone to a midwife, she may have been advised to adopt a knees to chest position (Figure 7.5), but this is not a practical position to transport her in an ambulance.

Assuming birth is not imminent, get the mother onto the ambulance trolley as quickly as possible. If you can get the trolley alongside, that is great; otherwise walk her to the ambulance. Do not use a carry chair as this can compress the cord.

Once on the trolley (in or out of the ambulance), place the mother in the right lateral position with hips raised, either with blankets or a vacuum splint under her hips (Figure 7.6), or by placing the trolley in the Trendelenburg position (that is, feet end of the trolley raised and head lowered).[8]

Make one attempt to replace a small loop into the vagina using a dry pad. If this is successful, cover with a dry pad to prevent further prolapse.[3] If this is not possible or a large loop of cord has prolapsed, handle the cord as little as possible; excessive handling can lead to cord spasm and fetal hypoxia.[14]

If there is a midwife or other suitably trained clinician present, they may elect to insert a urinary catheter and fill the bladder with 500–750 mls of normal saline before clamping it off. The filled bladder applies pressure to the presenting part, lifting it off the cord which is why midwives are advised to carry a urinary catheter for this purpose.[10]

You know the last bit … prompt transport to a consultant-led obstetric unit, with a clear pre-alert stating you are bringing in a visible cord prolapse.

Shoulder dystocia

A shoulder dystocia is a term applied to vaginal cephalic births where the baby's

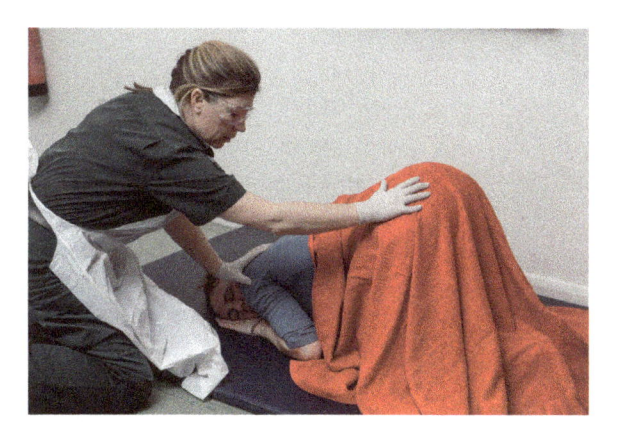

Figure 7.5 The knees to chest position. Not suitable for ambulance transport.

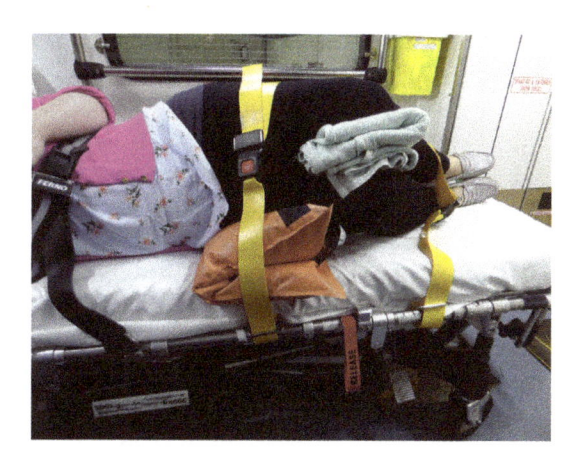

Figure 7.6 Right lateral with hips raised.

anterior shoulder becomes impacted on the maternal symphysis pubis, requiring specific manoeuvres in order to facilitate the birth.[11] Shoulder dystocia is difficult to predict prior to birth, with around 50% of cases having no risk factors and in babies of normal birth weight.[14]

In the late second stage of labour, a clue that shoulder dystocia is a possibility is head bobbing, where the fetal head is visible during contractions, but retracts in between. At the time of delivery, you may see the 'turtle neck sign', where the fetal chin retracts tightly onto mother's perineum and the fetal neck is not visible at all.[11]

Management

First and foremost in this situation, it is important to remember to keep calm. If the clinician is panicking, the effect of adrenaline on their actions is more likely to result in damage to the fetus from the application of excessive downward traction. This is where human factors often play a part, as becoming task-fixated can negatively impact on the situation. The brain can become overwhelmed at this point and this is when crucial errors can be made.

Considering the following when managing a shoulder dystocia:[3]

- Shoulder dystocia is diagnosed if the baby fails to be born in two contractions following the complete birth of the head. But remember there is normally a break after the birth of the baby's head before the body is born. Don't jump in too soon.
- First, keep your emergency operations centre (EOC) updated: call in and state your emergency and request the presence of a midwife.
- Do not panic. This is easy to say, but the most common injury caused to the baby during a shoulder dystocia is a brachial plexus injury or Erb's palsy, where there is hyperextension of the brachial plexus nerve causing damage to the nervous control of the baby's arm. This is caused by the hyperflexion of the fetal head being pulled downwards during attempts to deliver the baby. This is avoided by only applying axial traction, that is, traction applied in the direction of the baby's axial skeleton, and definitely not downwards (Figure 7.7).
- Do not cut or interfere with the baby's umbilical cord. Cutting of the cord will deprive the baby further of oxygen.
- Do not put pressure or push on the top of the uterus, the fundus, as this will just cause further impaction on the shoulder.
- Lay the mother flat with one pillow under her head and bring her knees up towards her chest. This causes the natural action of abduction around the abdomen into the McRoberts' position. This should ideally be conducted with a minimum of three persons, two taking a leg each and then the third delivering the baby. If you do not have three members of staff then utilise any persons who happen to be on scene, such as a mother or partner. If there is no one then the mother may be able to hold her own legs, but remember that the idea of

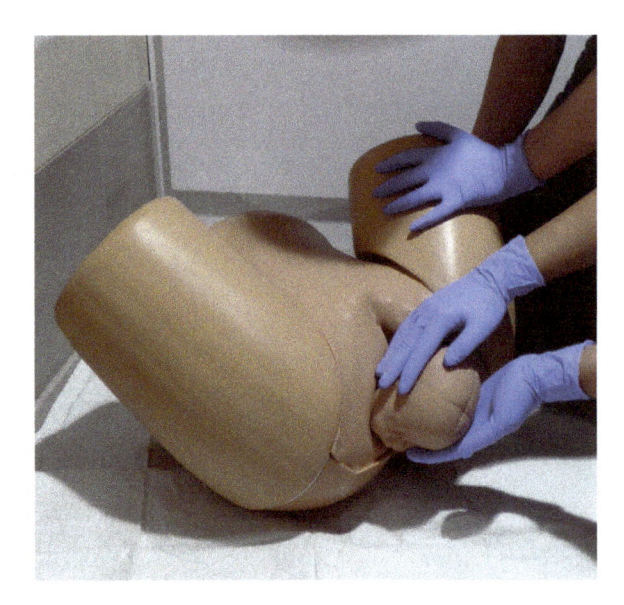

Figure 7.7 Axial traction.

Childbirth Complications

this posture is that the hips are abducted and the pelvis tilted and if the mother tires then the position will be ineffective. For lone workers it is recommended to use the all-fours position first, as detailed later.
- If you are lucky enough to have two crews and four clinicians, then two clinicians will each take one of the legs while the third attempts to deliver the baby and the fourth person sets up the newborn resuscitation area.
- For 30 seconds attempt to deliver the baby's body in the McRoberts' position with axial traction applied to the baby's head. If the baby has failed to deliver, then the next step is to apply suprapubic pressure. This should be applied in combination with McRoberts' and axial traction.
- To apply suprapubic pressure, first identify the fetal back – this should be the side where the occiput is – then ask your assistant to apply steady constant pressure with the heel of the hand, using the same hand position as when performing CPR, two fingers above the symphysis pubis in the direction of the fetal face. The objective is to reduce the shoulder diameter in order for the anterior shoulder to be delivered under the symphysis pubis (Figure 7.8).
- Perform this for 30 seconds with the direct pressure being applied. If this has not facilitated the birth of the baby, another 30 seconds should be performed with a gentle 'rocking' motion. If after 30 seconds of pushing using intermittent pressure the shoulders have still not delivered, then the mother should be turned in the all-fours position, sometimes referred to as the Gaskin manoeuvre.
- Position the mother on her hands and knees with her hips well flexed and bottom elevated and her head as low as possible. Apply axial traction to the baby's head in order to try and deliver the posterior shoulder from the sacral hollow first. In some studies this has been shown to have a success rate of 83% when used.
- If after 30 seconds the shoulders still fail to deliver, undertake a time-critical transfer to the nearest consultant-led obstetric unit. Do not await the arrival of the midwife.

If the mother is upstairs in the house, she cannot sit on a carry chair for extraction, so she will have to walk. The best way to assist this is to get her dressing gown, ask her to put it on and tie the cord over her abdomen. This will not only protect her modesty, but by getting her to pull the tails of the dressing gown through her legs it can form a sling. She will then need to walk backwards down the stairs, which helps to move the pelvis and may help to dislodge the shoulder. The sling effect of the dressing gown may help to catch the baby if it is born halfway down the stairs – remember that this movement may facilitate and precipitate the birth, so do not move your hands too far away from baby's head.

Once the mother is on the stretcher lay her on her side and fully strap her in – her safety is paramount. Place a pillow or blanket between her knees to prevent her leg crushing the baby's head. Allow her to keep using the

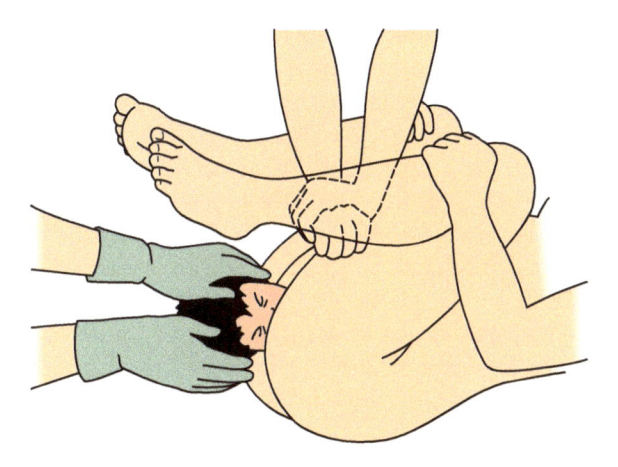

Figure 7.8 Applying suprapubic pressure with a woman in the McRoberts' position.

Chapter 7 Obstetrics and Gynaecology

Entonox, and if she needs to keep pushing don't discourage her but if it has not worked with the manoeuvres just mentioned, then it will probably not work now.

A pre-alert should be placed to the nearest consultant-led obstetric unit and an estimated time of how long the head has been born should be given.

There is no evidence as to how the baby will respond after a period of extended dystocia. The delay between the birth of the head and the body can lead to cord compression and hypoxia. The healthy well-grown baby will initially compensate well, but as the delay time increases so will the degree of acidosis, and a hypoxic brain injury can develop. However, this risk is small if the delay interval is less than 5 minutes. If the baby is born after a period of dystocia, then newborn resuscitation is very likely to be required.

Documentation

Documentation is key with any patient contact. Don't forget that if it's not written down (or typed!) then it didn't happen. It is also worth remembering that any documentation relating to a maternity care episode should be kept for a minimum of 25 years.

With this in mind, there are a few key points that are essential to include along with your standard documentation of primary and secondary surveys, for example:

- Time the head was born
- The direction that the baby's back was positioned, for example, the fetal back was located on the maternal right with the face pointing towards the mother's left leg
- That gentle axial traction was applied
- Which manoeuvres were employed and the order in which they were utilised
- The time of the birth of the baby's body
- Any apparent injuries at the time of birth
- The condition of the baby at birth

Breech presentation

In a breech presentation, the fetus enters the birth canal with buttocks or feet first, rather than the more usual, head first. The most common presentations are shown in Table 7.4.[13]

Breech presentations are similar to normal labour except that you may see buttocks, feet or the soles of the feet during your assessment of the introitus. In addition, the genitals may look bruised and swollen, and meconium may be present (looking a bit like black toothpaste).[15]

Management

A woman who is in labour with a baby in the breech position will experience the same normal contractions with her labour progressing in the same way as a head-down or cephalic presentation; however, on inspection at the vaginal opening, the following may be visible:

- The buttocks
- Feet or soles of the feet
- Swollen or bruised genitalia (because of the pressure on the genitals)
- Frank meconium, in a string like black toothpaste (because the lower abdomen is squeezed during the birth).

If the woman has a known breech presentation and birth is not imminent, but the patient is in labour, the clinician must decide whether there is time to transfer the woman to her booked unit. If labour is too far advanced, then the baby must be born on scene. This is a difficult decision to make as the clinician needs to avoid the birth taking place on the ambulance at all costs, although – as we all know – births do not always go according to plan and labour can progress rapidly without warning.

When dealing with a birth of any kind the clinician must have a full situational

Childbirth Complications

Table 7.4 Common breech presentations.

Presentation	Incidence	Explanation	
Frank	65%	Bottom-first with legs flexed at the hip and extended at the knees.	
Complete	25%	Hips and knees are flexed resulting in the fetus sitting cross-legged, with feet beside the bottom.	
Footling	10%	One or both feet come first, with bottom higher up. Rare presentation at term, but common in premature births.	

Adapted from: MacDonald & Johnson, 2017.

awareness, must be aware to request help when required, and must have a clear grasp on time frames as these can so easily slip out of hand. Don't forget to request a midwife to assist on scene. In many areas a community midwifery service is unavailable; however, you don't know unless you ask!

This not only gives you a valuable resource on scene but also may negate the need for conveyance to hospital if the woman can be discharged to the midwife on scene. One thing that must never happen with ANY birth, whether head- or bottom-first, is for a woman in the second stage of labour to be moved. Birth on the ambulance must always be avoided where possible.

There are several factors that you should consider when making a decision to transport a woman in labour (Table 7.5).

The stages of a breech birth

The recommended position to assist the birth of a breech baby is the all-fours position (see Figure 7.5 on page 211).[16–19] This position allows gravity to play a really important role and allows the clinician to remain completely hands off when necessary. The mother should be encouraged to move into this position, but if she prefers, she can be positioned on the edge of a chair or sofa or bed, ensuring that there is no touching of the baby but that the baby has sufficient space to be able to hang and allow gravity to perform most of the birth.

Once the presenting part is visible (for example, the bottom), it will advance and withdraw in a similar way to a head. You will typically see a line of meconium appearing from the bottom like a string of black toothpaste. Do not touch this or wipe it, just

Chapter 7   Obstetrics and Gynaecology

Table 7.5 Factors to consider when considering transport.

Gestation	A pre-term infant is harder to manage in the pre-hospital environment, so whether the baby is cephalic or breech, if you can get to the hospital safely then (as with all births) transfer. The pre-term infant is also more likely to need some assistance with its transition and possibly even resuscitation.
Parity	The higher the parity of the woman, the more rapid the birth is likely to be; always evaluate with great caution if the baby is not the woman's first.
Location – close to hospital or isolated	Your geographic location is really important as you will know how long it will take you to reach an appropriate care facility. Remember it may be much quicker to get a midwife to you than to take the woman to the midwife!
Weather conditions – thick snow or ice	The weather will have a large impact on your decision to move. Fine weather will obviously make any journey run more smoothly; inclement weather will add time to your journey and will increase danger factors, such as skidding off the road in icy conditions.
Driving conditions, for example, rush hour traffic	This again will depend on your location: if you are in a very rural area, then rush hour may not apply to you. However, trying to get across busy cities in the height of traffic will again add those precious minutes to your journey time, even with blue lights and sirens.
Is a midwife available or can one be summoned?	As previously stated, it may be quicker and safer to get the midwife to you instead of trying to transfer a woman in labour. Even if you have not had success in the past, it is always worth a telephone conversation with your local maternity unit or midwife-led unit to try and get the midwife out. This also means that if the birth is straightforward there is no need to transfer the woman and her newborn to hospital at all, and they can be left in the care of the midwife in their own home. However, never leave a woman at home without having a midwife physically there with you to accept the direct handover.
How difficult the extraction from the house will be	If you are on the 20th floor of a block of flats you need to consider again whether it is actually safer to remain there on scene than to risk having a baby born in a stairwell or stuck in a lift.
What are the home conditions/environmental factors?	Not everyone lives in good-quality housing and has a good quality of living. If the environmental factors are such that you feel it safer to be in the vehicle, for example, you are presented with a squat or a shared house with no privacy, then the vehicle may be a safer option – just remain stationary!
Is the room warm/clean?	If the room is not warm and has no method of heating, then the vehicle may be a better alternative. The cleanliness may not be up to your standards but remember they will be living there with the baby afterwards. However, as before, if the woman is in the second stage you will have to stay put and make the best that you can of the situation. Keeping the newborn dry and warm is your primary priority.

Childbirth Complications

allow it to fall. When the widest part of the bottom is born, this is known as the 'rumping' – like the crowning as the head is born, just the opposite way round!

Once the rumping has occurred then the bottom will twist clockwise and the legs should now be directly facing you (Figure 7.9). This is where you need to remember the mantra 'baby's tum to mum's bum' or 'baby's bum to mum's tum' as this will help you to remember the way the baby should be positioned: they should always be looking at one another.

Once the baby is born up to the umbilicus (Figure 7.10), then a timer should be started. The baby should be born within 3–5 minutes of the umbilicus becoming visible, so these births are a lot quicker than a head-down birth. Do not touch the baby at this point, nor should you pull or touch the cord for any reason. Most definitely do not cut or clamp the umbilical cord until the head is born.

If the baby is in the frank breech position, with the legs fully extended upwards, then the legs will normally birth together or just after each other (Figure 7.11). Encourage the mother to bear down and push with her contractions and don't touch the baby.

As the birth progresses there are several signs you can look for that will indicate a healthy baby at this point:

- The baby will have good tone.
- The baby will be a good colour, that is, purple/blue.
- The cord will be full.
- The valley of the cord is visible (the crease that runs up the chest wall will be like a valley).
- The baby will do the characteristic 'tummy crunches' movement that is normal to encourage the birth of the arms and head.

Don't interfere with the baby during the crunches. These are the natural movements that the baby will make in order to get them into the position needed to allow the arms and head to be born. Don't worry if the baby doesn't crunch but this will lead to a slower descent and the baby will be more likely to need resuscitation.

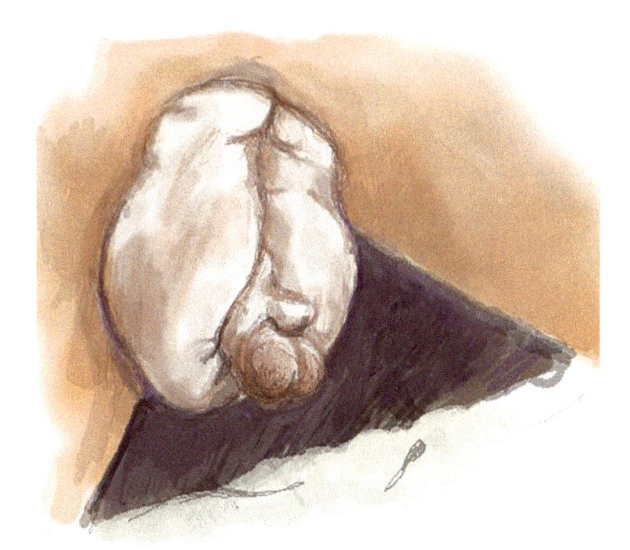

Figure 7.9 Following rotation this is the 'tum to bum' position.

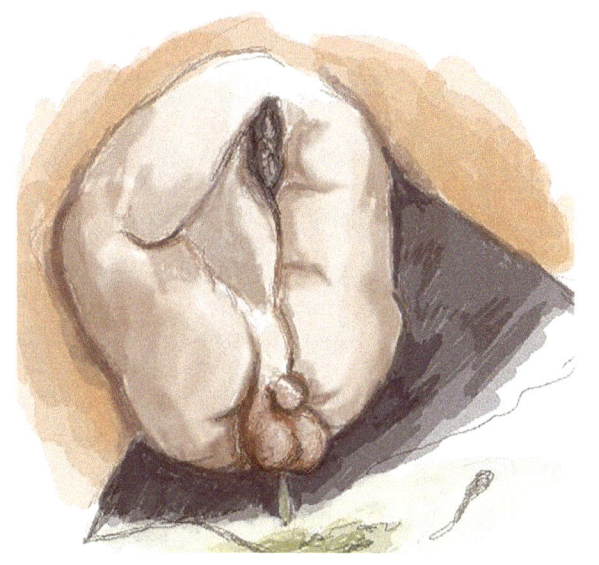

Figure 7.10 Once the baby has been born up to the umbilicus, start the timer.

217

Chapter 7 Obstetrics and Gynaecology

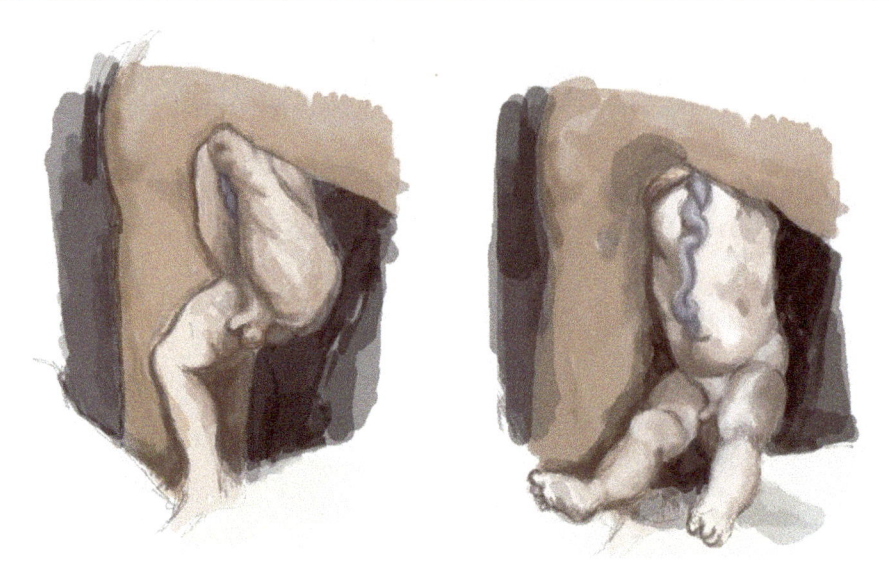

Figure 7.11   The legs will normally birth together or just after each other.

Do not pull on the baby's abdomen in an attempt to expedite the birth as this may cause the baby to raise its arms in utero causing nuchal arms (arms which are raised over the head).

Once the arms are free, then again, leave the baby and do not interfere with the natural physiology. This is often the most unnerving time and the point at which most clinicians want to take hold and hold the baby upward as they fear it will damage the neck. This is the worst thing you can do right now! If you hold the baby at this point the head will not engage in the pelvis and it may stop the baby from being born at all.

Once you see the chin, the head is almost there (Figure 7.12). The head has to contend

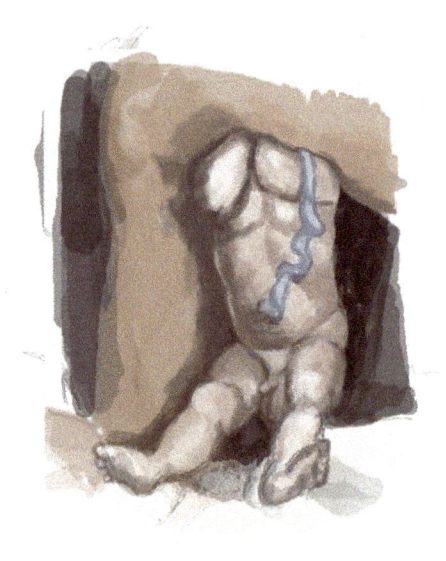

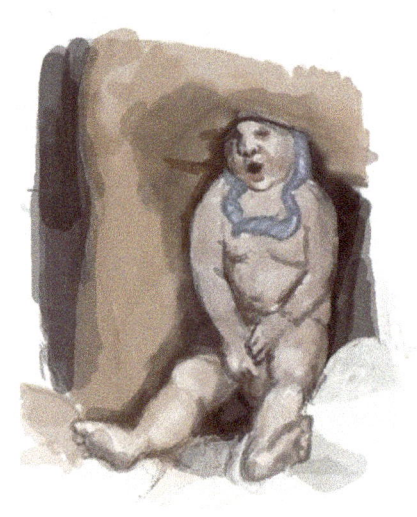

Figure 7.12   The head is born.

with the curve of the vagina just as it does in a head-down birth, but the opposite way round. So the first time that you have to touch the baby is as the head emerges and you are there to catch the baby as the head is freed from the birth canal.

If a slow descent is happening, there are a few key tips recommended by the Breech Birth Network (https://breechbirth.org.uk):

1. Encourage movement: get the mother to rock her hips from side to side to shake the baby downwards.
2. Get the mother to adopt the 'running start' position like a runner in the blocks of a race with one knee lifted; this will open the outlet of the pelvis.
3. A gentle shoulder press when the chin is born, pushing the baby backwards, can facilitate the birth of the head.

The baby born in the breech presentation is more likely to be covered in meconium and is also more likely to require some form of resuscitation. As well as this, they are at risk of getting cold as they have hung out wet and without wrapping.

If there is any other body part presenting, other than head, buttocks or feet (for example, a hand or arm), then this requires an immediate rapid transfer to an obstetric facility with pre-alert placed.

Chapter 7   Obstetrics and Gynaecology

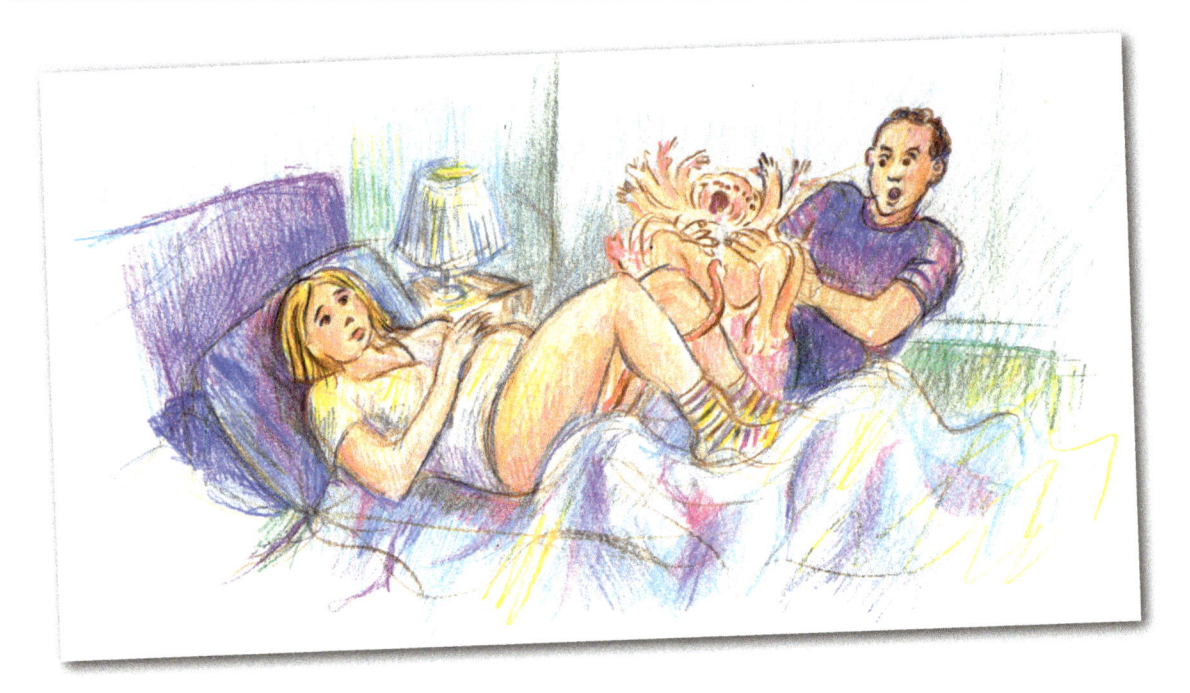

Postpartum Haemorrhage

You are on standby, trying to get your feet to thaw out when the MDT passes you details of your next job. "Female, 37, in labia, connections 2 minutes apart." Your colleague guffaws at the errors in the message before moaning about how they "can't be bothered to get in the car in case their waters break on the velour seats."

The address is at least 20 minutes away, even on blue lights and with your former rally driving colleague at the wheel, but you head off, tyres screaming and lights and sirens blazing. You call up the emergency operations centre (EOC) and ask if a rapid response vehicle (RRV) has been dispatched. "Sorry, you're the nearest, and only, response," the dispatcher cheerfully replies, "oh, and they're giving birth instructions on the line too." Your colleague catches your eye and gives you an 'I'm glad you're attending' look.

You pull up at the address and find the front door open, with an anxious woman just inside who mutters "Quick, up the stairs! I've never seen anything like this." You grab the response bag and the maternity pack, and shout at your colleague to leave the heater running and bring the monitor up. As you ascend the stairs you can hear the beautiful sound of a newborn roaring. At least that's one open airway! You give a brief knock on the bedroom door and say, "Hello, ambulance service." "Quick, in here, she's bleeding bad!" says a voice from inside the room. As you enter the small back bedroom, you can't help thinking that having a sneaky peek at the postpartum haemorrhage guidelines would have been more useful than newborn life support. Patricia, the new mum, is on the bed, propped up with several pillows and naked apart from her top. Her partner, Dom, is holding a beautiful baby boy but looking rather scared. The baby is crying with good tone and is pink all over, and you assign a top APGAR score of 10. There is a towel at the bottom of the bed, which you pass to Dom and ask him to dry the baby, before wrapping it in a clean one. There is a pool of blood, approximately 300 ml, collecting between Patricia's legs and the cord is still attached.

> What are you going to do: **Cut the cord** (read on) or **Leave it intact until it has stopped pulsating** (skip the next paragraph)?

Cut the cord

Your colleague arrives just as you are wielding the cord scissors. "Hold on," she exclaims, "the cord is still pulsating." She patiently explains to you that cutting the cord immediately at birth is no longer standard practice and although the exact duration of the delay has not been determined,[20] ambulance guidelines state that there should be a minimum delay of one minute following birth.[3]

Leave it intact

You remember an article you read recently about the benefits of delayed cord clamping. Allowing the baby to receive all the blood from the cord resulted in a number of benefits including:[20]

- Improving iron and ferritin levels
- Increased blood volume
- Providing antibodies
- Providing stem-cells
- Providing an oxygenated blood supply.

You place the baby skin-to-skin with Patricia as you seem to remember this causes the release of oxytocin to aid in placental delivery, and also helps the newborn adjust to the extra-uterine environment and the regulation of breathing, heart rate and temperature.[21]

Five minutes has now elapsed, and on checking the cord, you notice that it has gone flat and opaque. Your colleague has helpfully checked Patricia's observations and found the following:

Airway

Patent

Breathing

Respiratory rate: 18 breaths/min
SpO_2: 98% on air

Circulation

Pulse: 88 beats/min and regular
Blood pressure: 110/62 mmHg.

Now that the cord has stopped pulsating you clamp and cut it, placing the clamps 2 cm apart and cutting between, taking care not to inadvertently amputate any fingers or genitalia. This done, you hand the baby to Patricia. As she tries to sit up a little, you notice a gush of blood (about 100 ml) and the cut end of the cord starts to lengthen, so you encourage Patricia to give a push. She can feel something coming out, so you grab a clinical waste bag and catch the placenta.

With the blood loss in the region of 400 ml, you ask your colleague to repeat Patricia's observations. You ask Patricia if you can palpate her uterus to give you an idea about where the bleeding is coming from. Starting just above her umbilicus, you palpate downwards, heading for the symphysis. As you reach the umbilicus, you feel a soft mass, which feels suspiciously like an atonic uterus. You recall a CPD session, where the midwife talked

Chapter 7 Obstetrics and Gynaecology

about 'rubbing up a uterus' and you struggle to picture her hands working in a circular motion, rubbing and squeezing the top of the fundus. With that vision in your mind, you do the same to Patricia and, after doing this for a brief period, notice the mass firming up and dropping just below the umbilicus. At the same time, Patricia expels a large clot, which the midwife said was normal, and you continue massaging for several more minutes until the uterus has contracted into a cricket ball.

You estimate that Patricia's blood loss has now reached approximately 500 ml, but her observations remain unchanged. Although you recall that the pregnant patient's physiological changes allow for a 50% loss of their circulating blood volume without a significant change in their observations, you decide that intravenous access would be a good idea.

You reach for the cannulation pack and, after assessing Patricia's veins, decide that the largest cannula you can confidently place is a 16 gauge. As you prepare to cannulate, Patricia asks if it is okay to breastfeed the baby. This is a great idea as it will produce more oxytocin to help keep the uterus contracted. As an added bonus, since this is Patricia's fourth baby, she is able to feed with one hand, while you cannulate the other.

Your colleague returns from her third trip up and down the stairs, having taken the kit back to the vehicle and fetched the carry chair. "I'm not sitting on that, I can walk," says Patricia loudly, attempting to get herself up out of bed while still breastfeeding, as if to prove the point. You explain with your patient voice, normally reserved for cantankerous elderly folk, that she has lost a significant amount of blood and a walk down the stairs and out to the ambulance is not a good idea. Patricia is not happy.

What are you going to do: **Allow her to walk** (read on), or **Carry her** (skip the next paragraph)?

Allow her to walk

Patricia detaches the baby from her breast and hands it to you, gets up off the bed and pulls on a long night dress while trying to find some underwear. Having gathered her things, packed her bag, given instructions to Dom about how to look after the remaining children, she announces that she is ready to go. You make a feeble attempt at asking her to go on the carry chair and she tells you to shush and stop faffing. Things go well until the fourth step down when she suddenly grabs the handrail and complains of feeling dizzy and lightheaded. You manage to sit her on the stairs and hand the baby to Dom, who has just appeared, wondering what the commotion is all about. Next, you succeed in getting Patricia to the bottom of the stairs by asking her to shuffle on her bottom, finally reaching the carry chair, which your colleague had the good sense not to return to the vehicle.

Carry her

Patricia puts up some resistance about sitting on the carry chair, but you know that that amount of blood loss is enough to risk her collapsing halfway down those stairs. She eventually relents when you put on your serious voice and look as grumpy as she does. Having relented, she turns her wrath on Dom, as he scurries about packing her hospital bag. Just to add to his workload, you hand the baby over for dressing and ask that he is placed in the car seat you almost fell over on the way in. Patricia pulls on a nightdress and her underwear and sits down in the carry chair. You are soon sitting her on the ambulance trolley and repeating her observations, which show a slight increase in heart rate and drop in blood pressure.

Dom appears with baby all snug and strapped into his car seat. You pull down the attendant's chair and strap the car seat on it securely. Keeping the baby close will help to keep that oxytocin flowing. You check her uterus to ensure it is still well contracted, which it is, but there is a large amount of blood on her maternity pad. She is secured onto the stretcher and all your kit is stowed securely. Your colleague clambers into the cab and asks if you have called the maternity unit?

You haven't, but don't tell your colleague and quietly make the call while she is tuning the radio. A cheerful sounding midwife answers the phone and you tell her what has been going on. She enquires about your estimated time of arrival (ETA).

> What type of transfer do you want: **Slow and steady** (read on) or **Blue light** (skip the next paragraph)?

Slow and steady

There's no rush, you are only 40 minutes away in normal traffic, and given your colleague's driving, the slow option is probably better. Patricia's blood pressure has fallen slightly to 101/60 mmHg and her pulse is around 90 beats/min. However, she is happily chatting about her other three children and the journey is uneventful. Just as you are turning into the maternity entrance, she starts to complain of feeling dizzy and lightheaded. Her pulse has risen to 110 beats/min and as you pull back the blanket, you notice that she has bled through her pads and underwear, and another 300 mls of blood is collecting on the stretcher. You palpate Patricia's uterus and find it back above the umbilicus again, soft and completely non-contracted. You massage her uterus to make it contract but seem to have lost your touch. You are still massaging her uterus as you roll through the maternity unit doors. The cheery midwife takes one look at the pale and tired-looking Patricia and chides you for not telling her she had bled so much. She catches a student midwife coming out of a delivery room and tells her to, "Run and get me an oxytocin drip, quickly."

Blue light

Given the blood loss so far, you are concerned about your ability to manage further significant bleeding in the back of an ambulance, and so elect for a 20-minute blue light journey. You pass on your concerns about the blood loss and the midwife assures you that she will have everything ready. With a slight drop in her blood pressure and a rise in pulse, you elect to set up an infusion of normal saline, but don't connect it to Patricia to avoid inadvertent infusion. You chat with Patricia on the way in, making regular checks to ensure the uterus remains contracted and enquire about her previous three pregnancies. She tells you that the last two required a drip to stop the bleeding after giving birth.

It takes only 15 minutes for you to reach the maternity unit, but you can see another 100 ml on Patricia's pads. As you make your way into the maternity unit you find the cheerful midwife, who greets you and indicates that you should enter a nearby room. A doctor comes in straight away to review Patricia and before you have even stripped and made up the stretcher, she has been started on an oxytocin infusion and is feeding the new baby again.

Scale of the problem

Primary postpartum haemorrhage (PPH) is defined by the World Health Organization (WHO) as a blood loss greater than 500 ml within 24 hours of birth.[22] It affects around 18% of vaginal births, although only a little over 1% involve major PPH, which is a blood loss of over 1000 ml.[23] The latest triennial report by MBRRACE-UK (Mothers and Babies: Reducing Risk through Audits and Confidential Enquiries across the UK) reported six maternal deaths that were caused by PPH, with a failure to measure routine observations a key contributing factor.[24] Globally, the problem is much greater, with 140,000 deaths each year. This equates to one woman dying every 4 minutes, making it the

Chapter 7 Obstetrics and Gynaecology

4th most common cause of maternal mortality worldwide.[25]

Anatomy and physiology

In a healthy adult, normal blood volume is approximately 5 litres, but in late pregnancy, physiological changes mean that in a healthy woman the circulating blood volume is closer to 6–7 litres, allowing for the blood loss that occurs with childbirth. In addition, there is an increase in clotting factors, which also provide physiological protection against haemorrhage at the time of birth.[23] However, although some women will tolerate losses of up to 1 litre with no apparent effect on their haemodynamic status, other women may be symptomatic with much smaller volumes, so it is important not to be complacent.

Risk factors

As with many aspects of obstetrics, there is no definitive list as to who will suffer a PPH and who will not, but there are a number of risk factors that make a PPH more likely:[14]

- Multiparity greater than 5
- Advancing maternal age
- Previous PPH or APH
- Long labour
- Obesity
- Anything that increases the size of the uterus (multiple pregnancy, large baby, excess liquor)
- Uterine fibroids
- Partial separation of the placenta.

Pre-hospital management

The management of the PPH depends on the cause of the bleeding, so it is important to determine this early in your assessment. There are four main causes of PPH, known as the four Ts:[26]

- Tone
- Tissue
- Trauma
- Thrombin.

Figure 7.13 can help you differentiate between the causes.

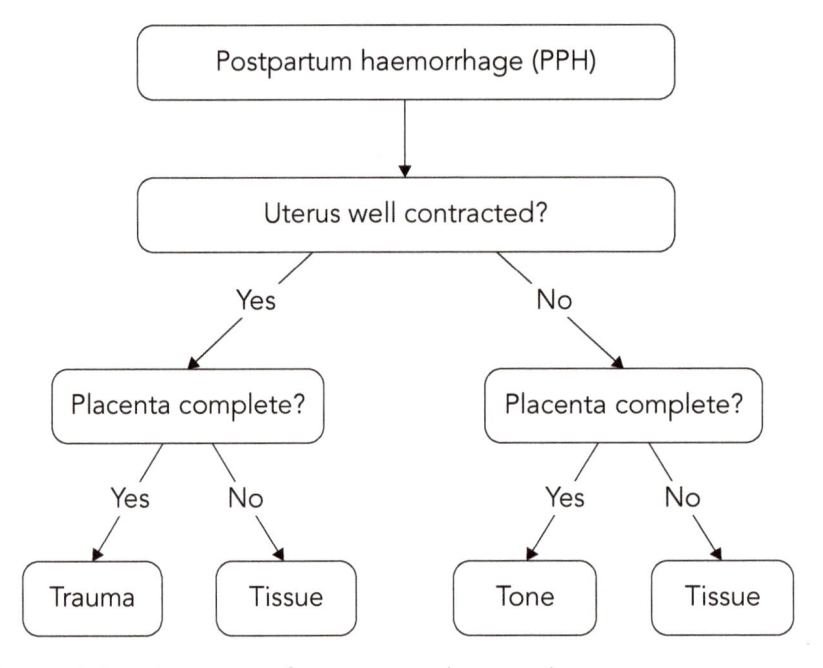

Figure 7.13 Determining the cause of postpartum haemorrhage.

Postpartum Haemorrhage

Tone

Uterine atony (poor tone of the uterus) is the cause of 70–90% of PPHs. Usually the uterus contracts after birth, occluding the spiral arteries that have provided the blood supply to the placenta during pregnancy (Figure 7.14).

In order to control the blood loss from an atonic uterus, the upper portion of the uterus (called the fundus) must be massaged to encourage the uterine fibres to contract. To perform fundal massage, start at the umbilicus and apply firm pressure backwards towards the aorta and then downwards towards the uterus in a circular cupping motion. This will encourage the contraction of the uterus (Figure 7.15). As this is an uncomfortable procedure, it is important to remember to inform the patient of what you are about to

Uterus and placenta before separation
- Muscle layer of uterus
- Maternal blood vessels
- 'Living ligatures'
- Plane of separation
- Membranes
- Umbilical cord

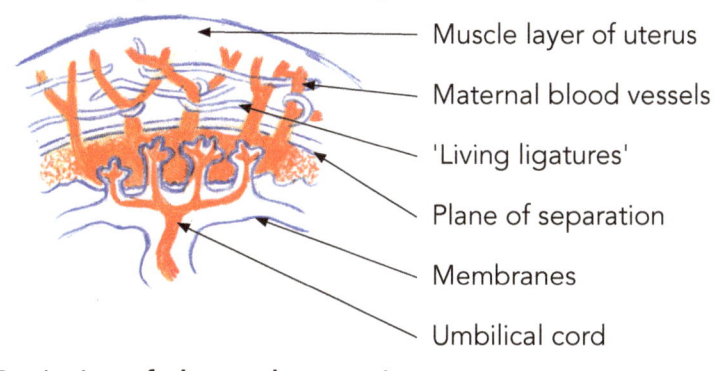

Beginning of placental separation
- Retraction causes fibres to shorten, clamping spiral arteries
- Septa torn, leading to separation
- Veins in spongy layer of decidua become tense and burst
- Villi collapse as blood is released

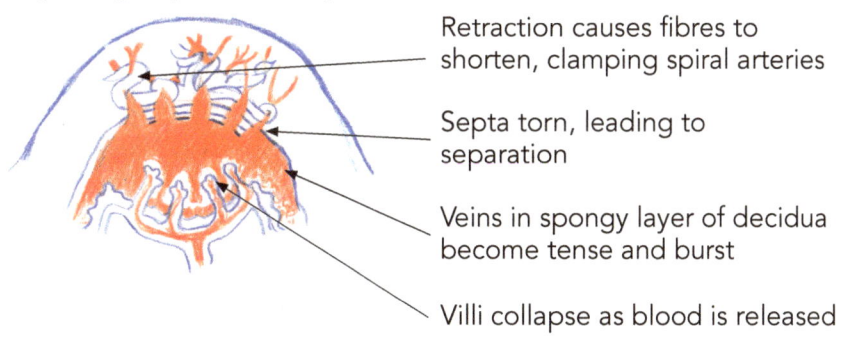

Placental separation almost complete
- Clamped spiral arteries collapse
- Blood tracks between placenta and decidua completing the separation

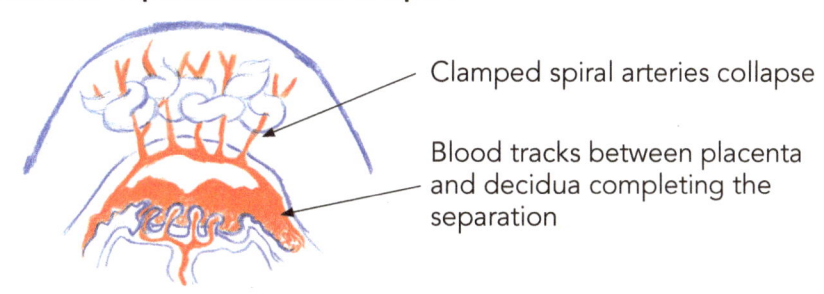

Figure 7.14   The placental site during separation.

perform and why, gain consent and ensure appropriate analgesia is utilised.

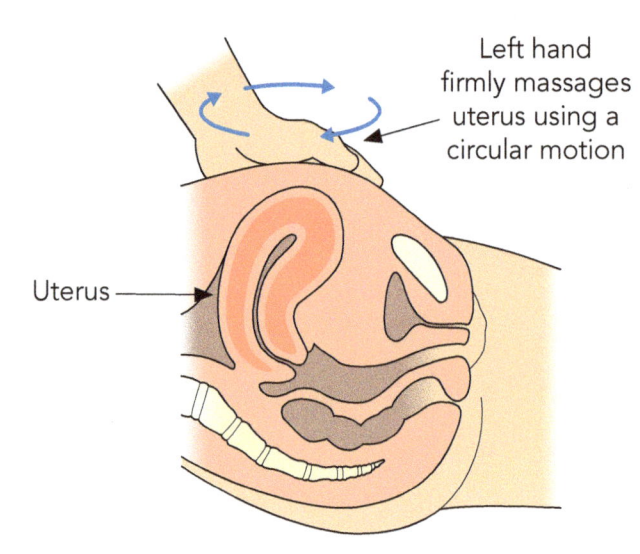

Figure 7.15 Fundal massage.

Trauma

Trauma to the genital tract during childbirth occurs in approximately 85% of births.[27] These are wide ranging in terms of severity, from small tears that only involve the skin of the perineum, to deeper tears that affect the muscle layers. Due to an abundant vascular supply, 20% of PPHs are caused by tears.[26] The bleeding can originate from the tear or ruptured vessels within the tissue. Definitive management is suturing of the perineum, but direct external pressure with a maternity pad or gauze is the mainstay of pre-hospital management.

Tissue

If there are any tissues left behind after the birth, such as the placenta or membranes, the uterus will continue bleeding in order to remove them. This mechanism is responsible for around 10% of PPHs.[26] Retained products may be expelled during fundal massage, causing clots and tissue to be expelled. This is nothing to worry about! The completeness of the placenta and membranes is important, so keep the placenta with the mother so it can be checked to ensure it is complete.

Thrombin

Clotting problems are rare, being responsible for 1% of PPHs. The most serious is disseminated intravascular coagulopathy (DIC), an extremely rare complication, where there is a systemic increase in coagulation and clot formation, with simultaneous impairment of fibrinolysis. This process consumes clotting factors and platelets, leading to abnormal and uncontrolled haemorrhage.

Extreme cases

In extreme cases there are some occasions where no therapy will stop the bleeding. In cases like this, bimanual compression may be life-saving. However, once this has been implemented, the clinician cannot remove their hands, so thinking ahead is essential. It is an invasive procedure, so clearly explain what it involves to both the patient and their partner/relatives and gain consent if possible. To perform bimanual compression, place your dominant hand into the vagina to form a fist, with the dorsum (the side you insert a cannula) facing downwards. Simultaneously, place your other hand onto the abdomen and apply pressure behind the fundus to compress the uterus between your hands (Figure 7.16).[22] The pressure exerted onto the bleeding site from the internal angle of the vagina is more effective than the external massage alone. This needs to be continued until a definitive care facility is reached. This intervention is recommended as a first-line treatment by RCOG in conjunction with pharmacological measures.[28]

Drug therapy

Syntometrine

Syntometrine is a synthetic version of the maternal hormone oxytocin combined with

Postpartum Haemorrhage

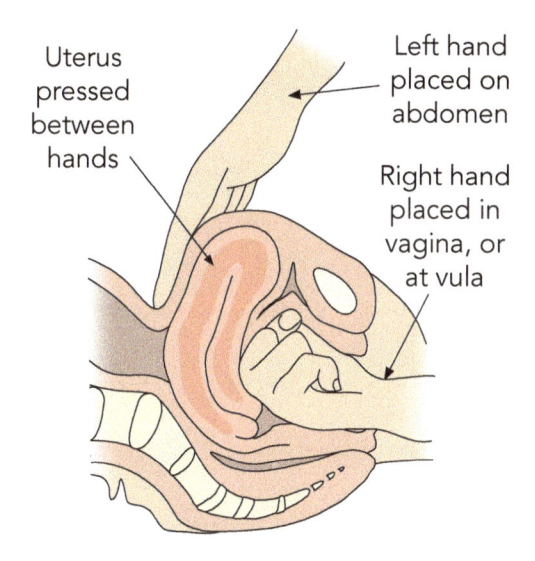

Uterus pressed between hands

Left hand placed on abdomen

Right hand placed in vagina, or at vula

Figure 7.16 Bimanual compression.

ergometrine, a fungus utilised for its uterotonic (increasing tone of the uterus) properties. It causes contraction of the uterine muscle fibres, stemming the blood loss from the placental bed and encouraging the placenta to shear off the uterine wall (Figure 7.17), whereby it can be removed using a process of controlled traction. Midwives and obstetricians administer Syntometrine prior to delivery of the placenta in order to conduct an active third stage. In paramedic practice, its intramuscular administration is reserved for the management of PPH, but note that the full effect of the drug takes around 7–10 minutes following administration.[3] There are several contraindications to Syntometrine:

- Hypertension – Syntometrine causes hypertension, so check maternal blood pressure prior to its administration and never give it to any woman with known hypertension or suspected pre-eclampsia.
- Multiple/concealed pregnancy – If there is no record of antenatal care or the pregnancy has been concealed, then be cautious administering Syntometrine. If there is a fetus in utero at the time of administration, their placenta will shear from the uterine wall and they will die.
- Cardiac disease – Syntometrine can cause coronary artery spasm, so avoid in women with a cardiac history.
- Kidney and liver disease – Syntometrine is rapidly metabolised and excreted by the liver and kidneys limiting its effects, so do not give to patients with severe kidney or liver disease.
- Known sensitivity – You did ask about drug allergies prior to administration, didn't you?

Common side-effects following administration of Syntometrine include nausea and vomiting, abdominal pain due to intense contraction of the uterus, headaches and hypertension.

Misoprostol

Misoprostol is another uterotonic drug which, unlike Syntometrine, can be given orally, vaginally and rectally. It is also a cheap drug and has made a significant impact in the developing world where maternal death rates due to haemorrhage are staggeringly high.[29] Misoprostol is not as effective as oxytocin in preventing the PPH, but is useful in settings where resources are limited, such as home births.[28] Oral administration of the drug results in a faster onset of action (typically 7–10 minutes), but a shorter action time, whereas the rectal route has a slower onset time, but is effective for a longer period. It works in a different way to Syntometrine, allowing the administration of both if the drug of choice has been ineffective after 15 minutes.[3] It is also useful in cases of hypertension, but does have side effects, including nausea, vomiting and diarrhoea, which occur in the majority of cases. Other common side effects include shivering and pyrexia.

Tranexamic acid (TXA)

The introduction of TXA to manage severe haemorrhage in trauma patients and its introduction into UK pre-hospital practice

Chapter 7 Obstetrics and Gynaecology

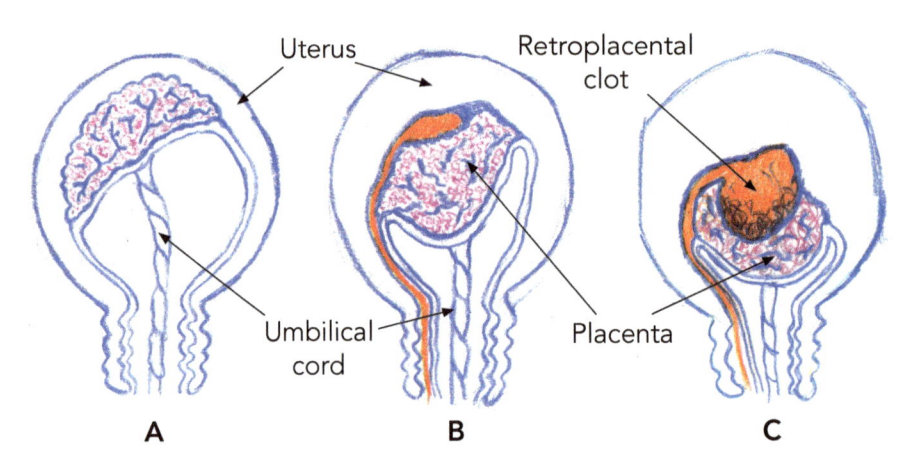

Figure 7.17 Placental separation from the uterine wall. **A** Uterine wall retracts but placenta still attached. **B** Uterine wall contracts and retracts further, leading to placental separation. **C** Placental separation complete and formation of retroplacental clot.

has heightened interest in the use of the drug for reducing mortality and the need for hysterectomy in PPH.[30] Since the publication of the WOMAN trial it is commonly used within the package of care for PPH. TXA will not control the haemorrhage as it has no uterotonic properties however, the study has proven that TXA reduces deaths due to bleeding from PPH.[31]

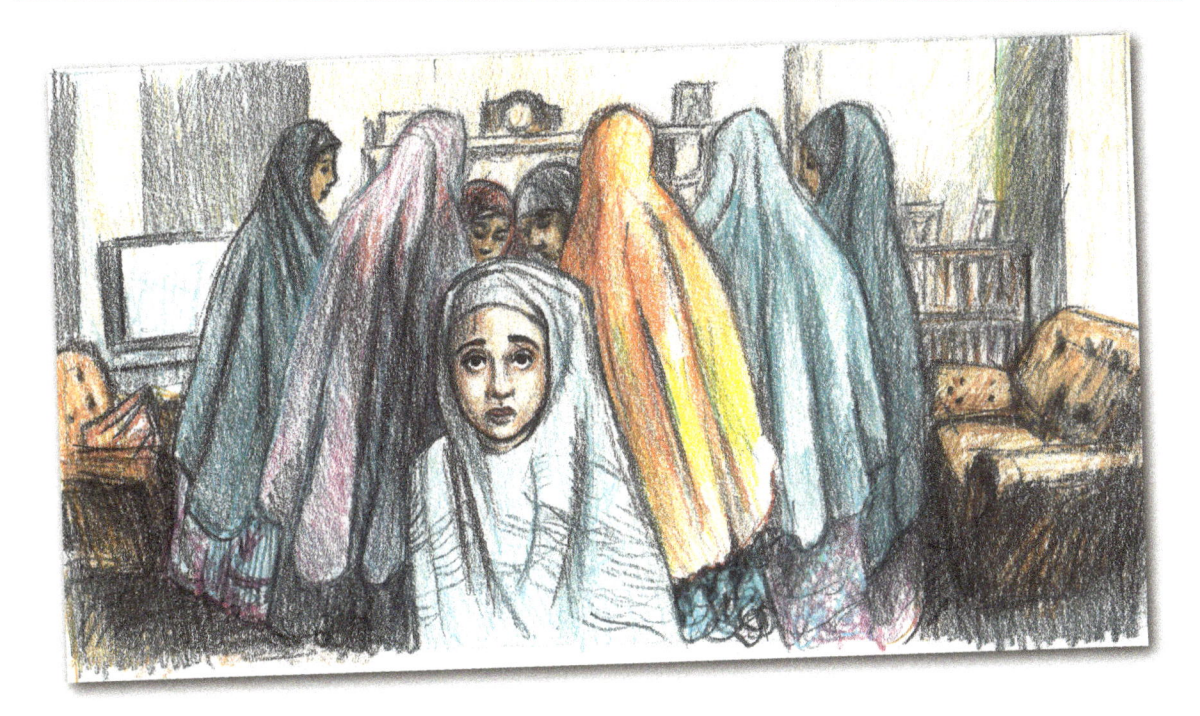

Female Genital Mutilation

You are on standby considering that overtime always seems like such a good idea when you book it. Your crew mate for the day is a fresh-faced, straight-out-of-university paramedic who is craving any knowledge you can give her. After a few calls you are just starting to think about lunch as you pass a sandwich shop, when the MDT flashes the next job: Female 21, in labour.

Great, another matern-a-taxi! However, your ever-keen crew mate exclaims, "Ahhhhhh, I love babies," while you salivate at the thought of the toasted sandwich you are now not going to be eating any time soon.

The address is only 5 minutes away, which proves to be short enough to be kept in the dark about the incident as no further updates are passed by the EOC. You pull up outside a small row of terraced houses and grab the response bag and maternity pack, while your colleague brings the Entonox and the monitor. You hear the patient before you see her, with her loud wailing, the unmistakeable sound of a woman in labour.

A young Somali girl greets you at the door and guides you to the front room. A crowd of women are surrounding the patient, and it quickly becomes apparent that the only English speaker is your 9-year-old guide. After you introduce yourself and ask her name, she tells you that she is called Elinah. She takes you over into the corner of the room towards the wailing woman and introduces you to her. She tells you that the patient is called

Chapter 7 Obstetrics and Gynaecology

Comfort, which is rather ironic, given how the patient is likely to be feeling at present.

Comfort appears to be full term but, as the little girl explains in her new role as your interpreter, she only arrived from Somalia three weeks ago and has not yet been registered with the doctor, let alone seen a midwife.

As you obtain the history, you determine that Comfort is primary survey negative, so you set about trying to determine which stage of labour she is currently in, as you are going to have to decide whether you can make a run for the local maternity unit, or if the baby is going to be born in the front room. Luckily for you, your colleague has a handy aide memoire to help differentiate the first and second stages of labour (Table 7.6).

Table 7.6 Differentiating between the first and second stages of labour.

First stage of labour	Second stage of labour
Regular contractions at a rate of 3–4 every 10 minutes	Regular contractions every 2–3 minutes
No pressure	Rectal pressure
No urge to push	Urge to push
No anal or perineal bulging	Anal or perineal bulging
	Heavy blood-stained show
	Evidence of a purple line from the anal margins to the natal cleft[1]
	Waters breaking (physiological time for them to break, but this can occur at any point)

Adapted from: MacDonald & Johnson, 2017.

You monitor Comfort's contractions and find they are approximately 2–3 minutes apart and appear expulsive in nature. During contractions, she cannot answer your questions about rectal pressure or the urge to push.

However, all of a sudden she gives the distinctive sound of a woman making a deep, instinctive push. "Looks like we're going to catch this baby here," you say to your colleague, who actually squeals with delight. You ask Elinah to get one of the other women to gather some towels. Despite the language barrier, your colleague seems to have established a good rapport with Comfort, so you step back, to allow her the privilege of bringing a new life into the world. She sets about making Comfort comfortable before indicating that she needs to remove her dress and underwear.

As you pass over the maternity pack, you see the look on the face of your colleague. The picture of happiness mixed with nervousness has been replaced by one of horror. She turns to you quickly and says in a clipped, stressed tone, "We need to go to the hospital NOW." Frankly, you are a little disappointed at her attitude and prepare to take over. However, you ask her why the need for a change of plan.

"Have you heard of the term 'FGM'?" she asks in a low hushed voice. You nod and the hairs on the back of your neck stand on end – a sure sign of trouble. "Comfort has a vaginal opening of only 2 cm. I'm not sure this baby will even be born without cutting her."

What should you do: **Stay on scene** (read on) or arrange a **Rapid exit** for the nearest consultant-led obstetric unit (skip the next paragraph)?

Female Genital Mutilation

Stay on scene

You reassure your colleague that babies have been born for generations and that this one will be no different: after all, pregnancy is a condition, not an illness. Comfort continues to push but refuses your repeated offers of analgesia. However, despite Comfort's best efforts, there is no sign of the baby and, after she has been pushing on scene for well over 30 minutes, there is still no baby visible. Comfort is quickly tiring and you come to the conclusion that your colleague was right. At the local maternity unit, you are given a dressing down by the matron, although luckily the baby appears to be unharmed from your procrastination on scene.

Rapid exit

You tell Comfort that she needs to come with you to the maternity hospital straight away. She manages to walk to the front door where your colleague has hastily prepared the ambulance trolley. Elinah introduces you to one of the women who were in the front room. She is Comfort's aunt and wants to travel with her, which you have no objection to. Since your colleague has built up a rapport with Comfort, you suggest that she travel in with the patient.

As you negotiate through traffic at speed, you can hear your colleague calling the obstetric unit with the patient's details. She relays to them that you are bringing in a 21-year-old female with an unbooked pregnancy, who appears to be full term, in advanced labour and has type 3 FGM.

On arriving at the obstetric unit you are greeted at the door by two midwives and a doctor. They open the back doors and jump into the ambulance before you've had a chance to lower the steps. The doctor introduces herself as Doctor Anu and asks Comfort's permission to remove the blanket.

She takes a quick look before announcing loudly: "Right team, inside pronto!"

You promptly transfer Comfort into the unit and wheel her along to one of the maternity rooms. She is starting to get rather distressed and you spot a band of sweat that is almost gluing her veil to her head. You assist her over onto the maternity bed and, as you are about to leave, she grabs hold of your colleague's hand and says, "Thank you."

You approach one of the midwives who was in the back of the ambulance, but who is not involved in Comfort's care, and ask about your decision to transport quickly. "It was a good call," she replies. "I haven't seen a type 3 like that in advanced second stage; most are reversed before they go that far to avoid doing it in labour." You are relieved that you made the correct decision, but feel even better as you walk back past Comfort's room and you hear the sound of a newborn baby crying.

Scale of the problem

Female genital mutilation (FGM) refers to the practice of deliberately harming a woman's genitals. The WHO defines FGM as 'all procedures that involve partial or total removal of the external female genitalia, or other injury to the female genital organs for non-medical reasons'.[32] It is classified into four types (Figure 7.18).[33]

- Type 1 Clitoridectomy: Removal of the prepuce (the fold of skin surrounding the clitoris) only (rare) or plus partial or total removal of the clitoris
- Type 2 Excision: Partial or total removal of the clitoris and the labia minora, with or without excision of the labia majora
- Type 3 Infibulation: Narrowing of the vaginal opening through the creation of a covering seal. The seal is formed by cutting and repositioning the inner, or outer, labia

Chapter 7 Obstetrics and Gynaecology

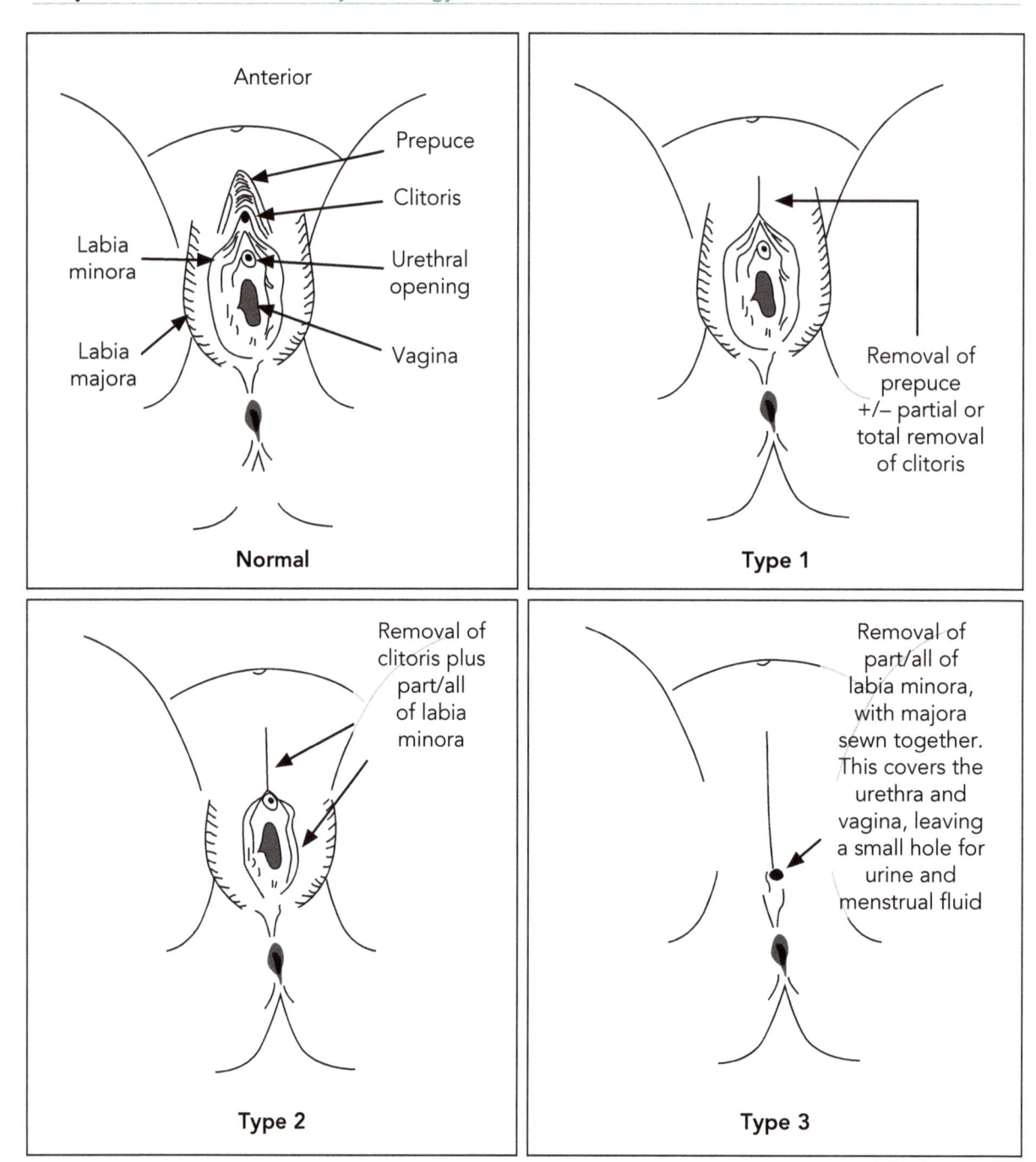

Figure 7.18 Types of FGM (Type 4 not shown).
Kaylima at en.wikipedia derivative work: Mouagip. Public Domain, via Wikimedia Commons.

(minora or majora, respectively), with or without removal of the clitoris
- Type 4 Other: All other harmful procedures to the female genitalia for non-medical purposes, for example, pricking, piercing, incising, scraping and cauterising the genital area.

It is estimated that more than 125 million women worldwide have undergone a form of FGM, but this is likely to be grossly underestimated due to the nature of the procedure, and the fact it is often carried out in communities and not talked about publicly.[34] In England and Wales it is estimated that there are 103,000 women aged 15–49 who are permanent residents, but were born in countries that practise FGM. Around 1.5% of all women giving birth each year in England and Wales have FGM.[35]

The 'culture' of FGM

There are a number of reasons why FGM is performed. However, the main aim appears to be the control of women. This is surprising, given that the instigators and keepers of the tradition are typically women and not men.[36] The justification women give for performing FGM varies from region to region. Many believe it is the wish of their ancestors and will protect the moral behaviour of women and their acceptance into adult society. There are also myths surrounding the genitals themselves, for example, that they are unclean or dirty, and that removing them will prevent premarital sex, thereby preserving virginity, and prevent adultery. Some believe that the clitoris is a dangerous organ and must be removed as it will damage their husband during sex. Religion is often given as a reason for FGM. However, there is no mention of the procedure in any religious texts.

The point at which the FGM is carried out varies greatly from community to community and depends upon well-established rituals.

In some areas the procedures are carried out during infancy, but most commonly FGM is performed on girls between the ages of 10 and 14, and is typically seen as a rite of passage. However, there are cases involving older women at times such as their engagement to be married or even in preparation for childbirth. Occasionally, FGM is actually performed during childbirth as it is believed that if the clitoris touches the baby it will be stillborn.[37]

The way the procedure is performed, just as the reasons for performing FGM, varies from area to area. It is predominantly carried out by women who have no formal medical training, but who are held in high regard within their community. Alternatively, FGM is performed by traditional midwives, healers, barbers, or nurses and with unsanitary equipment. Knives, scissors, scalpels, glass and razor blades are all common implements used, typically without sterilisation or an anaesthetic. Girls often have to be forcibly restrained in order to carry out the mutilation, which will often lead to flashbacks and post-traumatic stress disorder (PTSD).

There are no known benefits to carrying out FGM and the consequences of its performance are often life-changing and sometimes even fatal. There are a number of immediate complications that can occur in the initial period after the procedure, including severe pain and haemorrhage, but as it is carried out in unsanitary conditions, infection is common and can lead to tetanus and sepsis. Retention of urine and problems with sores in the genital region can also occur.

In the longer term, girls and women can suffer from:[38]

- Recurrent bladder and urinary tract infections (UTIs)
- Dermoid cysts as well as keloid scarring
- Fistula formation
- Chronic pelvic pain

Chapter 7   Obstetrics and Gynaecology

- Infertility and menstrual problems
- Mental ill-health including PTSD and flashbacks.

FGM can also have serious consequences for childbirth, particularly type 3 FGM, and is associated with increased maternal and newborn mortality. Difficult childbirth and obstructed labour often occur as a result of the narrowing of the vaginal opening. Depending on the degree of narrowing, obstructed delivery occurs as the fetus presses upon the scar tissue. This can arrest the labour and/or rupture the scar, uterus, vulva and perineum. These injuries may be repeatedly repaired following successive childbirths, further increasing the immediate and long-term risks.

Management during childbirth

The issues that can arise during childbirth are very much dependent upon the type of FGM that is performed. There will not only be the physical scars to deal with, which will be greater in type 3, but there are the mental scars that will be present in every woman no matter which type she had performed. Women who declare at booking that they have any form of FGM will be assessed by a specialist to ensure that they are able to give birth vaginally and prevent the situation that happened to the woman in the case study.

Within the UK there are 15 specialist centres that receive women with FGM, provide counselling and can perform a procedure known as de-infibulation. This procedure can be performed on any woman with type 3 FGM, not just those who are pregnant. The procedure is done under local anaesthetic and involves cutting upward through the scar tissue and then stitching back over the edges to reform the labia which would have been removed during FGM.[39] The procedure is done antenatally in preference to during labour as there is risk of damage to the underlying structures and complications such as increased haemorrhage and increased incidence of perineal and vaginal tears.[40]

If you are called to a woman with FGM, follow their care plan where possible. If the woman has received no antenatal care, then management will depend on the type of FGM. Type 1 and 2 FGM are unlikely to cause any problems with childbirth. However, a woman with type 3 FGM cannot give birth without de-infibulation and so should be transported to the nearest consultant-led obstetric unit without delay.

The Law

The Female Genital Mutilation Act came into force on 3rd March 2004, meaning that FGM is illegal in the UK. In the Act, FGM is a collective term for a range of procedures which involve partial or total removal of the external female genitalia for non-medical reasons.[41] It is also an offence to take a girl out of the country for the purpose of enabling her mutilation. The maximum sentence is 14 years and/or an unlimited fine.

Safeguarding

If you have any suspicions or concerns over FGM, relating either to your patient or to the other women and girls within the household, you are legally bound to report these concerns via safeguarding referral pathways. In addition, it is important that any concerns you may have are passed on to the hospital staff so that they can ensure that the appropriate follow-up care is in place.

References

1. Morton S, Brodsky D. Fetal physiology and the transition to extrauterine life. Clinics in Perinatology, 2016 Sep;43(3):395–407.
2. Hooper SB, te Pas AB, Lang J, van Vonderen JJ, Roehr CC, Kluckow M, et al. Cardiovascular transition at birth: a physiological sequence. Pediatric Research, 2015 May;77(5):608–614.
3. Joint Royal Colleges Ambulance Liaison Committee, Association of Ambulance Chief Executives. JRCALC Clinical Guidelines. Cited from JRCALC Plus (Version 1.2.13) [Mobile application software]. Bridgwater: Class Publishing Ltd; 2021.
4. Madar J, Roehr CC, Ainsworth S, Ersdal H, Morley C, Rüdiger M, et al. European Resuscitation Council Guidelines 2021: Newborn resuscitation and support of transition of infants at birth. *Resuscitation*, 2021 Apr 1;161:291–326.
5. Tappero E, Honeyfield M. *Physical assessment of the newborn: a comprehensive approach to the art of physical examination*, 4th edition. Santa Rosa: NICU Ink Book Publishers; 2010.
6. Güemes M, Rahman SA, Hussain K. What is a normal blood glucose? *Archives of Disease in Childhood*, 2016 Jun 1;101(6):569–574.
7. National Institute for Health and Care Excellence. Intrapartum care for healthy women and babies [Internet]. NICE; 2017. Available from: https://www.nice.org.uk/guidance/cg190
8. Royal College of Midwives. Parental Emotional Wellbeing and Infant Development – An updated good practice guide [Internet]. 2019. Available from: https://www.rcm.org.uk/media/4645/parental-emotional-wellbeing-guide.pdf
9. Office for National Statistics. Births in England and Wales: 2019 [Internet]. 2020. Available from: https://www.ons.gov.uk/peoplepopulationandcommunity/birthsdeathsandmarriages/livebirths/bulletins/birthsummarytablesenglandandwales/2019
10. Royal College of Obstetricians and Gynaecologists. Umbilical Cord Prolapse (Green-top Guideline No. 50) [Internet]. Royal College of Obstetricians & Gynaecologists. 2014. Available from: https://www.rcog.org.uk/en/guidelines-research-services/guidelines/gtg50/
11. Royal College of Obstetricians and Gynaecologists. Shoulder Dystocia (Green-top Guideline No. 42) [Internet]. Royal College of Obstetricians & Gynaecologists. 2017. Available from: https://www.rcog.org.uk/en/guidelines-research-services/guidelines/gtg42/
12. Royal College of Obstetricians and Gynaecologists. Management of Breech Presentation. BJOG: An International Journal of Obstetrics & Gynaecology, 2017;124(7):e151–177.
13. Macdonald S, p G, editors. *Mayes' midwifery*, 15th edition. Edinburgh; New York: Elsevier; 2017.
14. Advanced Life Support Group, editor. *Pre-obstetric emergency training: a practical approach*, 2nd edition. Hoboken: Wiley-Blackwell; 2018.
15. Advanced Life Support Group. *Pre-hospital obstetric emergency training*. Chichester: Wiley-Blackwell; 2010.
16. Louwen F, Daviss B-A, Johnson KC, Reitter A. Does breech delivery in an upright position instead of on the back improve outcomes and avoid cesareans? *International Journal of Gynecology & Obstetrics*, 2017;136(2): 151–161.
17. Reitter A, Halliday A, Walker S. Practical insight into upright breech birth from birth videos: a structured analysis. *Birth*, 2020;47(2): 211–219.
18. Walker S, Parker P, Scamell M. Expertise in physiological breech birth: a mixed-methods study. *Birth*, 2018;45(2):202–209.
19. Walker S, Scamell M, Parker P. Deliberate acquisition of competence in physiological breech birth: a grounded theory study. *Women and Birth*, 2018 Jun 1;31(3):e170– e177.
20. McDonald SJ, Middleton P, Dowswell T, Morris PS. Effect of timing of umbilical cord clamping of term infants on maternal and neonatal outcomes. *Cochrane Database of Systematic Reviews*, 2013;(7):1–92.
21. Reed R, Peetze J, Barnes M. Birth: an evidence-based approach. *Journal of Paramedic Practice*, 2010;2(1):6–11.

22. World Health Organization. WHO recommendations for the prevention and treatment of postpartum haemorrhage [Internet]. Geneva: World Health Organization; 2012. Available from: http://apps.who.int/iris/bitstream/10665/75411/1/9789241548502_eng.pdf?ua=1
23. Prompt Maternity Foundation. *PROMPT course manual*. Cambridge: Cambridge University Pres; 2018.
24. Knight M, Bunch K, Tuffnell D, Shakespeare J, Kotnis R, Kenyon S, et al. Saving Lives, Improving Mothers' Care – Lessons learned to inform maternity care from the UK and Ireland Confidential Enquiries into Maternal Deaths and Morbidity 2016-18 [Internet]. 2020. Available from: https://www.npeu.ox.ac.uk/assets/downloads/mbrrace-uk/reports/maternal-report-2020/MBRRACE-UK_Maternal_Report_Dec_2020_v10_ONLINE_VERSION_1404.pdf
25. Edhi MM, Aslam HM, Naqvi Z, Hashmi H. Post partum hemorrhage: causes and management. *BMC Research Notes*, 2013;6:236.
26. American Academy of Family Physicians. *Advanced life support in obstetrics provider manual*. Kansas: AAFP; 2012.
27. Smith LA, Price N, Simonite V, Burns EE. Incidence of and risk factors for perineal trauma: a prospective observational study. BMC Pregnancy & Childbirth, 2013;13(1):59.
28. Royal College of Obstetricians and Gynaecologists. Green-top Guideline No. 52: Prevention and Management of Postpartum Haemorrhage. Obstetrics & Gynecology, 2017;19(2):189–189.
29. Hofmeyr GJ, Gulmezoglu AM, Novikova N, Linder V, Ferreira S, Piaggio G. Misoprostol to prevent and treat postpartum haemorrhage: a systematic review and meta-analysis of maternal deaths and dose-related effects. *Bulletin of the World Health Organization*, 2009 Sep;87(9):666–677.
30. Cook L, Roberts I. Post–partum haemorrhage and the WOMAN trial. *International Journal of Epidemiology*, 2010 Jan 8;39(4):949–950.
31. Shakur H, Roberts I, Fawole B, Chaudhri R, El-Sheikh M, Akintan A, et al. Effect of early tranexamic acid administration on mortality, hysterectomy, and other morbidities in women with post-partum haemorrhage (WOMAN): an international, randomised, double-blind, placebo-controlled trial. The Lancet. 2017 May 27;389(10084):2105–2116.
32. World Health Organization. Female genital mutilation [Internet]. WHO. 2014. Available from: http://www.who.int/mediacentre/factsheets/fs241/en/
33. World Health Organization. Care of girls and women living with female genital mutilation [Internet]. WHO. World Health Organization; 2018. Available from: http://www.who.int/reproductivehealth/publications/health-care-girls-women-living-with-FGM/en/
34. UNICEF. Female Genital Mutilation/Cutting: A statistical overview and exploration of the dynamics of change [Internet]. 2013. Available from: https://data.unicef.org/wp-content/uploads/2019/04/UNICEF_FGM_report_July_2013.pdf
35. Alison Macfarlane BA, Stat F. Female Genital Mutilation in England and Wales: Updated statistical estimates of the numbers of affected women living in England and Wales and girls at risk Interim report on provisional estimates. 2014 Available from: https://openaccess.city.ac.uk/id/eprint/3865/
36. Lee KS. *Female genital mutilation: multiple-case studies of communication strategies against a taboo practice*. ProQuest; 2008. 126 p.
37. Momoh C. *Female genital mutilation*. 1st edition. Oxford: Radcliffe Publishing Ltd; 2005. 184 p.
38. Bieber E. *Clinical gynecology*, 2nd edition. Cambridge: Cambridge University Press; 2015. 1102 p. (Medicine).
39. United Kingdom. Female genital mutilation (FGM) [Internet]. 2015. Available from: https://www.gov.uk/female-genital-mutilation
40. Paliwal P, Ali S, Bradshaw S, Hughes A, Jolly K. Management of type III female genital mutilation in Birmingham, UK: a retrospective audit. *Midwifery*, 2014 Mar;30(3):282–288.
41. UK Government. Female Genital Mutilation Act 2003 [Internet]. Statute Law Database; 2003. Available from: https://www.legislation.gov.uk/ukpga/2003/31/contents

8　　　　　　　　　　　　　　　　Paediatrics

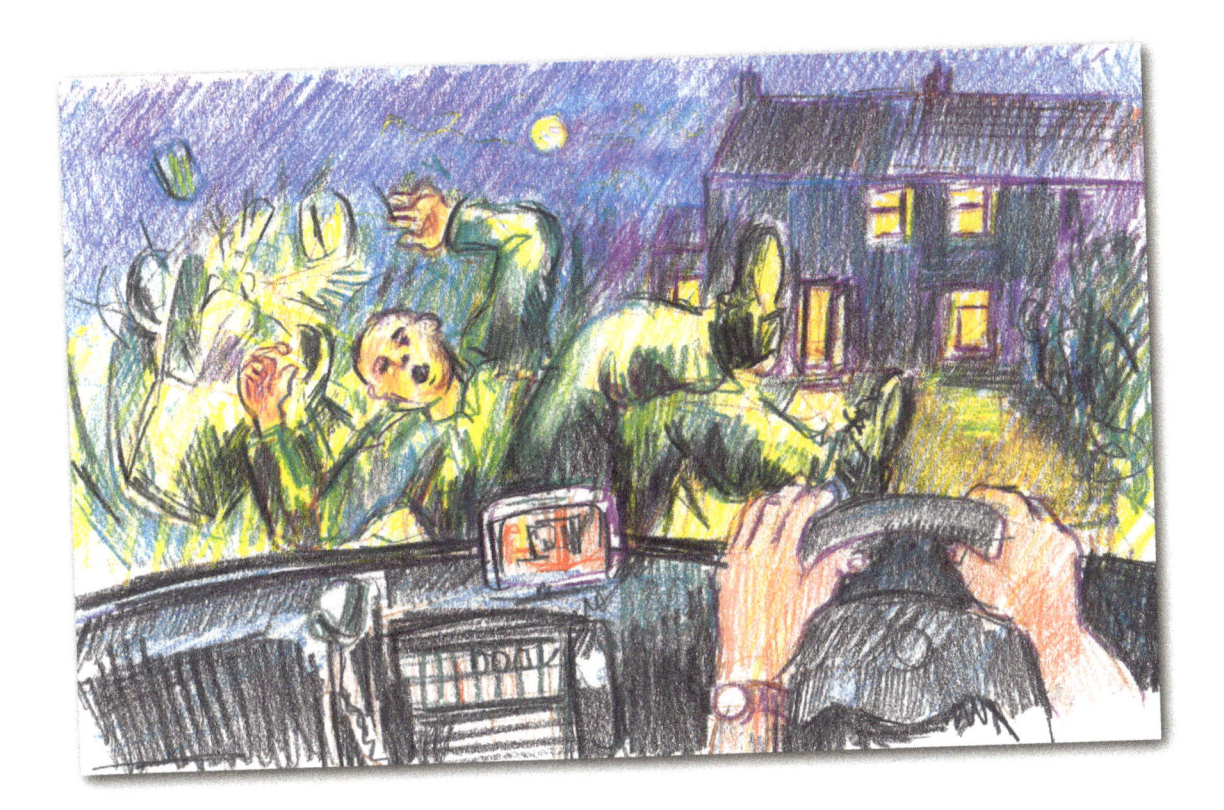

Croup

You are on standby with a young colleague, SMS, so-called due to his tendency to use acronyms. He seems to be busy updating his Instagram, but is interrupted by the MDT providing details of your next job; a 3-year-old with difficulty breathing.

As you set off, you note the time (22:15) and, thanks to the absence of traffic, are soon turning into the patient's street. It hasn't been gritted and you feel the ambulance lose traction as you negotiate the turn. Pulling up outside the house, SMS leaps out, and before you can say "I think it's icy," he has already slipped on the road and ended up on his bottom. "OMG!" he yelps. After carefully exiting the vehicle and grabbing some gear, you head to the house. The front door is wide

Chapter 8 Paediatrics

open and you can hear the distressed chatter of the mother on the phone to the emergency operations centre.

You knock and enter the house. The mother notifies the call handler of your arrival and then hangs up. "Thank goodness you are here, it's Karina," she says hurriedly. You are lead through the house to the living room. Karina watches you warily as you enter and you give her a smile as the mother explains that she has been suffering from a cold for the past week, but had deteriorated over the weekend.

Her parents had done the right thing and visited the general practitioner (GP), and the patient appeared to improve after the visit, until this evening. Mum had checked on Karina after hearing her crying and found her panicking (the patient that is, although mum admitted she wasn't particularly calm either) and saying she could not breathe. "She was turning blue," the mother exclaims, clearly reliving that moment.

In keeping with previous episodes, dad had taken her outside and Karina seemed to improve. They had come back inside and sat her on his lap, put on the TV and things seemed to improve slightly. Apart from several bouts of croup in the past, the patient is usually fit and well, with no allergies. She had paracetamol 3 hours ago and ibuprofen 1 hour ago, as the patient's temperature refused to drop below 38.0°C.

> SMS is keen to examine the patient, judging by the impatient twirling of his stethoscope. What are you going to do: **Let SMS assess the patient** (read on) or **Assess her from the doorway** (skip the next paragraph)?

Let SMS assess the patient

SMS moves in with arms outstretched, his stethoscope already in his ears and a loud "Heeeeyyyy!" by way of introduction. However, his approach doesn't wash with the little girl and she tries to recoil from SMS by burying herself into her father's arms. She also starts crying, and then coughing. In seconds she is centrally cyanosed and you pull SMS back to the edge of the living room. Karina's father is not impressed and takes her back out into the garden to calm her down.

Assess from the doorway

You know that you are going to have to gain the trust of this little girl but want to get a feel for how sick she is, so use the paediatric assessment triangle to assess her from the edge of the room. You review your findings:

Appearance

Sat in father's arms, but is quiet
Nods in response to questions asked by parents, but is not speaking
Is appropriately suspicious of you and SMS

Work of breathing

Respiratory rate: 36 breaths/min
Substernal and intercostal recession and accessory muscle use while at rest
Audible stridor on inspiration and expiration

Circulation to skin

Pale, cyanosed when crying

The patient is clearly unwell with respiratory and cardiovascular involvement, although her brain seems well-enough perfused at present. SMS pipes up, "Hot and steamy?" It takes you a moment to get what he is on about, then recall a common treatment for croup is to place the child in a steamy/moist environment.

> What are you going to do: **Steam up the bathroom** (read on) or **Take her outside** (skip the next paragraph)?

Steam up the bathroom

You suggest that the patient might feel better if she breathes in some steam. "We were told that was a waste of time by the paediatric doctor last time we went to hospital," the father retorts, "talking of which, shouldn't we be going to hospital?"

Take her outside

You know there is little evidence that steamy environments make any difference in croup and given how sick she is, the patient needs to go to hospital. "I think an expeditious departure to the local paediatric hospital is required," you tell SMS, who gives you a blank look. You sigh and translate, "SCH, ASAP." SMS recognises the acronym for the local children's hospital and flies out the door, clearly having forgotten that it is icy. Still, he does make it to the ambulance having only fallen over twice.

Karina's father carries her onto the ambulance and you set off. As the senior clinician you elect to stay in the back with the patient. With some gentle coaxing, you manage to auscultate her chest and attach an SpO$_2$ probe to Karina's finger.

You find the following:

Airway

Patent, but audible inspiratory/expiratory stridor

Breathing

Respiratory rate: 36 breaths/min
Marked substernal, subcostal and intercostal recession
Decreased air entry in bases
SpO$_2$: 90% on air

Circulation

Palpable radial pulse at a rate of 155 beats/min

Disability

Alert and orientated, but quiet and looking tired
Blood sugar: Not performed to avoid upsetting Karina

Exposure/Environment

Skin: pale, cyanosed when coughing/crying
Temperature: 38.0°C

It's a 20-minute blue light run to the emergency department (ED) and you can hear SMS making a pre-alert call. You set up a non-rebreathing mask and give it to Karina's father, encouraging him to place it as close as he can to her face. The child starts to well up, however after a couple of minutes, her oxygen saturations increase to 95% and you can see the relief in her face as she realises that the plastic mask with blowing air is making her feel a little better. With her father's help, you also manage to administer 2 mg of dexamethasone to Karina.

> Ten minutes into the journey and the child's stridor is getting quieter and her respiratory rate is dropping. Are you reassured: **Yes** (read on) or **No** (skip the next paragraph)?

Yes

These steroids are great, despite being orally administered they have taken less than 10 minutes to work. You elect to complete some paperwork as everything seems under control, and it is several minutes until you casually glance up at the monitor to see how the patient is doing. Her oxygen saturations are 88% and you quickly check the oxygen mask, but find it still in situ. The patient is looking vacantly towards the back of the ambulance, with eyes half open. You move into the patient's field of vision, but there is no response. Examining her chest, you guess her respiratory rate is 36 breaths per minute, but

Chapter 8 Paediatrics

are of inadequate depth. You yell through to SMS to pull over.

SMS leaps into the back, "OPA and BVM?," he enquires and you nod. Karina tolerates the oropharyngeal airway (OPA) and you commence bag-valve-mask (BVM) ventilations. Her oxygen saturations slowly increase to 92% by the time you arrive at the ED, but she is still unresponsive. You find out later that she was moved to the paediatric intensive care unit (PICU).

No

Oral steroids are unlikely to have worked that fast and you suspect impending respiratory failure. You prepare for the worst by selecting a range of OPAs and connect the paediatric BVM to the oxygen supply while wondering if there is something else you can do.

> What can you do: **Tell SMS to drive faster** (read on) or **Contact the ED** and ask to speak to a consultant (skip the next paragraph)?

Tell SMS to drive faster

You stick your head into the bulkhead window, "SMS, she's deteriorating," you say. SMS gives you a quizzical look in the rear-view mirror, so you translate. "ED, ASAP," you say and he nods in comprehension. The patient continues to decline and you gently release her from her father's grasp and lay her flat on the trolley, insert an OPA and commence ventilations with the BVM. On arrival at the ED, the patient is descended upon by the resus team and later transferred to PICU.

Contact the ED

Nebulised adrenaline. It comes to you in a flash of inspiration. It buys time in croup. It's not in your ambulance clinical guidelines but you know that Karina is unlikely to make it to the ED conscious if she continues to go downhill. You call the ED and explain your predicament and the patient's current condition. The consultant agrees that the situation is grave and advises that you administer 5 mg of 1:1,000 adrenaline. You empty the entire ambulance supply of 1:1,000 adrenaline into a nebuliser chamber and swap it for the non-rebreathing mask. Within five minutes, you can see the effects of the adrenaline. Her work of breathing has decreased slightly and the SpO_2 is holding at 96%.

You are met at the doors of the ED by the consultant, who after looking at the patient gives you a nod of approval.

You find out later that the patient was admitted for observation, but thanks to your prompt intervention, did not require ventilation or a stay on PICU. As you get back into the cab, SMS is rifling through the ambulance clinical practice guidelines. "ADX via NEB for DIB?" he enquires. "It's AWOL, LOL," you reply and push clear.

Scale of the problem

Croup is a common childhood disease in infants and children aged between 6 months and 6 years of age, although it can occur in babies as young as 3 months and in adolescents.[1] The peak age incidence is 2 years and it is one and half times more common in boys. The largest number of cases occur in the autumn and lowest in summer.[2] Over 95% of cases are caused by viruses, with parainfluenza virus the most common. However, other culprits include metapneumovirus, respiratory syncytial virus (RSV) and influenza.[1]

Anatomy

Children are not small adults and there are a number of important anatomical differences between the airways of adults and children that are significant in croup (Figure 8.1). Firstly, the narrowest portion of a child's

Croup

Child

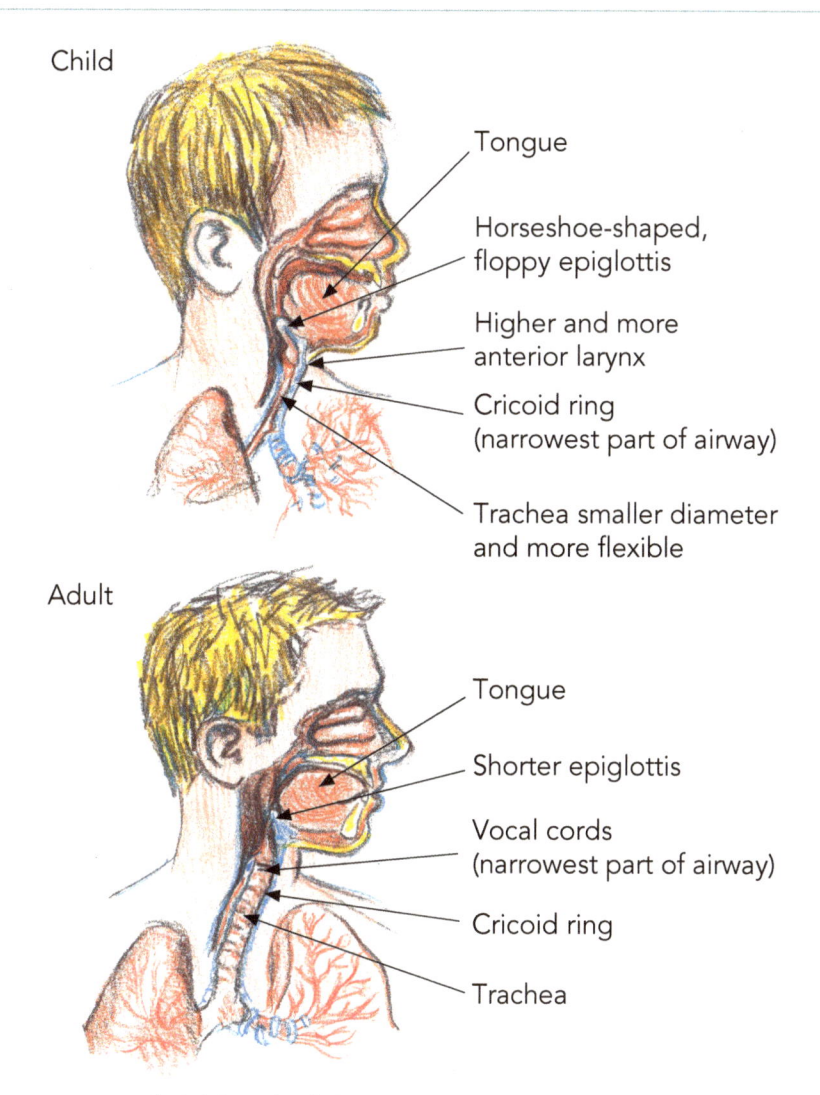

- Tongue
- Horseshoe-shaped, floppy epiglottis
- Higher and more anterior larynx
- Cricoid ring (narrowest part of airway)
- Trachea smaller diameter and more flexible

Adult

- Tongue
- Shorter epiglottis
- Vocal cords (narrowest part of airway)
- Cricoid ring
- Trachea

Figure 8.1 Comparison of child and adult airways.

airway is subglottic, at the cricoid ring. Secondly, the small diameter of the airways means that minimal oedema can lead to airway compromise (Table 8.1).[3]

Table 8.1 The effect of 1 mm of oedema on airway diameter and resistance.

Age	Cross-sectional area	Airway resistance
Infant	Decreases 44%	Increases 200%
Adult	Decreases 25%	Increases 40%

Source: Brown et al., 2017.

Pathophysiology

Croup can be broadly divided into two types: acute laryngotracheitis and spasmodic croup. As the name suggests, laryngotracheitis is characterised by erythema and swelling of the lateral walls of the trachea, just below the vocal cords.[2]

In croup caused by parainfluenza viruses, there is chloride secretion and inhibition of sodium absorption across the tracheal epithelium, which leads to oedema and subglottic narrowing causing a barking cough, turbulent airflow and stridor.[4] This is sometimes referred to as spasmodic croup, since the oedema is not caused by an inflammatory process.

However, in bacterial croup, the tracheal wall is infiltrated by inflammatory cells, which lead to the production of thick pus in the trachea and lower air passages. In addition, the infection results in generalised airway inflammation and oedema of the upper airway mucosa, including the larynx, trachea and bronchi, causing epithelial necrosis and shedding.[5]

The symptoms of croup are typically worse at night and although the actual cause is not known, it has been suggested that it is linked to circadian fluctuations in cortisol secretion, which peak around 08:00 and trough between 23:00 and 04:00.[5] In addition, research into nocturnal asthma, has identified nocturnal airway cooling and gastro-oesophageal reflux as factors in night-time exacerbation of that disease,[6] which might also provide a physiological explanation for the exacerbation of croup.

Recognition and differential diagnoses

The classic presentation of croup is that of the night-time appearance of a barking cough, often accompanied by stridor, a hoarse voice and intercostal/subcostal recession, depending on severity. These acute symptoms are usually preceded by coryzal symptoms (nasal discharge and obstruction, sore throat, headache … think common cold or man flu) in the 12–48 hours leading up to acute presentation. Croup symptoms typically resolve within a couple of days, although in some cases they can last for up to a week.[1]

In children with the classic signs and symptoms previously mentioned, you are unlikely to get the diagnosis of croup wrong, and most differential diagnoses are uncommon, but include:[1]

- Allergic laryngeal oedema
- Bacterial tracheitis
- Diphtheria
- Epiglottitis
- Inhalation of smoke and hot air from fires
- Measles
- Retropharyngeal abscess
- Trauma to the throat.

Arguably the most important differentials to exclude are epiglottitis and bacterial tracheitis. Both are true airway, and thus life-threatening, emergencies. Fortunately, thanks to the *Haemophilus influenzae* type b (HiB) vaccine, epiglottitis in children is now very uncommon in the United Kingdom.[7] The most important differences between croup and epiglottitis are the presence or absence of coughing and drooling.[8] In croup, patients will typically have a cough, but not drool, whereas in epiglottitis, the opposite is true, that is, the patient will drool but have no cough!

Bacterial tracheitis has a similar clinical picture to severe croup, except the child usually has a high fever and looks very sick. It is usually caused by either *Staphylococcus aureus* or *Haemophilus influenzae* and leads to the production of large amounts of thick secretions, which can occlude the airway, necessitating intubation and ventilatory support.[9] Treatment consists of broad-spectrum intravenous antibiotics. Nebulised adrenaline (discussed a bit later on) is ineffective.[5]

Assessment

Based on the history and clinical examination, you should be fairly confident with your diagnosis of croup. However, it is important to gauge the severity in order to adopt the most appropriate management plan. There are a range of tools to aid in the assessment of croup severity, most of which have been designed as research tools.

The most commonly used tool is the Westley scoring system (Table 8.2), which consists of five elements to gauge severity: recession, stridor, cyanosis, level of consciousness and air entry, with croup classed as mild with a score of less than 4, moderate with a score of 4–6 and severe if the score is greater than 6.[10] This is useful in clinical trials, but is less helpful in routine clinical practice.

Table 8.2 The Westley scoring system for croup.

Measure	Severity	Score
Chest wall recession	None	0
	Mild	1
	Moderate	2
	Severe	3
Stridor	None	0
	With agitation	1
	At rest	2
Cyanosis	None	0
	With agitation	4
	At rest	5
Level of consciousness	Normal	0
	Disorientated	5
Air entry	Normal	0
	Mildly decreased	1
	Markedly decreased	2

Source: Westley et el., 1978.

A more pragmatic choice is the modified Taussig score, which only requires the recording of two variables, stridor and recession (Table 8.3).[11] Croup is classed as

Table 8.3 Modified Taussig score.

	Stridor	Recession
None	0	0
Only on crying	1	1
At rest	2	2
Biphasic (inspiration and expiration)	3	3

Source: Sparrow and Geelhoed, 2006.

mild with a score of 1–2, moderate with a score of 3–4 and severe if over 4. In addition, there are a number of ominous signs, which signify that a child is heading for respiratory failure.

These include:[12]

- Oxygen saturations less than 95% on air
- Cyanosis
- Physical exhaustion, evidenced by reduced stridor and recession in an increasingly sick child
- Restlessness, irritability and an altered level of consciousness

Management

All children with significant illness should receive high levels of supplemental oxygen.[12] Nebulisers have been de-emphasised in early management of croup due to concerns over the distress they may cause in a child who already has respiratory compromise. Crying can dramatically increase airway resistance and thus work of breathing, so try to avoid upsetting the child if you can.[13]

Steroids are the mainstay of treatment and the current *JRCALC Clinical Guidelines* advocate oral dexamethasone, with doses of 0.15 mg/kg (luckily calculated for you).

Although absent from the *JRCALC Clinical Guidelines*, it is common practice in hospitals to administer nebulised adrenaline in cases of severe croup to 'buy time' while oral steroids get to work. This typically involves the administration of 400 mcg/kg (up to a maximum of 5 mg) of adrenaline 1:1,000, which lasts around 30 minutes.[14] It appears that concerns over rebound stridor following the administration of nebulised adrenaline are unfounded.[15] If you have a child with severe croup and are able to speak directly to the receiving hospital when making a pre-alert call, for example, you may be able to get authorisation from a senior doctor to administer adrenaline in this fashion. Follow local guidance to avoid getting yourself in trouble.

Chapter 8   Paediatrics

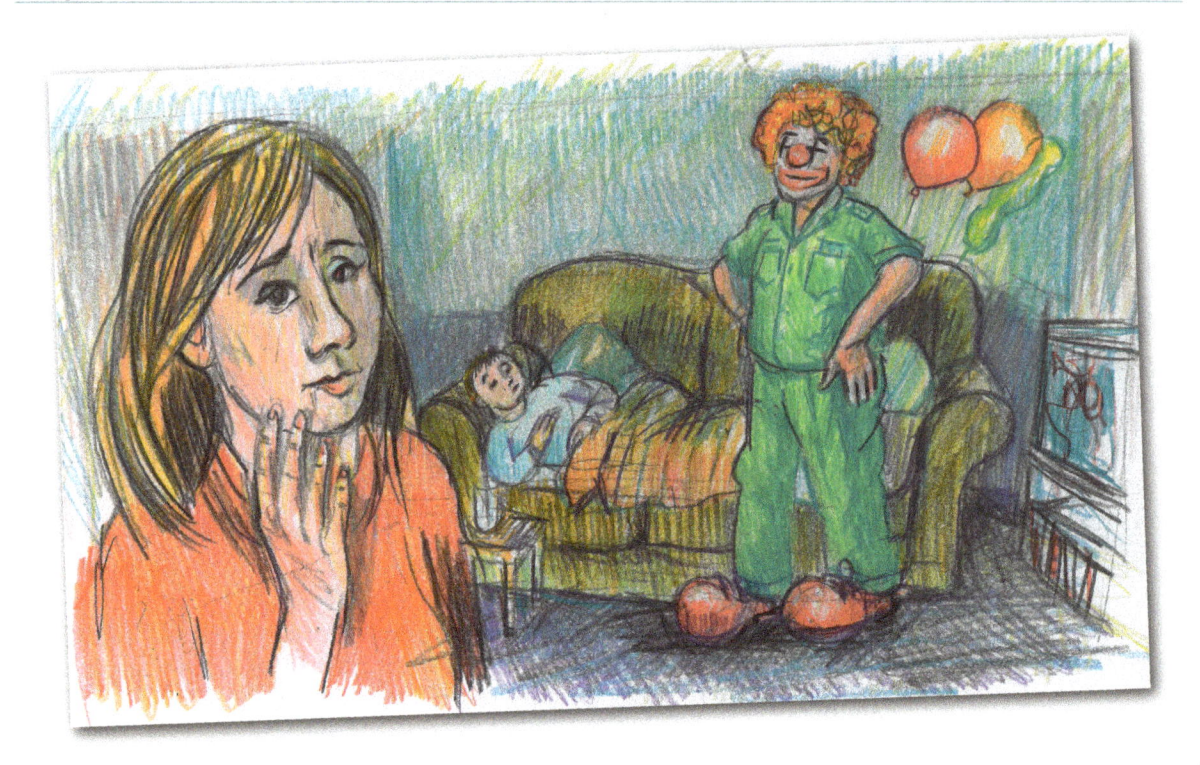

Feverish Illness in Children

You are on standby with the station clown. At least, everyone agrees that his clinical practice is a joke. Sadly, his practical joking is proving to be wearing, particularly since you are stuck with him for the entire shift.

The MDT flashes into life, passing you details of a redirected 111 call relating to a 4-year-old boy. The patient has a six-day history of fever, rash and cough. "Oh dear, another worried mother," your colleague chuckles to himself, "probably just run out of paracetamol." He gives two honks of the ambulance horn and sets off to the address.

The incident location is a terraced house in a rundown part of town, which seems to affirm your colleague's "worried mother" hypothesis. He parks up and skips round to the house, despite the fact that it is your turn to attend. Without being invited in, he steps past the mother who has opened the door and disappears inside.

You find him in the living room, where the mother is trying to provide a history, but keeps getting interrupted by your colleague:

"It started a week ago. He got a fever which I just couldn't get down …" starts the mother.
"Perhaps you should give him paracetamol," interrupts your colleague.
"I have been, every four hours and …"
"He could have ibuprofen at the same time too, you know."
"I was told not to give them together, but stagger them …"
"Well, perhaps you should go and see your GP."
"I did, two days ago, and he gave me these antibiotics, but they're not working …"
"Well, they can take several days to work, dear."

Feverish Illness in Children

"The doctor told me that, but Thomas is not eating or drinking and just lies on the sofa …" "Sitting about watching TV, eh? It's a good life for some."

Having apparently finished with the mother, your colleague slumps himself down next to the child, Thomas, who is curled up on the sofa. "Watcha watching?" giggles your colleague. Thomas turns to face him but does not speak. He is also apparently unimpressed by your colleague's repertoire of 'funny faces'. The boy does stick his tongue out when asked and it looks strawberry red, which seems odd. "Whoa there, cowboy, you need to take it easy on the blackcurrant squash." The mother looks incredulous, "What? He's only been drinking water." "Well, I don't see that there's much to worry about, mum. Keep up with the paracetamol and those antibiotics will get to work soon. If not, you can always go and see your GP … again."

> What should you do: **Leave** (read on) or **Do some obs** (skip the next paragraph)?

Leave

You offer to fetch the non-conveyance form, but your colleague isn't keen. "All that paperwork just gets in the way of saving lives, don't you think?" "Aren't you going to at least check him out?" asks the mother, who is fast losing faith in your colleague. "Well, if it would put your worries to bed," says your colleague condescendingly, "my chum here will get the monitor, won't you?"

Do some obs

Your colleague's hands-off approach is getting rather worrying, so you troop back to the ambulance and fetch the monitor/defibrillator and blood glucose meter. Once back in the house, you introduce yourself to Thomas and explain what you'd like to do. He is quiet and compliant, which makes you suspicious. He doesn't even flinch when you obtain a blood glucose from his very red hands. The results of your primary assessment are as follows:

General impression

Lethargic child lying on sofa

Airway

Patent

Breathing

Respiratory rate: 30 breaths/min
SpO_2: 96% on air

Circulation

Heart rate: 130 beats/min
Capillary refill time: 3 seconds
Looks pale

Disability

GCS score: 14/15
Pupils: Equal and round, reacting to light
Conjunctivae are reddened
Blood glucose: 3.8 mmol/l

Exposure/Environment

Temperature: 39.2°C
Wong-Baker pain score: 6/10
Blanching rash on torso

Your colleague looks triumphant: "See? No red traffic light symptoms, he'll be fine." The mother, however, does not look the least bit reassured.

> What are you going to do: **Contact the GP** (read on) or **Transport** (skip the next section)?

Contact the GP

You point out that any amber traffic light symptoms in children under 5 should have serious consideration given to being transported to hospital. At the very least, you need to contact the patient's GP. "If it will stop you worrying," responds your colleague sarcastically. You contact the GP, but have to wait 15 minutes for a call back, while putting up with your colleague's comments.

The GP does call back and you retell the history and outline your concerns about leaving the patient at home. The GP agrees and wonders aloud, "What idiot would leave that child at home." You see this as the perfect time to hand over the phone to your colleague. The GP sees this as an ideal opportunity to provide your colleague with some distance learning, and the cheesy grin on your colleague's face soon disappears as the GP lays out in no uncertain terms the seriousness of the consequences had the child been left at home. After the call ends, your colleague sheepishly turns to the mother and advises her that a trip to hospital is probably the best way to proceed.

Transport

Although the child is still flagging up as an amber on the traffic lights for feverish illness, the history and symptoms are worrying you. In the darkest recess of your mind a Japanese-sounding disease is trying to escape, but it takes a quick internet search to remind you – Kawasaki disease. It's a form of vasculitis that can cause aneurysms to form on children's coronary arteries.

You show the webpage to your colleague, which soon wipes the smug look off his face. "We'd better go to the ED, eh?" you suggest. You explain to the mother that although Thomas doesn't seem to be in any immediate danger, he needs to see a paediatrician urgently. She is grateful that someone has taken her concerns seriously and quickly gathers up items that she needs for Thomas and the trip to hospital.

Once at the hospital, the diagnosis of Kawasaki disease is confirmed and the patient is treated with immunoglobulin and aspirin, which comes as a surprise to you given the risk of Reye's syndrome that makes it a contraindication in your ambulance clinical practice guidelines.

Scale of the problem

Fever is defined by the National Institute for Health and Care Excellence (NICE) as an elevation of body temperature above normal daily variation.[16] There is no actual temperature value specified in the guidelines for fever, although temperatures of 38°C and above in infants under three months are classed as high risk. For older infants, temperatures of 39°C and above are classed as an intermediate risk.

Feverish illness in children is one of the most common reasons for a GP visit, and is responsible for up to half of paediatric emergency department (ED) attendances. About a quarter of these ED attendances involve infants and half, children aged 1–3 years. Between 5% and 25% of feverish illness is due to a serious bacterial infection.[17]

Although NICE provide a technical definition, in reality fever is perceived in three main ways by parents and healthcare professionals:[18]

- As a disease
- As a diagnostic sign
- As a symptom.

There is considerable anxiety around fever in children and the natural tendency is to aggressively relieve it, despite the fact that fever on its own is not dangerous. Clinically, it is indicative of infection, but not a reliable indicator of the severity of the underlying disease.[16]

Physiology of fever

Fever (also often referred to as pyrexia) is caused by cytokine-induced resetting of the hypothalamus thermostatic set-point, but temperatures in excess of this are possible

Feverish Illness in Children

during prolonged convulsions, hyperthermic states and impairment of the hypothalamus.[19]

Although fever is mainly associated with infection, non-infectious illnesses can also cause fever, including myocardial infarction, pulmonary embolism, cancer and overdose of certain drugs, such as ecstasy. In addition, central nervous system trauma and intracranial haemorrhage involving the hypothalamus can also lead to increased body temperature.[19]

For this explanation, however, we are going to focus on the most common cause, that is, an infection. For the visual learners, this process is shown in Figure 8.2:

1. Infection that induces fever can be local or systemic. It starts with the shedding of bacterial cell-wall substances known as exogenous pyrogens, which then enter the general circulation.

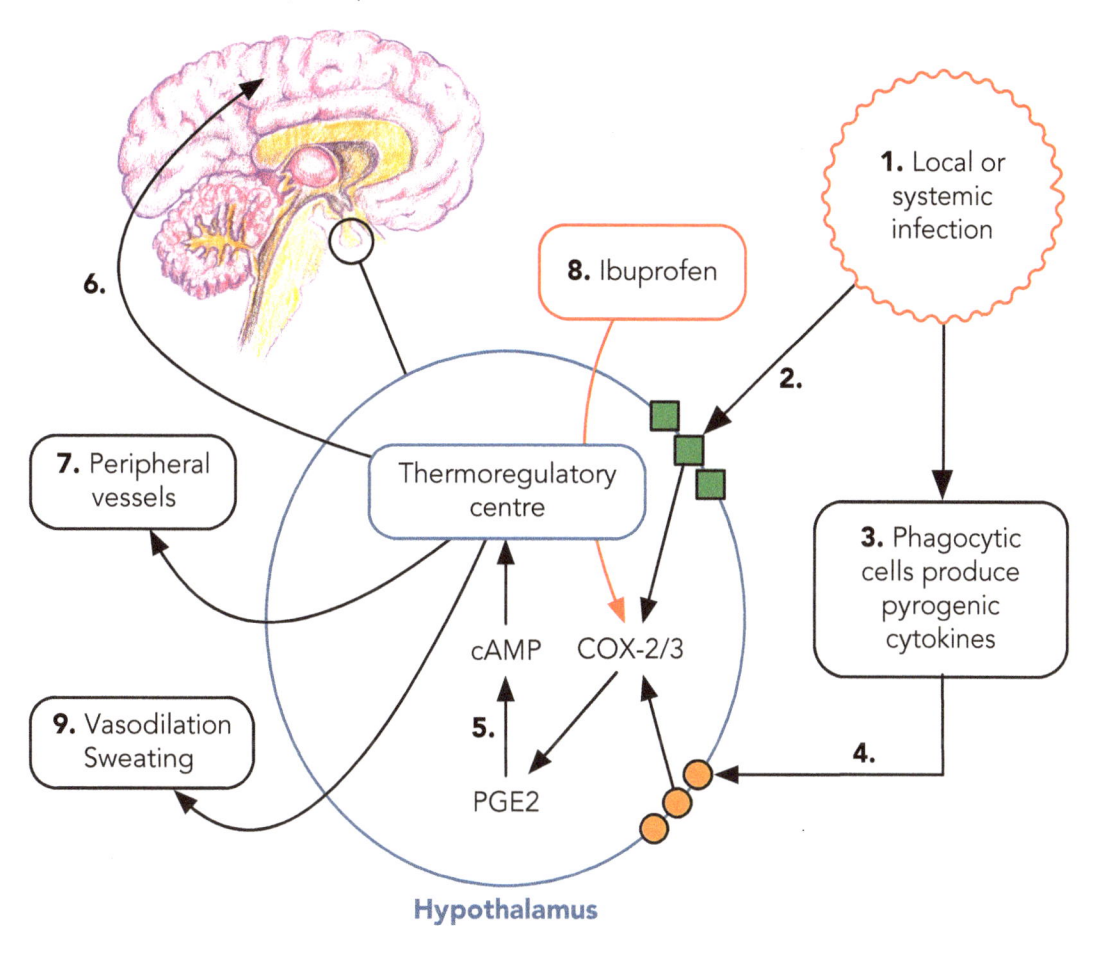

Figure 8.2 The physiology of fever.

2. Exogenous pyrogens do not cross the blood–brain barrier, but instead bind to toll-like receptors (TLR) and activate the endothelium of the hypothalamus.
3. In addition, exogenous pyrogens also bind to the body's phagocytic cells (such as neutrophils and macrophages) and blood vessel endothelial cells. This causes the synthesis of pyrogenic cytokines (sometimes called endogenous pyrogens) including interleukin-1 (IK-1) and tumour necrosis factor alpha (TNF-a), which are released into the blood.
4. The pyrogenic cytokines are transported by the general circulation to the hypothalamus, where they bind to cytokine receptors.
5. In the hypothalamus, activation of TLR and cytokine receptors activate cyclo-oxygenase-2 (COX-2) and possibly COX-3, leading to synthesis of prostaglandin E2 (PGE2). This in turn stimulates the release of the secondary messenger cyclic-adenosine monophosphate (cAMP), increasing the thermoregulatory centre set-point.
6. Increasing the set-point results in signalling to the cerebral cortex to initiate behavioural change (such as wrapping yourself in the thickest duvet you can find) to promote heat conservation. This stage can also be accompanied by violent shivering and teeth chattering (rigors).
7. At the same time, efferent nerves utilise the sympathetic nervous system to signal the peripheral vessels to constrict, further decreasing heat loss and increasing the core body temperature.
8. The increase in body temperature continues until the levels of PGE2 in the hypothalamus fall, either due to the administration of anti-pyretics, usually non-steroidal anti-inflammatory drugs (NSAIDs) such as ibuprofen that inhibit COX-2/3, or COX-2/3 synthesis decreases as a result of reduced activation of TLR and cytokine receptors as the infection resolves.
9. Once the PGE2 levels return to normal, the set-point returns to its baseline and temperature-lowering strategies are implemented, such as vasodilation, sweating and increasing the respiratory rate.

The purpose of fever is not fully understood, but with every 1°C rise in body temperature, the body's metabolic rate increases by 10%.[20] This is useful as this leads to increased motility and activity of white blood cells and activation of T-cells, to fight infection. In addition, many microbes replicate best at normal body temperature and increasing body temperature slows this process. Finally, fever causes a shift from glucose metabolism to lipolysis and proteolysis, reducing the amount of free glucose that can be utilised by invading microbes.[19]

Assessment

Conduct an initial paediatric assessment triangle and ABCDE assessment to identify immediate life-threatening conditions. Once this has been undertaken, obtain a history, ensuring that you cover the following:[12]

- Duration of illness
- Associated symptoms
- Urinary symptoms
- Abdominal pain
- Headache, photophobia, neck stiffness
- Painful joints, sore throat, ear pain
- Adequacy of fluid intake
- Existing medical problems
- Current medication
- Other illness in the family/school/nursery
- Recent foreign travel.

NICE have produced a table utilising a 'traffic light' system to stratify signs and symptoms according to risk (Table 8.4).[16]

Children with fever who have any of the signs and symptoms in the red column should be considered to be high risk. Similarly, children with fever and signs and symptoms only in the yellow column are classed as intermediate risk and for signs and symptoms in the green

Table 8.4 NICE traffic light system for identifying risk of serious illness.

	Green (Low risk)	**Amber (Intermediate risk)**	**Red (High risk)**
Colour (of skin, lips or tongue)	Normal colour	Pallor reported by parent/carer	Pale/mottled/ashen/cyanosed
Activity	Responds normally to social cues Content/smiles Stays awake or awakens quickly Strong normal cry/not crying	Not responding normally to social cues No smile Wakes only with prolonged stimulation Decreased activity	No response to social cues Appears ill to a healthcare professional Does not wake or if roused does not stay awake Weak, high-pitched or continuous cry

Respiratory		Nasal flaring
		Tachypnoea:
		  RR >50 breaths/min, age 6–12 months
		  RR >40 breaths/min in children
		Oxygen saturations 95% or less in air
		Crackles on chest auscultation
			Grunting
			Tachypnoea:
			  RR >60 breaths/min
			Moderate or severe recession

Circulation and hydration	Normal skin and eyes
	Moist mucous membranes
		Tachycardia:
		  >160 beats/min, age >12 months
		  >150 beats/min, age 1–2 years
		  >140 beats/min, age 2–5 years
		CRT 3 seconds or more
		Dry mucous membranes
		Poor feeding in infants
		Reduced urine output
			Reduced skin turgor

Other	No amber or red signs or symptoms	Age 3–6 months, temperature 39°C or higher Fever for 5 days or more Rigors Swelling of a limb or joint Non-weight bearing limb/not using an extremity	Under 3 months of age, temperature 38°C or higher Non-blanching rash Bulging fontanelle Neck stiffness Status epilepticus Focal neurological signs Focal convulsions

Key: RR – respiratory rate; CRT – capillary refill time

Source: NICE, 2019.

Chapter 8 Paediatrics

column only, low risk.[16] Although it is not always clear what has caused the fever, there are some signs and symptoms that are associated with specific diseases, which are worth keeping in mind, particularly if you are considering leaving the child at home (Table 8.5).

Table 8.5 Summary table for symptoms and signs suggestive of specific diseases.

Disease	Signs and symptoms
Meningococcal disease	Non-blanching rash, especially if one or more are present: 　Ill-looking child 　Spots >2 mm in diameter (purpura) 　Capillary refill time of 3 seconds or more 　Neck stiffness
Bacterial meningitis	Neck stiffness Bulging fontanelle Decreased level of consciousness Convulsive status epilepticus
Herpes simplex encephalitis	Focal neurological signs Focal convulsions Decreased level of consciousness
Pneumonia	Tachypnoea: 　>60 breaths/min, age 0–5 months 　>50 breaths/min, age 6–12 months 　>40 breaths/min, age 　>12 months Crackles on auscultation Nasal flaring Chest recession Cyanosis SpO_2 95% or less in air
Urinary tract infection	Vomiting Poor feeding Lethargy Irritability Abdominal pain or tenderness Urinary frequency or dysuria
Septic arthritis	Red, swollen joint Not using an extremity Non-weight bearing
Kawaswaki disease	Fever >5 days and at least 4 of: 　Bilateral conjunctival injection ('red eyes') 　Dry, cracked lips and/or strawberry-coloured tongue 　Change in extremities such as oedema or erythema 　Polymorphous rash 　Cervical lymphadenopathy

Adapted from: NICE, 2019.

Thermometers

Oral thermometers are not suitable for children aged 5 years or under. Forehead thermometers are not accurate and should not be used at all. In infants under 4 weeks, NICE recommend recording axillary temperature (that is, in the armpit). For older infants and children up to 5 years of age, there are a number of acceptable options:[16]

- Electronic or chemical dot thermometer in the axilla
- Infrared tympanic thermometer (although note that tympanic thermometers typically cannot be used in infants under 3 months).

Management

Anti-pyretics

Giving a patient anti-pyretics such as ibuprofen or paracetamol for fever is not necessary, if the child is otherwise asymptomatic. However, they are useful for treating other symptoms associated with infection such as aches, pains and generally feeling unwell, and may also reassure concerned parents, who in turn can relay their anxiety to the child.[21,22] There is no evidence that anti-pyretic drugs prevent febrile convulsions occurring, or are beneficial in preventing further episodes when a child has suffered from a convulsion.[23]

Transport vs safety netting

All febrile children meeting the following criteria should be transported to hospital:[12]

- Any child under 5 years who has a single red traffic light sign or symptom
- Any febrile infant less than 1 month old
- Any febrile child under 3 months who does not have an obvious cause for their fever
- Any child under 3 years who does not have an obvious cause for their fever and who cannot have a urine sample analysis arranged via the GP at the time the crew are on scene
- Any child with signs/symptoms of a serious illness or where there is any concern that they might be seriously ill
- Any child with a significant fever who has received antibiotics in the last 48 hours
- Any child on steroids or other immuno-suppressant drugs
- Any child where there is concern about the provision of adequate supervision
- Those with a medical protocol stating admission is necessary.

Safety netting

A safety net in healthcare is verbal and/or written advice about when to re-contact or access further healthcare advice and provision, or follow-up consultations to ensure further assessment and treatment, if required.[24]

If you decide not to transport a feverish child, make sure you provide written information on warning symptoms and advice about how further healthcare can be accessed.

Any child with amber traffic light signs and symptoms requires a follow-up with a GP or paediatric healthcare professional. Obtain a specific time-frame and location for this follow-up when making the referral.[12]

Chapter 8   Paediatrics

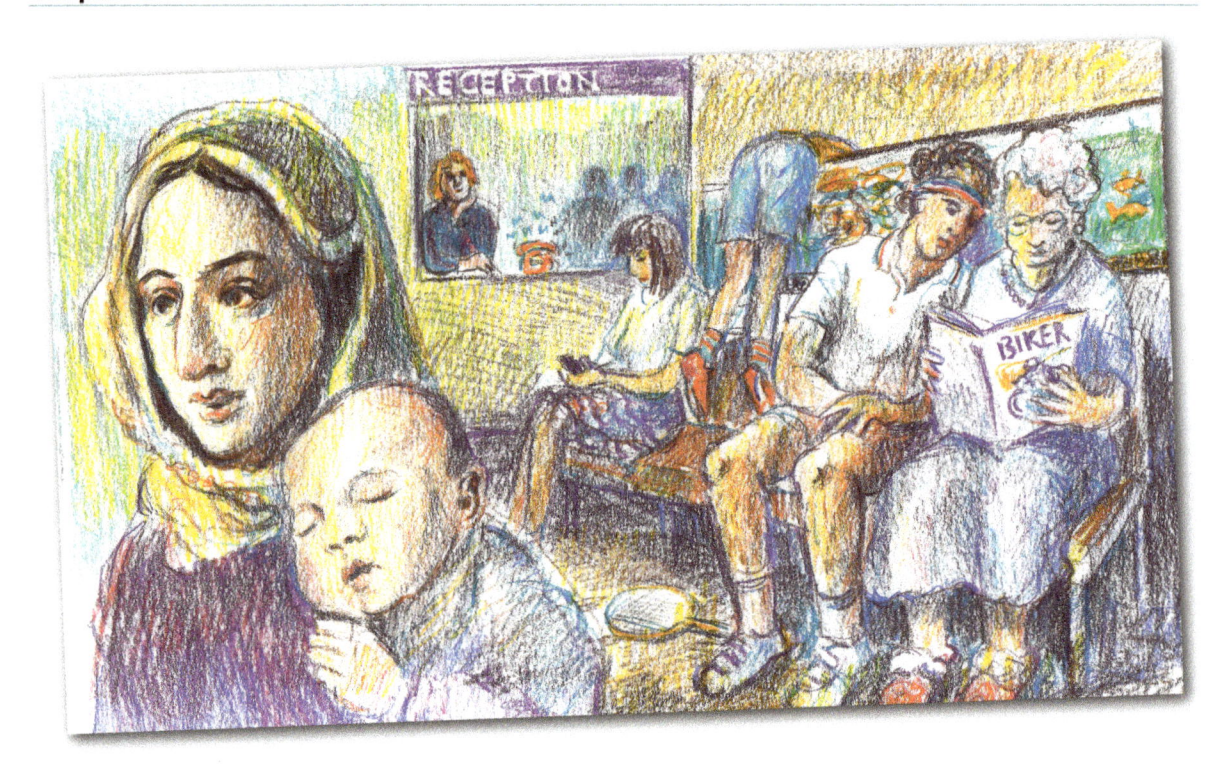

Meningococcal Disease

You are on standby, trying to book a routine appointment with your general practitioner (GP). The phone is answered by your least favourite receptionist, and after unsuccessfully trying to get the purpose of your visit out of you, she states that there are no appointments until next month.

The MDT cuts short your discussion as you are passed an emergency call at another GP surgery nearby. The patient is a 6-month-old girl with possible meningitis. Four minutes later, you arrive at the surgery and are directed to the GP's consulting room by a flustered-looking receptionist. The GP looks rather pleased to see you and briefly outlines the history. He explains that the infant has been generally unwell and not feeding properly since yesterday. "She was not her normal self," adds the mother, who had called the out-of-hours GP deputising service and was advised over the phone to keep up oral fluids.

This morning, the mother had awoken to find her daughter still asleep in the cot, which was unusual. She initially thought her daughter was dead, as she looked pale and was floppy when picked up, so rushed around to the GP surgery, and demanded to see a doctor. "The receptionist told me there were no appointments, can you believe it?" spits the mother. You nod in agreement, but decide that this is not the right time to share your own frustrations with GP receptionists. Fortunately, a passing GP came to investigate the fuss and on spotting the child, called 999 straightaway.

The patient is clearly unwell and looks lifeless in her mother's arms. You enquire about a rash and are told that there is a blanching, maculopapular rash under the armpits and in the groin. She feels hot and the GP informs you that her temperature is 39.3°C.

> What should you do next: **Relax and administer paracetamol** (read on) or **Stay alert and leave now** (skip the next two paragraphs)?

Relax and administer paracetamol

You have lost count of the number of febrile children you have been called to. You direct the mother to remove the infant's clothes, including the nappy, and ask the doctor if there is any paracetamol in the surgery. The rash is blanching, so she can't be suffering from meningococcal septicaemia, right?

The GP returns with the paracetamol, but the infant is not alert enough for you to administer it. You take the infant from the mother and return to the ambulance. After placing the infant on the stretcher, you take a look at the infant and to your horror, you can clearly see the marks left by your hands where you picked her up. You start to mumble an apology to an equally aghast mother, but before your eyes, a petechial rash starts to form. You realise too late, that this infant does indeed have meningococcal septicaemia. Despite your colleague driving the ambulance as if he had stolen it, the infant is covered in purpura by the time you arrive at hospital and in the panic, you fail to administer benzylpenicillin. Despite the best efforts of the hospital team, the patient suffers a cardiac arrest and dies.

Stay alert and leave now

The blanching rash is little comfort to you, given how sick the infant is. You rapidly exit the surgery with mum and the little girl. As you place her on the stretcher, you note the appearance of petechiae, where you had been holding her. They appear to be growing before your eyes.

> What is your next move: **Administer benzylpenicillin** (read on) or **Do something else** (skip the next paragraph)?

Administer benzylpenicillin

You know that early administration of antibiotics is important, so you set about drawing it up. The situation is not made any easier by erratic swaying of the ambulance, as your colleague curses their way through traffic and after a particularly tight corner, the vial slips from your grasp and rolls into a dark recess. By the time you have drawn up a second dose, the ambulance is pulling into the hospital and as you approach the infant to administer the drug, you realise that she is not breathing. The doors spring open as soon as the vehicle stops. You see the concerned faces of the hospital team turn to disgust, when they spot the apnoeic infant lying on the stretcher.

Do something else

Benzylpenicillin is important, but you know you need to address the ABCs first. You open the infant's airway and insert an oropharyngeal airway, which she accepts. Her breathing is rapid, but appears adequate at present, so you apply a non-rebreathing mask and turn up the oxygen. After instructing your colleague to set off for hospital, you draw up the benzylpenicillin and administer it intramuscularly.

The infant is clearly shocked and requires fluid resuscitation. You take a brief look at her arms and can see no obvious veins, so elect to gain intraosseous access. However, while preparing the necessary kit, you reassess the infant and realise that she is no longer ventilating adequately, prompting you to abandon your attempt at gaining vascular access, and instead commence bag-valve-mask ventilations. The ambulance squeals up to the hospital doors and as soon as the vehicle stops, the ambulance doors spring open and the concerned faces of the hospital team come into view. You enquire about the patient several days later and find out that she has survived, but unfortunately had to have one of her legs amputated.

Incidence and definition

Meningococcal disease is an umbrella term for a systemic bacterial infection caused by *Neisseria meningitidis* (meningococcus). It presents as meningitis, septicaemia or a combination of both.[25] Although uncommon, 5% of those affected will die, and up to 36% may have long-term physical, cognitive, and psychological consequences.[26] It is most common in infants, followed by children aged 1–4 years and young adults (15–19 years).[27]

Meningococci are classified according to the antigenic properties of their capsule (serogroup).[26] There are at least 13 different types, but the most common are A, B, C, W and Y. Type A causes epidemics in sub-Saharan Africa and W135 is most commonly found in Hajj pilgrims visiting Mecca and in the Middle East generally. In the UK, the most prevalent serogroup is B.[27]

Pathophysiology

Meningococci can inhabit the nasopharynx without causing a problem. However, if the meningococci manage to penetrate the protective mucosa of the nasal passages and enter the bloodstream, they rapidly multiply, doubling in number every 30 minutes.

The outer wall of the meningococcus contains lipopolysaccharides (endotoxin), which are shed by the meningococcus in vesicles (blebs). The endotoxin binds with lipopolysaccharide binding protein (LBP), which amplifies its effect and aids attachment to monocytes and endothelial cells. The endotoxin and LBP complex attach to toll-like receptors on the cells, usually with the aid of an intermediary binding molecule (CD14).[28] This causes the release of pro-inflammatory cytokines, including tumour necrosis factor alpha (TNFα), interleukin 1 (IL-1) and interleukin 8 (IL-8 or interferon-γ). In addition, anti-inflammatory cytokines (IL-4 and IL-10) are released and the clotting cascade is activated via the expression of tissue factor.[19]

In response to endotoxin activation, neutrophils produce toxic oxygen species, inflammatory proteins, proteases and other enzymes, which can damage tissues.[29]

Complement cascade

The complement system plays a key role in host defence mechanisms, including:[30]

- Destruction/dissolution (lysis) of bacteria
- Increasing phagocytosis by macrophages and neutrophils
- Neutralisation of endotoxin
- In addition, it is also important in the coagulation and fibrinolysis systems, as well as helping to maintain vascular permeability and tone.

Endotoxin can activate all three pathways of the complement system, resulting in cleavage of complement factor C3 to C3b, which binds to the surface of pathogens and marks them for elimination through phagocytosis or cell lysis, via the formation of the membrane attack complex through the microbial plasma membrane.[31]

However, some endotoxins can avoid being marked for destruction by being structurally related to human blood group antigens (and so be considered to 'belong' to the host), or by synthesising sialic acid, usually produced by endothelial cells and erythrocytes, which inhibits the complement cascade.

Vascular endothelium

The endothelial cells in the vasculature are in direct contact with the blood and maintain an uninterrupted blood flow by promoting anticoagulation and fibrinolysis. Collectively, the cells have a huge surface area, estimated to be 4,000–7,000 m^2.[32] Anti-coagulation is achieved by the presence of heparan sulphate, a glycosaminoglycan (GAG) related to heparin on the cell surface, and thrombomodulin receptors, which bind thrombin. Heparan activates circulating antithrombin III (ATIII), which inactivates a number of clotting factors, including factor X, and removes free thrombin from the blood, preventing the formation of fibrin. The combined thrombin-thrombomodulin complex activates protein C, another anti-coagulant, which combines with protein S to inactivate factors Va and VIIIa in the clotting cascade (Figure 8.3) as well as inactivating plasminogen activator inhibitor (PAI-1).[33] Finally, endothelial cells release tissue plasminogen activator (tPA) to promote fibrinolysis.

Endothelial cells play an important role in the regulation of vasomotor tone, including the synthesis of nitric oxide (a potent vasodilator and platelet and endothelin inhibitor) and endothelin (a potent vasoconstrictor). In sepsis, there is an early compensatory vasoconstriction in some vascular beds, such as the skin, but generalised vasodilation. Although peripheral vasoconstriction is a protective mechanism, if it persists, the extremities can become ischaemic.[30]

If endothelial cells are activated due to cytokine or endotoxin exposure, the structure and function of the cells change to a pro-coagulant state. There is loss of surface heparans and thrombomodulin and release of tissue factor, von Willebrand factor (vWF) and plasminogen activating inhibitor (PAI-1). Active separation of the tight junctions between the cells occurs, leading to the loss of high molecular weight proteins (such as albumin) into the interstitial tissues, resulting in profound hypovolaemia as fluid and electrolytes follow the albumin out of the vessels (Figure 8.4).[32]

The clotting cascade

Tissue factor released by monocytes and endothelial cells leads to activation of the extrinsic pathway of the clotting cascade. In addition, damage to endothelial cells, caused by the release of enzymes from neutrophils which adhere to the endothelium, can trigger the intrinsic pathway (Figure 8.3). This coincides with a general reduction of tissue factor pathway inhibitor and so activation of the clotting cascade proliferates in the absence (or reduction) of anti-coagulant mechanisms, such as antithrombin III, heparan and activated protein C. Activated platelets adhere to the endothelial cells, thanks to expression of von Willebrand Factor (vWF). This is compounded by the reduction in endothelial tissue plasminogen activator (tPA) and circulating plasmin, and an increase in endothelial plasminogen activator inhibitor (PAI-1).

Overall, this results in an increase in coagulation and clot formation at the same time that fibrinolysis is impaired. The formation of microthrombi ensues and is most clearly seen in the skin. In severe meningococcal sepsis, widespread purpura fulminans can be seen due to thrombosis and haemorrhagic necrosis in large areas of the skin. In some cases, this can lead to infarction and gangrene of digits and even whole limbs. The widespread thrombosis by this mechanism is known as disseminated intravascular coagulation (DIC).[29]

Chapter 8 Paediatrics

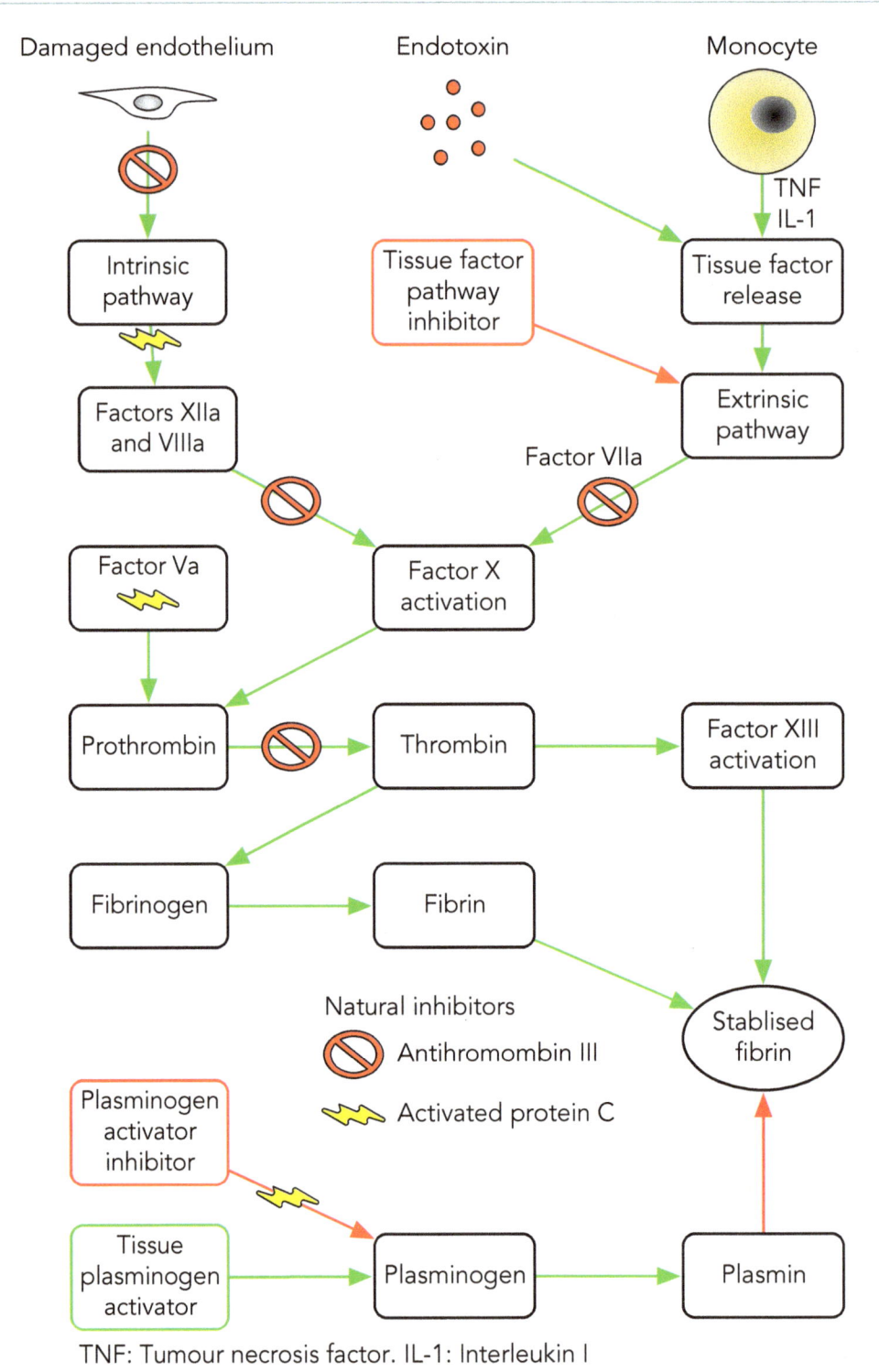

Figure 8.3 The clotting cascade.

TNF: Tumour necrosis factor. IL-1: Interleukin I

Meningococcal Disease

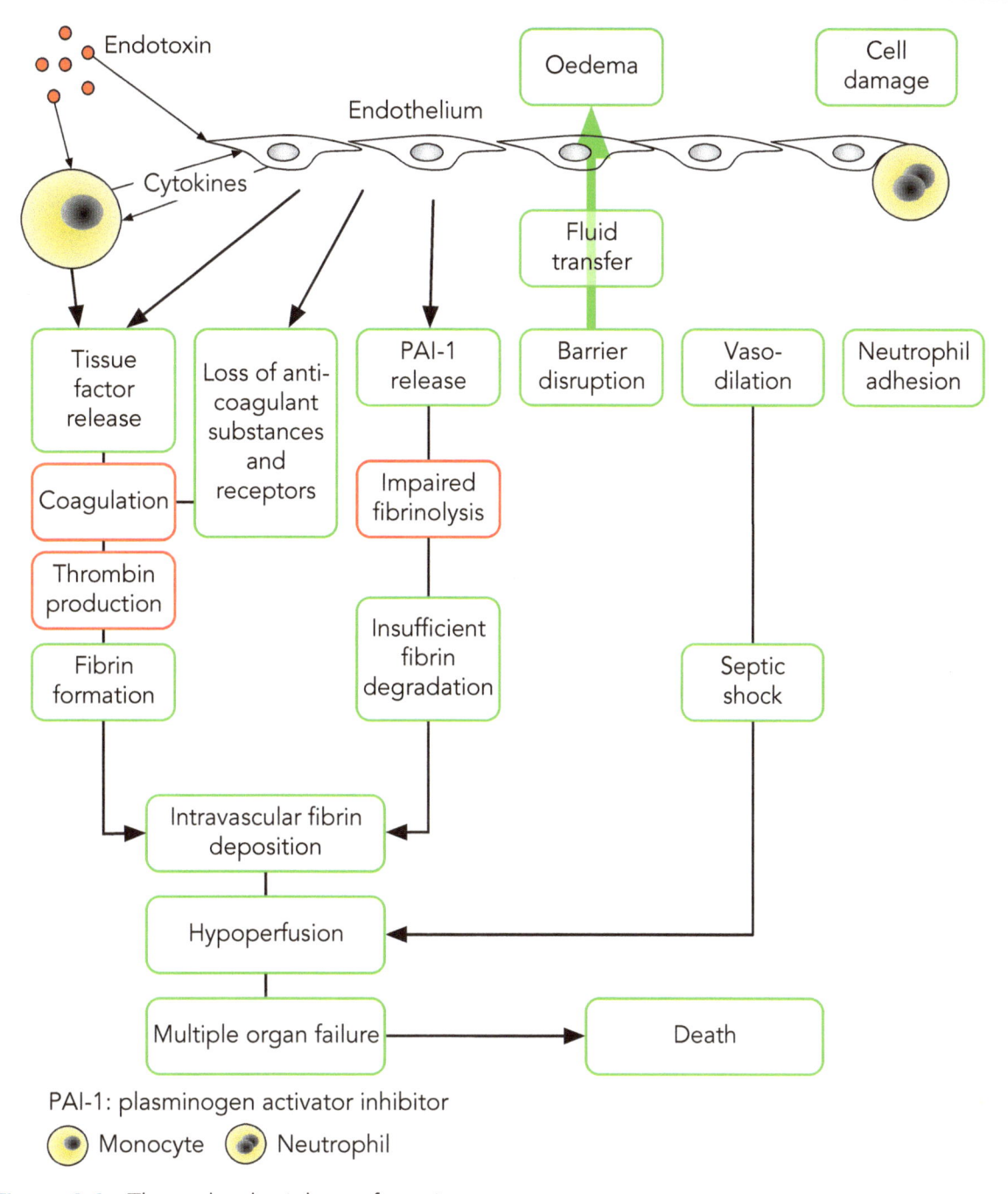

Figure 8.4 The pathophysiology of sepsis.

PAI-1: plasminogen activator inhibitor

Myocardial dysfunction

Hypovolaemia as a result of capillary leak, is a major contributor to the myocardial dysfunction seen in meningococcal septicaemia. A pro-inflammatory cytokine, interleukin 6 (IL-6), has been identified as a direct myocardial depressant. This, coupled with the hypoxia, acidosis, hypoglycaemia and electrolyte imbalances found in meningococcal sepsis all adversely affect the myocardium, which may persist even after initial volume resuscitation.[34]

Meningococcal meningitis

The exact mechanism by which meningococci manage to penetrate the blood–brain barrier is not entirely understood. However, in areas of very low blood flow (such as the cerebral microcirculation), the meningococci adhere to endothelial cells of the blood–brain barrier and over the course of several hours, create an intercellular space, in effect posing as an endothelial cell.[35,36] Once this has been achieved, the bacteria are free to multiply inside the cerebrospinal fluid. The subsequent release of endotoxin and cytokines cause leakage of proteins and fluid out of the cerebral vasculature. This increases the brain water content and intracranial pressure. As with septicaemia, microthrombi can form, further reducing cerebral perfusion and leading to ischaemia and infarction.[37]

Signs and symptoms

A major issue in the recognition of meningococcal disease is the non-specific nature of the signs and symptoms in the initial stages of the disease. These include:[38]

- Fever
- Nausea/vomiting
- Lethargy
- Irritable/unsettled
- Ill appearance
- Refusing food/drink
- Headache
- Muscle ache/joint pain
- Respiratory signs and symptoms or breathing difficulty.

However, the diagnosis window is short. Many children will have non-specific signs and symptoms in the first 4–6 hours, but can be close to death after 24 hours.[39]

Sepsis and shock

The first specific clinical signs to appear are likely to be those of sepsis and shock and include leg pain, abnormal skin colour, cold hands and feet and, in older children, thirst. Parents of younger children may also report drowsiness and difficulty in breathing (described as rapid or laboured).[39] Don't forget to enquire about how much urine a child has been passing or if they have had a wet nappy recently. Oliguria is an early sign of shock.[37]

Fever

Many children with septicaemia will become acutely ill with a fever. This can be complicated by a trivial viral illness that precedes this, but look for a sudden change in the history. Remember that not all children with meningococcal disease have fever and you should not dismiss a fever responsive to anti-pyretics (such as paracetamol and ibuprofen) as of viral origin.[37] Rather counter-intuitively, infants can actually develop hypothermia in sepsis.[40]

Rash

The classic sign is a petechial non-blanching rash. However, only 10% of children presenting with the rash will have meningococcal disease. The remainder will have a viral infection. On the other hand, febrile and ill children with a purpuric rash (a non-blanching rash of greater than 2 mm in diameter), are very likely to have meningococcal disease.[40] Care needs to be taken with blanching rashes, such as a maculopapular rash, as up to 30% of children may initially present with this, although careful examination will generally yield some non-blanching elements.[41] On dark skin, you may have to check the soles of the feet, palms of the hand, abdomen or conjunctivae and palate. You must fully undress the child and be thorough in your search. Petechial rashes may not be widespread initially and can be easily missed.

Meningism

The signs of meningococcal meningitis can be complicated by concurrent septicaemia in the child, making it difficult to differentiate an altered mental state due to sepsis-induced hypoperfusion, and that caused by raised intracranial pressure.

In younger children (particularly those under 2 years of age), there is less likely to be neck stiffness or photophobia. Babies with meningitis sometimes have a full or bulging fontanelle due to raised ICP and present with paradoxical irritability, that is, they become more distressed when handled than when left alone.[37]

Management

Given the complexity of the pathophysiology of meningococcal disease and the often-subtle presentation of early meningococcal septicaemia, the management of a sick child with meningococcal disease is relatively straightforward.[12,38]

- Ensure a patent airway
- Administer high-flow oxygen and look for signs of failing ventilation. You may need to assist ventilations in this case.
- Once A and B have been addressed, you need to leave scene. Everything else can be done en route.
- If meningococcal septicaemia is suspected and there is a non-blanching rash, administer benzylpenicillin. If there is no rash and the journey to hospital is short, then benzylpenicillin should not generally be administered. If transport is delayed or there is a long-journey time, administer benzylpenicillin, irrespective of whether the patient has a non-blanching rash.
- Obtain vascular access (one or two wide-bore cannulae, either intravenous or intraosseous).
- Treat signs of shock with 20 ml/kg fluid boluses, up to a maximum of 40 ml/kg. Fluid administration over 40 ml/kg will result in pulmonary oedema requiring intubation and ventilation at the receiving hospital.
- Remember DEFG, don't ever forget glucose. Obtain a blood glucose measurement en route to hospital and correct hypoglycaemia with 5 ml/kg of 10% glucose.
- Don't forget in all the excitement to pre-alert the receiving hospital. Continue to frequently reassess your patient.

Chapter 8 Paediatrics

References

1. National Institute for Health and Care Excellence. Croup [Internet]. 2019. Available from: https://cks.nice.org.uk/topics/croup/
2. Cherry JD. Croup. *New England Journal of Medicine*, 2008 Jan 24;358(4):384–391.
3. Brown CA. *The Walls manual of emergency airway management*, 5th edition. Sakles JC, Mick NW, editors. Philadelphia: Lippincott Williams and Wilkins; 2017.
4. Kunzelmann K, König J, Sun J, Markovich D, King NJ, Karupiah G, et al. Acute effects of parainfluenza virus on epithelial electrolyte transport. Journal of Biological Chemistry, 2004 Nov 19;279(47):48760–48766.
5. Bjornson CL, Johnson DW. Croup. *The Lancet*, 2008;371(9609):329–339.
6. Shigemitsu H, Afshar K. Nocturnal asthma. *Current Opinion in Pulmonary Medicine*, 2007 Jan;13(1):49–55.
7. Guldfred L-A, Lyhne D, Becker BC. Acute epiglottitis: epidemiology, clinical presentation, management and outcome. Journal of Laryngology & Otology, 2008; 122(08):818–823.
8. Smith DK, McDermott AJ, Sullivan JF. Croup: Diagnosis and Management. *American Family Physician*, 2018 May 1;97(9):575–580.
9. Kuo CY, Parikh SR. Bacterial tracheitis. Pediatrics in Review, 2014 Nov;35(11):497–499.
10. Westley CR, Cotton EK, Brooks JG. Nebulized racemic epinephrine by IPPB for the treatment of croup: a double-blind study. *American Journal of Diseases in Childhood*, 1960. 1978 May;132(5):484–487.
11. Sparrow A, Geelhoed G. Prednisolone versus dexamethasone in croup: a randomised equivalence trial. *Archives of Disease in Childhood*, 2006 Jan 7;91(7):580–583.
12. Joint Royal Colleges Ambulance Liaison Committee, Association of Ambulance Chief Executives. JRCALC Clinical Guidelines. Cited from JRCALC Plus (Version 1.2.13) [Mobile application software]. Bridgwater: Class Publishing Ltd; 2021.
13. Wheeler DS, Wong HR, Shanley TP. *Pediatric critical care medicine: basic science and clinical evidence*. London: Springer; 2007.
14. Bjornson C, Russell K, Vandermeer B, Klassen TP, Johnson DW. Nebulized epinephrine for croup in children. *Cochrane Database of Systematic Reviews*, [Internet]. 2013;(10). Available from: https://www.cochranelibrary.com/cdsr/doi/10.1002/14651858.CD006619.pub3/full
15. Sakthivel M, Elkashif S, Al Ansari K, Powell CVE. Rebound stridor in children with croup after nebulised adrenaline: does it really exist? *Breathe*, 2019 Mar;15(1):e1–e7.
16. National Institute for Health and Care Excellence. Fever in under 5s: assessment and initial management [Internet]. NICE; 2019. Available from: https://www.nice.org.uk/guidance/ng143
17. De S, Williams GJ, Hayen A, Macaskill P, McCaskill M, Isaacs D, et al. Accuracy of the 'traffic light' clinical decision rule for serious bacterial infections in young children with fever: a retrospective cohort study. *British Medical Journal*, 2013 Feb 13;346(feb13 1):f866–f866.
18. Purssell E. Fever in children – a concept analysis. Journal of Clinical Nursing, 2013 Sep 1;1–8.
19. Porth C. *Essentials of pathophysiology: concepts of altered states*, 4th edition. Philadelphia: Lippincott Williams and Wilkins; 2014.
20. Broom M. Physiology of fever. *Journal of Pediatric Nursing*, 2007 Jul;19(6):40–44.
21. Bont EG de, Francis NA, Dinant G-J, Cals JW. Parents' knowledge, attitudes, and practice in childhood fever: an internet-based survey. *British Journal of General Practice*, 2014 Jan 1; 64(618):e10–e16.
22. Williams C, Roland D. Does the use of antipyretics prolong the duration of fever or illness? Archives of Disease in Childhood – Education and Practice, 2014 Jan 21; edpract-2013-305796.
23. Offringa M, Newton R, Cozijnsen MA, Nevitt SJ. Prophylactic drug management for febrile seizures in children. *Cochrane Database of Systematic Reviews*, [Internet]. 2017;(2). Available from: https://www.cochranelibrary.com/cdsr/doi/10.1002/14651858.CD003031.pub3/abstract
24. Roland D, Jones C, Neill S, Thompson M, Lakhanpaul M. Safety netting in healthcare

settings: what it means, and for whom? *Archives of Disease in Childhood – Education and Practice*, 2014 Apr;99(2):48–53.
25. Public Health England. Meningococcal disease: guidance on public health management [Internet]. GOV.UK. 2019. Available from: https://www.gov.uk/government/publications/meningococcal-disease-guidance-on-public-health-management
26. Public Health England. Meningococcal: the green book, chapter 22 [Internet]. 2016. Available from: https://www.gov.uk/government/publications/meningococcal-the-green-book-chapter-22
27. Public Health England. Invasive meningococcal disease in England: annual laboratory confirmed reports for epidemiological year 2019 to 2020 [Internet]. 2021. Available from: https://assets.publishing.service.gov.uk/government/uploads/system/uploads/attachment_data/file/951142/hpr0121_imd-ann.pdf
28. Daniels R, Nutbeam T. ABC of sepsis [Internet]. Chichester: BMJ/ Wiley-Blackwell; 2010 [cited 2012 Oct 23].
29. Pathan N, Faust SN, Levin M. Pathophysiology of meningococcal meningitis and septicaemia. *Archives of Disease in Childhood*, 2003 Jul;88(7):601–607.
30. de Kleijn ED, Hazelzet JA, Kornelisse RF, de Groot R. Pathophysiology of meningococcal sepsis in children. European Journal of Pediatrics, 1998 Nov;157(11):869.
31. Marieb E, Hoehn K. Human anatomy & physiology, 11th edition. Pearson; 2019.
32. Knoebl P. Blood coagulation disorders in septic patients. *Wiener Medizinische Wochenschrift*, 2010 Mar;160(5–6):129–138.
33. Ritter JM, Flower RJ, Henderson G, Yoon Kong Loke MB BS MRCP MD, MacEwan D, Rang HP. *Rang & Dale's pharmacology*, 9th edition. Edinburgh: Elsevier; 2019.
34. Cathie K, Levin M, Faust SN. Drug use in acute meningococcal disease. *Archives of Disease in Childhood – Education and Practice*, 2008 Oct 1;93(5):151–158.
35. Coureuil M, Nassif X. [The trick of the meningococcus]. *Médecine/sciences*, 2010 Jan;26(1):15–17.
36. Coureuil M, Join-Lambert O, Lécuyer H, Bourdoulous S, Marullo S, Nassif X. Mechanism of meningeal invasion by Neisseria meningitidis. *Virulence*, 2012 Mar 1;3(2):164–172.
37. Ninis N, Nadel S, Glennie L. *Lessons from research for doctors in training*, 4th edition. Bristol: Meningitis Research Foundation; 2018.
38. National Institute for Health and Care Excellence. Meningitis (bacterial) and meningococcal septicaemia in under 16s: recognition, diagnosis and management [Internet]. 2015. Available from: https://www.nice.org.uk/guidance/cg102
39. Thompson MJ, Ninis N, Perera R, Mayon-White R, Phillips C, Bailey L, et al. Clinical recognition of meningococcal disease in children and adolescents. *The Lancet*, 2006 Feb;367(9508):397–403.
40. Wells LC, Smith JC, Weston VC, Collier J, Rutter N. The child with a non-blanching rash: Low likely is meningococcal disease? *Archives of Disease in Childhood*, 2001 Sep;85(3):218.
41. Hart CA, Thomson APJ. Meningococcal disease and its management in children. *British Medical Journal*, 2006;333(7570):685–690.

9 Mental Health

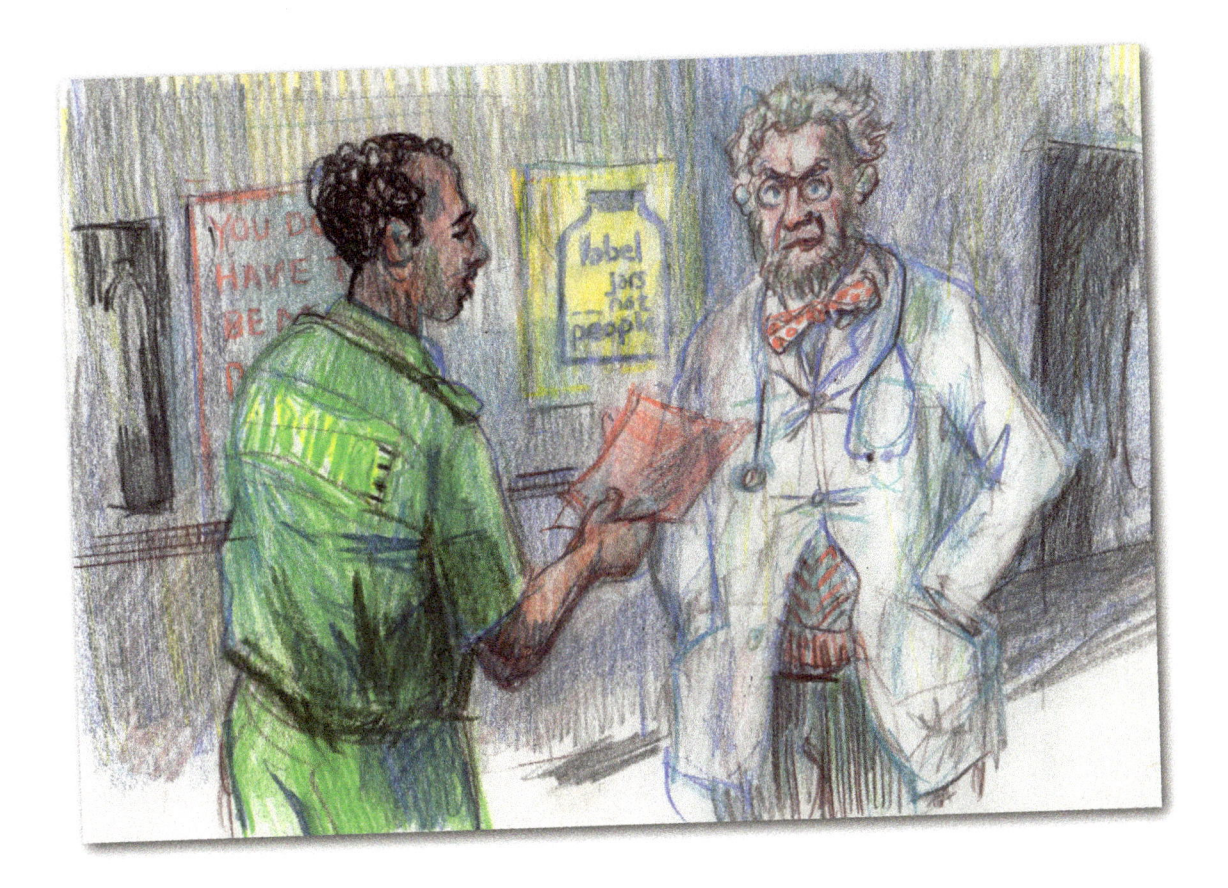

Mental Disorders and the Mental Health Act
By Sid Fletcher

You are technically not on standby, since you are waiting for the emergency operations centre (EOC) to let you know about your current incident. However, the delay has resulted in a 20-minute respite from a busy shift. The patient you have been called to has been detained under Section 3 of the Mental Health Act (MHA) and requires transport to the local psychiatric hospital. However, there is no one at the address, which is rather puzzling. The EOC has contacted the police, who deny having any incident logged to the address. The most helpful resource turns out to the be a neighbour who has watched you walking around the property and informs you that

Chapter 9   Mental Health

a police car took his neighbour away some hours ago.

This is your second mental health-related job so far. The shift started when a woman with a personality disorder decided to plunge a neon green plastic knife into a surgical wound (created a couple of weeks before when she had used a kitchen knife). The live-in carer looked rather sheepish as you quizzed her about the chain of events that led the patient to locking herself in the bathroom with the knife. Still, the patient had been no trouble and, apart from applying a couple of bulky dressings to secure the knife, the patient was stable en route to the local emergency department (ED).

After a pleasant wait, the EOC get back in touch and inform you that the police have, in fact, already transported the patient. However, just so you don't feel left out, they pass you details of another patient requiring transport to the local psychiatric hospital. The address is not far away, and your colleague sets off.

Things look promising as you arrive on scene, as you are flagged down by a dishevelled-looking individual. Luckily, you don't put your foot in it by assuming he is the patient as he introduces himself as Imran, an approved mental health professional (AMHP), who has assessed the patient and determined that a detention under Section 3 of the MHA is appropriate.

The patient (or client) is Richard, a 50-year-old male who has suffered from schizophrenia for 25 years and has been in the local psychiatric hospital on numerous occasions in the past, both informally and under the MHA. He also has hypertension and type 2 diabetes. "But is he violent?" your colleague asks, concerned. Imran assures you that there is no history of physical violence, although Richard can be verbally aggressive and truculent when unwell. Further, he has not taken any drugs or alcohol today. Richard's mental health has been declining for the past 5–6 weeks, despite intervention by the community mental health team. However, Richard has become convinced that the community team are actually foreign agents and so has become increasingly distrustful. In the last 2 days, he has been drinking only bottled water as he believes that the tap water is contaminated by the government. However, as he is on a low income (sickness benefits) this only amounts to three 500 ml bottles per day.

You follow Imran up the path towards the property, but your colleague does not move. You turn around and give him your 'what's up' look. "Aren't we going to wait for the police to come?" he enquires.

> What are you going to do: **Wait for the police** (read on) or **Follow Imran** (skip the next paragraph)?

Wait for the police

Your colleague is right, these 'mental' patients are dangerous, aren't they? Turn your back for a second and you'll likely have an axe in your head!

Actually no, you won't; Imran has already given you a full appraisal of the situation and he knows the patient far better than you do. You decide to follow him.

Follow Imran

The police have not been requested by Imran and his colleague and following their assessment, they are confident that they can persuade Richard to go to hospital. Criminalising a patient with mental health problems is not helpful.

You ascend a flight of stairs and are greeted by Imran's colleague, Lila, who is sitting with

Mental Disorders and the Mental Health Act

Richard. Richard looks up at you and, having decided you are not foreign agents, explains the conspiracy that is unfolding in the flat. He is very convincing, and only when he confides in you that his thoughts are being broadcast to the White House after his neighbour installed a satellite dish in the loft, are you reminded that Richard is seriously unwell.

Fortunately, he relishes the chance of escaping the surveillance in his flat and even takes a bottle of water from you, after you have drunk some yourself. Imran is satisfied that you are up to the task and passes you the relevant paperwork relating to the detention, electing not to travel as he has another client that requires his attention. The journey is uneventful and you see Richard safely onto the ward at the hospital. He is escorted into a room by one of the staff and the door has just closed when another person in a white coat approaches. He tells you he is Dr Kildare and would like to see the paperwork relating to Richard.

What are you going to do: **Hand it over** (read on) or **Ask to see some ID** (skip the next paragraph)?

Hand it over

You know better than to argue with a doctor, so you pass him Richard's paperwork. Fortunately, the staff member is just exiting the room and witnesses the transaction. "David, you know better than to read other client's notes." He mumbles an apology and slumps off. It turns out that "Dr Kildare" is actually an in-patient, not a member of staff.

Ask to see some ID

Having been to a psychiatric hospital before, you know that it can sometimes be hard to tell the difference between staff and in-patients, so you ask to see some ID. The doctor produces his bus pass, which identifies him as David Dickinson. Cover blown, he slinks away as the member of staff re-appears. After checking her ID, you hand over the paperwork and return to the ambulance.

Scale of the problem

Almost 40% of adults aged 16–74 years in England are accessing mental health treatment for a common mental disorder such as anxiety, depression, phobias and obsessive compulsive disorder (OCD).[1]

Diagnoses and interventions in relation to mental health are not sequential. Unlike other physiological measurements, such as heart rate, blood pressure and blood sugar, which are all easily recordable, the process of assessing mental health and its perceived risk is based upon a patient's collateral history in conjunction with a sound and robust mental state examination.

The vast majority of mental disorders are episodic in nature in the same way some physical illnesses are. It's perfectly feasible for a person to suffer a psychotic episode for a few weeks, or even months, and completely recover. These presentations are highly unlikely to be classed as schizophrenia.

The Mental Health Act 1983 (as amended 2007)

If a person has a mental disorder (defined as any disorder and disability of the mind) and is required to be detained against their wishes, specific sections of the MHA will be used to admit patients without their agreement.[2] You will commonly hear these patients referred to as being 'sectioned' or 'detained' under the MHA. This is in contrast to patients who agree to attend a psychiatric ward, whose admission may be referred to as 'informal' or 'voluntary'.[3]

Chapter 9 Mental Health

The MHA specifies a number of important roles relating to the decision to detain patients using the MHA. These include the approved mental health professional (AMHP), Section 12 doctor and nearest relative.

AMHP

An AMHP is usually a social worker (although since the amendment to the MHA in 2007, nurses, occupational therapists and psychologists, for example, can also become an AMHP)[4] who has been approved by the local social services authority to carry out a number of activities specified in the MHA.[5]

Their role includes the following:[6]

- Informing the nearest relative about the admission of the patient and their right to discharge
- Consulting the nearest relative about admission for treatment or guardianship and discontinuing the application (in the case of detention under Section 3 of the MHA) if the relative objects
- Applying for admission or guardianship if they are satisfied that the application is necessary
- Interviewing patients to determine that detention in hospital is the most appropriate way to care for the patient
- Reporting on the patient's social circumstances.

Section 12 doctor

This is a senior doctor (typically a middle-grade or higher psychiatrist) who is an approved clinician, that is, has been approved by the Secretary of State (England) or Welsh minister (Wales).[3]

Nearest relative

This is a really important role in the MHA. The nearest relative is defined as the highest in the following hierarchy:[2]

- Relative who usually resides with or cares for the patient
- Husband, wife or civil partner
- Child
- Parent
- Sibling
- Grandparent
- Grandchild
- Uncle or aunt
- Nephew or niece.

They have a range of powers including:[6]

- To apply for admission of the patient for assessment, treatment and guardianship (although this is unlikely: this is virtually always undertaken by an AMHP)[5]
- To object to an AMHP's proposed application for treatment under Section 3
- To discharge the patient having given 72 hours' notice in writing to hospital managers
- To apply to a mental health review tribunal.

Guiding principles

When deciding on a course of action to take using the MHA, AMHPs must take into account five guiding principles. Essentially, in real terms these principles ensure that all other avenues have been exhausted and admission under section is the only intervention that is likely to be successful and stabilise this particular episode of mental ill health. They are:[5]

- The **purpose** of an admission, i.e. why is the patient being admitted? Usually, this is to assess and/or stabilise their mental disorder
- Is there a **less restrictive** alternative available?
   - This may include home treatment, staying at a crisis house, staying with a relative or friend, for example
   - Would the patient be willing to go into hospital informally?

Mental Disorders and the Mental Health Act

- Will the assessment and admission process **respect** the wishes of patients and families/carers?
  - For example, the patient may have to be admitted promptly in order to prevent them further embarrassing themselves or putting themselves at risk
- The **participation** of the patient involved
  - Does the patient have capacity to be consulted and take part in the decision?
- The **efficacy/potential effectiveness** of the admission
  - Is admission likely to be effective?
  - Is it a proportionate response to the presentation, or a sledgehammer to crack an egg?

Section 2

This section provides the power to admit a patient to hospital and detain them for up to 28 days for the purposes of assessment on the grounds that they are suffering from a mental disorder severe enough to warrant the admission and that detention is appropriate for maintenance of the health and safety of the patient and others. The applicant needs to be an AMHP or the nearest relative and requires the agreement of two doctors, one of whom must be approved under Section 12 of the MHA.[2]

Section 3

This section provides the power to admit a patient to hospital and detain them for a period of 6 months initially (although it can be renewed) for the purposes of treatment, on the grounds that they are suffering from a mental disorder severe enough to receive treatment in hospital, that detention is appropriate for maintenance of the health and safety of the patient and others, and that an appropriate treatment is available. As before, the applicant needs to be an AMHP or nearest relative and requires the agreement of two doctors, one of whom must be approved under Section 12 of the MHA.

Section 4

This section is rarely used as it is viewed as an incomplete Section 2 or 3 by mental health professionals. It allows for the emergency admission of a patient for the purposes of assessment, requires the applicant to be an AMHP or nearest relative, but only requires one Section 12 approved doctor to recommend detention. The criteria for admission are the same as for Section 2.

Section 135

If a patient believed to have a mental disorder is being ill-treated, neglected or not kept under proper care, or is unable to care for themselves and living alone, an AMHP can obtain a warrant from a magistrate to enter any property where the patient is believed to be located, and, if necessary, remove them to a place of safety. This requires a police officer to execute the warrant and gain access to a property, with force if necessary, but they must be accompanied by a doctor and AMHP.[3]

Section 136

If a police officer encounters a person in a public place who appears to be suffering from a mental disorder and in immediate need of care or control, they can remove that person to a place of safety.[2] This should not normally be a police station and you are likely to be called to assist in transporting the person to a suitable location, such as a Section 136 suite at a local psychiatric hospital.[5]

Transporting a patient who has an application made under the MHA

You will have no doubt spotted a potential problem with the Sections of the MHA previously outlined. They typically require three healthcare professionals, including an AMHP to make the application and two doctors, one Section 12 approved, to detain a patient under Sections 2 and 3 of the MHA. This is usually impractical in the community, so there is provision in the MHA for the detention (if necessary) and transport of patients for whom an AMHP has made an application under the MHA.

This limbo period in-between deciding upon detention to the patient arriving at the ward is covered by Section 6 of the MHA. This allows the applicant (that is, the AMHP) or someone (such as you) authorised by the applicant, to take the patient to hospital, forcibly if necessary.[2] Under Section 137,[2] as an authorised person, you have the same powers, authorities, protection and privileges as a police officer! In reality, if there is a risk of physical violence then the police are likely to be involved following a risk assessment by the AMHP. You are also protected from civil and criminal proceedings (i.e. prosecution) under Section 139 (1) of the MHA unless you act in bad faith or do not take reasonable care. Always make sure you take the documentation relating to the application for admission and treatment under the MHA with you, even if (in most cases) the AMHP does not travel with the patient.

Generally, it falls to the ambulance service to transport patients, as use of police personnel and vehicles has been highlighted as bad practice, and their use should be reserved for physically violent patients.[7]

Mental disorders

Personality disorders

Personality disorder (PD) patients make frequent contact with emergency services (police and ambulance), GPs and emergency departments. Although making up around 5% of the general population, prevalence is closer to 40% in psychiatric in-patients. They can be a chaotic and challenging patient as they have a tendency to experience many pseudo-psychiatric symptoms, hence the term 'borderline', which implies a condition that is fleeting in nature but not chronic. They are usually worse when there is some form of social/relationship stressor as a backdrop.[8]

The best way to understand personality disorder is in terms of an entrenched extremely maladaptive and rigid coping mechanism (can't cope/won't cope). The best outcomes for PD patients are achieved with consistent, long term, therapeutic relationships and a readiness by the patient to address their coping mechanisms, typically with talking therapy. Medication has minimal effect, and repeated emergency service responses with subsequent hospital admission is not beneficial.[9]

The nature of the personality disorder is about frantically avoiding perceived isolation and abandonment, which typically manifests as becoming engaged in risky behaviour in order to prompt rescue. This can elicit 'knight in shining armour' behaviour in emergency services personnel and is in stark contrast to mental health staff who are likely to be more consistent and stick to the patient's care plan, becoming unpopular in the process. A common strategy adopted by patients with PD is to 'divide and rule' (known as splitting) to help them take control of a seemingly intolerable situation. Watch for comments relating to a comparison between how caring and understanding you are versus how bad mental health or ED staff are.

Psychosis

Psychosis refers to misperception of thoughts and perceptions that arise from the patient's own mind/imagination as reality, and includes delusions and hallucinations.[8] Two types of psychotic disorders are schizophrenia and bi-polar affective disorder.

Schizophrenia

The most common type of schizophrenia is the paranoid subtype, which includes delusions and auditory hallucinations. Delusions are frequently:[8]

- Persecutory – Someone or some group is out to harm the patient
- Delusions of reference – The patient is mentioned on the TV news or in a newspaper.

Disorders of thought can occur including:

- Derailment – Seemingly random connections between verbal statements in conversation
- Neologisms – The patient uses made up words, or uses words in a special way
- Word salad – Jumbled nonsense
- Concrete thinking – Inability to deal with abstract ideas.

Symptoms are often split into:

- Positive – Hallucinations and delusions
- Negative – Withdrawn, uncommunicative, unemotional, for example, monotonic speech.

Bi-polar affective disorder

This disorder (formerly called manic depression) is characterised by recurring episodes of altered mood and activity, typically swinging between depression and mania.[8]

The classic features of a manic episode are an elevated mood (although the patient can become irritable too) and the presence of the following associated features:[8]

- Exaggerated optimism and inflated self-esteem
- Decreased social inhibition, for example, sexual over-activity, reckless spending, dangerous driving
- Rapid thinking and speech (flight of ideas)
- Lack of insight into disorder.

Managing risk in mental health

Patients with mental disorders are not normally dangerous. You are much more likely to be assaulted by a member of your own family than by your next patient with a mental disorder. Actually, patients with long-term mental health problems are much more likely to be the victim of assault and exploitation themselves.

Suicide and deliberate self-harm (DSH)

In the UK, there are just over 6,500 suicides each year, the majority of whom were male. People who regularly self-harm will continue to be at risk of future self-harm, but not typically suicide. Although DSH is regarded as taboo and unfathomable by many people, including clinicians, it may help you to think of DSH as a method of coping with incredibly difficult feelings rather than as a serious wish to die.[10] People who regularly overdose and/or engage in risky behaviour that is designed to elicit a response are more at risk via misadventure or accidental death and it is not uncommon for a coroner to give a narrative verdict in such cases. Predicting who will commit suicide is very difficult, and scales, such as the SAD PERSON scale, do not accurately predict the risk of death by suicide.[11]

IPAP suicide risk assessment

Although suicide risk assessment tools are not recommended, it is helpful to have some guidance relating to the factors that suggest your patient is at risk and appropriate actions to take. Current UK Ambulance Services Clinical Practice Guidelines recommend using 'IPAP' and also provide suggested actions to take based on the outcomes of this tool:[12]

- **Intent:** Any thoughts of killing self?
- **Plans:** Does the patient have a plan about how they would kill themselves?

Chapter 9 Mental Health

- **Actions:** Has the patient ever attempted suicide before?
- **Protection:** Does the patient have any support, such as family and friends? Are there any factors that would stop the patient taking their own life, such as family, pets, work, religion?

Tips for the management of patients with mental health problems

- Don't panic – Remain calm, professional and in control. Patients are often incredibly astute at sensing any uneasiness and will try to press your buttons or force your hand.
- There is no rush – Making and implementing a plan can take hours.
- Do consider their medical health – An overdose of 1 g of amitriptyline, for example, can cause serious harm and needs addressing prior to their mental health.[13]
- Consider their mental health – If patients state that their mental health is not good, consider whether an ED attendance will really benefit anyone here, apart from relieving your own anxieties (and responsibility) about this patient group. In most cases, a risk assessment can be conducted by mental health staff over the phone and a contingency plan put in place.
- Frontline mental health staff are not there just to 'have a chat' with patients – Several national helplines are available for that purpose such as Rethink, Saneline and the Samaritans.
- Unless patients are detained under the MHA or they haven't got mental capacity they cannot be made to go to the ED – If patients refuse to travel despite your kind words and advice then make a thorough note of this, then make it clear you are leaving and GO. You may find that it's at this point they decide to travel.
- Desperate attempts and pleas to engage can indicate you're out of your depth – If you are struggling, speak to mental health staff and see if the patient is known, if there are any current concerns and/or if there is a care plan that needs to be adhered to.
- Many mental health patients have a care plan – Of course you aren't going to know this because you can't see it and patients may not be happy with it or may feel it doesn't address their needs 24/7. This is often the case with frequent callers who challenge the out-of-hours services when offered a different response from that which they receive during the daytime.
- Don't tell people to pull themselves together – It can reinforce any negativity or feelings of hopelessness.
- Be objective – It can be helpful to see how patients can contradict themselves, not so you can point it out to them and make them feel stupid, but more as a reassurance that what they're saying and what they're actually doing are two different things. For example:
  - "I feel like killing myself tonight, but I'm seeing my GP the day after tomorrow."
  - "I feel like killing myself, but I'm worried about the impact it would have on my children."
  - "I feel like killing myself, but I'm worried I'll fail and end up disabled or in pain."
  - These are common statements people make, which paradoxically protect them from suicide and are statements that mental health professionals look out for during an assessment. Ensure they are documented on your patient report form.
- Its okay to be human and personable – However, don't disclose too much about yourself, or try to solve their problems. Their issues may be long-term problems and it's highly unlikely you'll solve them at 03:00 with excessive personal self-disclosing.
- Don't feel you have to fill the void – Silences of a minute or two do not mean you're not being helpful. Be comfortable

with silence; it's not up to you to have all the answers.
- Don't just do something, stand there! – Don't confuse movement with action.
- There are no absolutes in mental health and it is never possible to state with absolute certainty that a patient isn't at risk.

Chapter 9 Mental Health

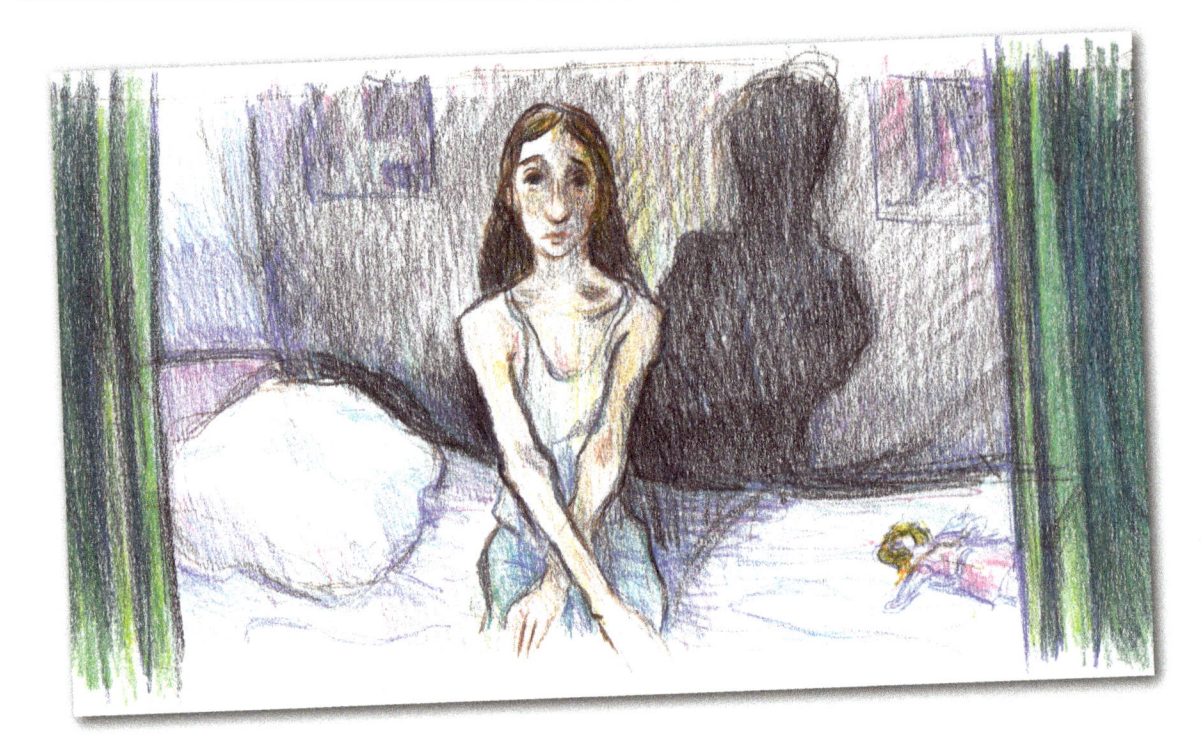

Eating Disorders

You are on standby listening to your colleague munching his way through a super-megaburger and chips. It's fine, he tells you, as calories don't count past midnight and you are well overdue your meal break. This presumably explains the tour of fast food outlets you have been subjected to throughout this set of night shifts.

The MDT passes you details of a 17-year-old 'sick person' at a clinic you don't recognise. Fortunately, the satellite navigation does know where it is and manages to take you on the most direct route. Fifteen minutes later you pull up outside a sweeping driveway guarded by two large metal gates. Your colleague struggles to lean out of the window to reach the intercom, but manages to press the button and, after a brief exchange, the gates slowly swing open, allowing you to enter.

The ambulance crunches up the gravelled driveway and your colleague brings the vehicle to a stop just outside the huge front door. As you exit the vehicle, a member of staff appears at the door. She walks over, introduces herself and thanks you for coming. She explains that this is an eating disorders clinic for women and girls. As you enter the tiled hallway, your colleague is drawn to a large tin of chocolates. The member of staff smiles and explains that they are for one of the clients. Your colleague's eyes light up when she offers him the tin, although they dull a little when you suggest that he just take one.

A side-door opens and you are ushered into a bedroom where your patient, Angela, is currently sitting on the edge of the bed. She is the thinnest person you have ever seen in real life. Your colleague has nonchalantly followed you in, preoccupied by his mission to find his favourite confectionery. He succeeds, raising the purple wrapped offering into the air just as he catches sight of the patient. The staff member who showed you in gently removes the tin from your colleague's grasp and he hurriedly places the chocolate in his pocket.

You approach Angela and introduce yourself. She acknowledges your presence by telling you she feels dizzy and wants to lie down. You assist her back into bed as the nurse looking after Angela explains that she was admitted to the clinic two weeks ago, following a significant drop in her weight. She is on a refeeding regime, but progress has been slow. Overnight, her blood pressure had dropped below 80 mmHg systolic and her heart rate had fallen below 40 beats/min. Following a discussion with the on-call doctor, it was decided that an urgent hospital admission was required.

You look around the room and determine that access is good and there is plenty of room. Angela is in no state to walk, so you need an alternative method of extrication.

> What are you going to do: Use a **Carry chair** (read on) or an **Ambulance trolley** (skip the next paragraph)?

Carry chair

You send your colleague for the carry chair, which cheers him up as the chocolate in his pocket is going rather soft. A staff member packs some of Angela's possessions to take with her. Your colleague returns, having managed to acquire a toffee, judging by the way he is now chomping and chewing. He casually flips out the chair and locks it into place, while you coax Angela up out of bed and assist her into the chair. No sooner has she sat on the chair than she complains of feeling dizzy and, as you are attempting to fasten the chest strap, promptly slumps over to one side. You manage to catch her and return her to the bed. An ambulance trolley looks like the better option.

Ambulance trolley

Given that access is good, and Angela's cardiac output is poor, you elect to bring in the ambulance trolley. You explain your plan to Angela and the staff and head off with your colleague to fetch it. On returning to Angela's room, you line up the ambulance trolley alongside her bed and she slowly clambers across onto it. After placing a blanket on top of her thin frame, you fasten her in.

Once Angela is loaded onto the ambulance, you ask your colleague to undertake some observations, while you have a chat with the nurse about the circumstances of admission. It transpires that Angela is currently not detained under the Mental Health Act and the staff are trying to use persuasion, rather than coercion. However, Angela's parents are involved and, indeed, will be meeting her at the hospital.

You jump on the back of the ambulance to find your colleague frowning at the monitor. He passes you a summary of the observations:

Airway

Patent

Breathing

Respiratory rate: 18 breaths/min, laboured
SpO_2: 96% on air

Circulation

Heart rate: 38 beats/min
Blood pressure: 80/50 mmHg
ECG: Sinus bradycardia

Chapter 9 Mental Health

Disability

GCS score: 15/15
Blood sugar: 3.7 mmol/l

Exposure

Temperature: 34.5°C

> What are you going to do: **Administer IV drugs** (read on) or **Something else** (skip the next paragraph)?

Administer IV drugs

You realise that a heart rate of under 40 beats/min is absolute bradycardia and an indication for atropine. You set about trying to gain IV access, but Angela does not have any veins. Defeated, you review the JRCALC guidelines and find that atropine is contra-indicated in hypothermia. In addition, after flicking through Angela's notes, you see a warning about limiting fluids due to severe cardiac atrophy. Your body gives a small involuntary shiver as you consider what might have happened if you had gained IV access and administered drugs and fluids as you originally planned.

Something else

Angela's observations are clearly deranged, but diving in with aggressive fluid and drug administration might be dangerous for her. You review her medical notes and discover that there is indeed a plan in place, including limited fluids and careful electrolyte monitoring during her refeeding. You flick on the ambulance heater and keep a close eye on Angela and her ECG on the way to hospital, but she remains stable.

Scale of the problem

The term 'eating disorders' has been described as a misnomer, since it encapsulates obsessive weight-loss disorders, such as anorexia nervosa, and body image-related disorders such as bulimia nervosa and binge-eating disorder.[14] Therefore, the umbrella term 'eating disturbance' has been advocated in the classification of these disorders. However, for simplicity, the term 'eating disorder' will be used in this chapter.

The definitions of the types of eating disorders are quite precise and laborious, but are worth having an appreciation of. Table 9.1 provides a summary of the differences between the various eating disorders.[15]

Table 9.1 Comparison of eating disorders.

	Anorexia nervosa	Bulimia nervosa	Binge-eating disorder
Over-evaluation of weight/shape	Yes	Yes	Can occur
Fear of fatness and/or behaviour preventing weight gain	Yes	Can occur	Uncommon
Underweight	Yes	No	No
Unmet nutritional and/or energy needs	Yes	Can occur	No
Overweight	No	Can occur	Common
Regular (weekly) binge eating	Can occur	Yes	Yes

	Anorexia nervosa	**Bulimia nervosa**	**Binge-eating disorder**
Regular (weekly) compensatory behaviour, for example, exercise	Can occur	Yes	No
Subtypes	Restrictive or binge–purge	None	None
Severity specifier	Body mass index	Frequency of compensatory behaviours	Frequency of binge eating

Source: Royal Australian and New Zealand College of Psychiatrists, 2014.

The definitions of anorexia nervosa, bulimia nervosa and binge-eating disorder are:[16]

Anorexia nervosa

- Restriction of energy intake relative to requirements, leading to a significantly low body weight in the context of age, sex, developmental trajectory and physical health
- Intense fear of gaining weight or of becoming fat, or persistent behaviour that interferes with weight gain, even though at a significantly low weight
- Disturbance in the way in which one's body weight or shape is experienced, undue influence of body weight or shape on self-evaluation, or persistent lack of recognition of the seriousness of the current low body weight.

Bulimia nervosa

- Recurrent episodes of binge eating. An episode of binge eating is characterised by both of the following:
  - Eating, in a discrete period of time (for example, within any 2-hour period), an amount of food that is definitely larger than what most individuals would eat in a similar period of time under similar circumstances
  - A sense of lack of control over eating during the episode
- Recurrent inappropriate compensatory behaviours in order to prevent weight gain, such as self-induced vomiting; misuse of laxatives, diuretics or other medications; fasting; or excessive exercise
- The binge eating and inappropriate compensatory behaviours both occur, on average, at least once a week for 3 months
- Self-evaluation is unduly influenced by body shape and weight
- The disturbance does not occur exclusively during episodes of anorexia nervosa.

Binge-eating disorder

- Recurrent episodes of binge eating. An episode of binge eating is characterised by both of the following:
  - Eating, in a discrete period of time (for example, within any 2-hour period), an amount of food that is definitely larger than what most individuals would eat in a similar period of time under similar circumstances
  - A sense of lack of control over eating during the episode
- The binge-eating episodes are associated with three (or more) of the following:
  - Eating much more rapidly than normal
  - Eating until feeling uncomfortably full
  - Eating large amounts of food when not feeling physically hungry
  - Eating alone because of feeling embarrassed by how much one is eating

- Feeling disgusted with oneself, depressed or very guilty afterwards.
- Marked distress regarding binge eating is present
- The binge eating occurs, on average, at least once a week for 3 months
- The binge eating is not associated with the recurrent use of inappropriate compensatory behaviour as in bulimia and does not occur exclusively during the course of bulimia or anorexia.

The prevalence of eating disorders in the UK is unknown, but the incidence for diagnosed cases in UK emergency departments is highest for girls aged 15–19 and boys aged 10–14 years.[17]

Aetiology (causes) of eating disorders

The causes of eating disorders are complex and multi-factorial. Socio-cultural, biological and psychological factors have all been implicated.[17] The most significant socio-demographic factors are being of female gender and living in the developed world where the 'thin ideal' prevails. Interestingly, migrants from the developing world are particularly vulnerable to this 'thin ideal'. Other socio-demographic risks include urban (as opposed to rural) living and activities/careers where body image is important, such as competitive gymnastics and fashion modelling.[15]

There is some evidence of a hereditary component in eating disturbances. For example, a family history of 'leanness' can predispose individuals to anorexia, whereas a personal or family history of obesity increases the risk of bulimia. Rather more mindblowing is the concept that events experienced by past generations (such as the Dutch famine in World War 2) can lead to changes in gene expression in subsequent generations, increasing their risk of developing eating disorders.[18]

A mixture of weight concern in a person's formative development years, as well as personality traits, make up the psychological factors in eating disorders. Low self-esteem is common to all eating disorders, whereas high levels of clinical perfectionism can increase the risk of anorexia, and high levels of impulsivity increase the risk of a person developing bulimia. In addition, adverse life experiences, such as emotional and sexual child abuse, increase the risk of developing an eating disturbance. Concurrent mental illness is common in people with eating disorders, particularly depression.[14]

Consequences of eating disorders

The consequences of an eating disorder can be divided into three categories:[14]

- Fasting and starvation with weight loss
- Weight control strategies: vomiting, and laxative and diuretic abuse
- Bingeing.

Fasting and starvation with weight loss

Chronic fasting and starvation has widespread, and multi-system, consequences for the person. Functional gastrointestinal disorders are common, such as irritable bowel syndrome, bloating, constipation and gastric ulcers. The metabolic rate reduces, leading to hypoglycaemia and impaired temperature regulation, which can cause hypothermia. Counter-intuitively, cholesterol is raised in around 50% of persons and a fatty liver is also common. Chronic malnutrition causes hypocalcaemia, which in severe cases can cause tetany and ECG changes. In addition, decreased phosphate impairs cardiac muscle function, while low levels of iron cause anaemia.

The cardiovascular system is severely affected, with cardiac muscle loss decreasing both its size and contractility, causing progressive falls in blood pressure and heart rate. In addition, arrhythmias increase the risk of sudden death, particularly in sufferers of anorexia, where QT prolongation is common at low weights. This is compounded if there is concurrent hypokalaemia because of laxative and/or diuretic abuse or the person suffers from the binge–purge subtype of anorexia, for example. Poor peripheral circulation can lead to cold, cyanosed extremities.

In the musculoskeletal system, muscle strength and stamina are reduced. Osteoporosis and pathological fracture are common causes of pain and disability in anorexia due to dietary deficiencies in calcium and vitamin D.

The immune system is adversely affected with reduced production of white and red blood cells and platelets. As a result, approximately a third of deaths in people with anorexia is due to infections such as bronchial pneumonia and sepsis.[19]

Psychologically, there is increasing preoccupation with food, leading to decreasing concentration on usual activities and increasingly obsessive behaviour. Consumption of even small amounts of food can result in considerable emotional distress and feelings of anger, shame and guilt. Feelings of hopelessness and depression contribute to high rates of suicide in sufferers of anorexia.[20]

There are also structural changes in the central nervous system, with cerebral atrophy in anorexia, which causes functional cognitive impairments, leading to poor performance in memory tasks and activities that involve having to adjust thinking or attention.

Finally, reproduction in women is affected, with amenorrhoea common once the body mass index (BMI) drops below 17.5. A decrease in fertility is common in anorexia and sufferers have significantly more miscarriages. Perinatal mortality is also six times higher than in the general population.

Weight control strategies

The most serious consequence of purging to control weight, either by vomiting and/or by laxative/diuretic abuse, are electrolyte abnormalities. Hypokalaemia secondary to vomiting or laxative/diuretic abuse leads to muscle weakness, arrhythmias, decreased gut motility and renal tubular dysfunction. This is common in lower-weight bulimia and the binge–purge type of anorexia, but not in pure restrictive anorexia.

Hyponatraemia can be caused by hypotonic dehydration as well as excess water consumption, leading to weakness and lethargy and, in severe cases, convulsions and death. In addition, chronic dehydration also causes a range of adverse effects, including renal insufficiency, which in severe cases can lead to renal failure and renal stones.

The most visual sign of gastrointestinal disorders in this group are dental changes in patients who persistently vomit, as this causes erosion of dental enamel, particularly the inner surface of the front teeth. Patients with bulimia who induce vomiting also suffer from a non-inflammatory swelling of their salivary glands, although the cause is unknown. Further down the gastrointestinal tract, repeated vomiting can lead to oesophagitis, Mallory-Weiss tears and bleeding.[14]

On the psychological front, shame and disgust are common feelings following vomiting. Sufferers are usually secretive about their behaviour.[21]

Bingeing

Weight gain and obesity are common in this group if there are no compensatory mechanisms, such as exercise. Bingeing with

Chapter 9 Mental Health

vomiting still leads to weight gain, since most calories are still absorbed. The large volumes of food consumed can lead to acute gastric dilatation and rupture and/or oesophageal rupture. In addition, the stomach can lose contractility, leading to venous occlusion and gastric perforation. These are irreversible unless corrected early, particularly in cases where the person is consuming large volumes of food after a period of fasting.

The psychological consequences are the same as for the other categories.

Assessment and management

You may think that patients with eating disorders are easy to spot. In cases of anorexia where sufferers have a low BMI, this may be true, but a normal BMI does not mean that your patient is not suffering from an eating disorder.

However, there are a number of external signs that may indicate an eating disorder:[22,23]

- Dry flaky skin with no collagen
- Lanugo hair (very fine and soft downy hair that is usually seen on the body of a newborn baby)
- Poor peripheral circulation
- Petechial rashes due to thrombocytopaenia
- Brittle nails
- Carotenaemia
- Russell's sign (callouses on the metacarpophalangeal joints due to inducing vomiting, Figure 9.1)
- Facial purpura (secondary to increased intrathoracic pressure associated with vomiting)
- Conjunctival haemorrhage (again, due to intrathoracic pressure changes related to vomiting).

If, during the course of a patient encounter, you suspect an eating disturbance, it may be helpful to use the SCOFF questionnaire,[24] although these are not suitable as the sole method to determine whether people have an eating disorder.[23]

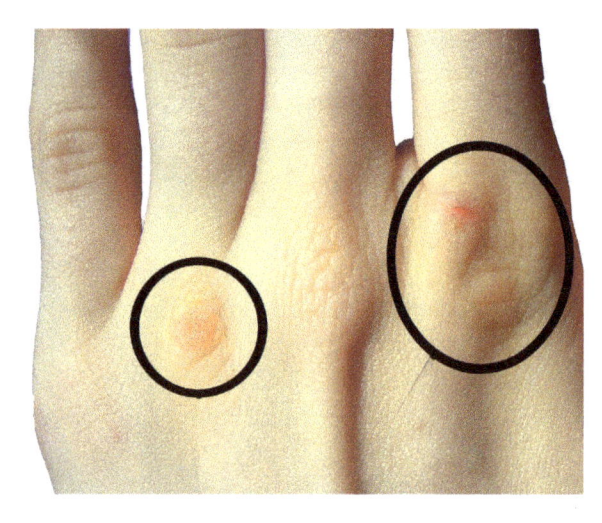

Figure 9.1 Russell's sign.
Source: Kyukyusha (Own work) [Public domain], via Wikimedia Commons.

- Do you make yourself **S**ick because you feel uncomfortably full?
- Do you worry you have lost **C**ontrol over how much you eat?
- Have you recently lost more than **O**ne stone (6 kg) in weight over a three-month period?
- Do you believe yourself to be **F**at when others say you are thin?
- Would you say that **F**ood dominates your life?

You should record the usual range of physiological observations, but do not rush to correct a low heart rate or blood pressure. The poor cardiac output in patients with anorexia, for example, is likely to be due to cardiac muscle atrophy and reduced contractility, which will not benefit from large volumes of fluid or doses of atropine.[25]

It is likely that you will be transporting patients who have been referred by their GP or another healthcare professional to a specialist eating unit. If they are available, review the patient's blood results, particularly the electrolytes. Patients with abnormal results should be closely monitored, including continuous ECG monitoring.[26]

References

1. NHS Digital. Adult Psychiatric Morbidity Survey: Survey of Mental Health and Wellbeing, England, 2014 [Internet]. NHS Digital. 2016. Available from: https://digital.nhs.uk/data-and-information/publications/statistical/adult-psychiatric-morbidity-survey/adult-psychiatric-morbidity-survey-survey-of-mental-health-and-wellbeing-england-2014
2. United Kingdom. Mental Health Act 1983 [Internet]. 1983. Available from: https://www.legislation.gov.uk/ukpga/1983/20
3. Mind. Mental Health Act 1983 [Internet]. 2018. Available from: https://www.mind.org.uk/information-support/legal-rights/mental-health-act-1983/about-the-mha-1983/
4. United Kingdom. Mental Health Act 2007 [Internet]. 2007. Available from: https://www.legislation.gov.uk/ukpga/2007/12/contents
5. Department of Health. Code of practice: Mental Health Act 1983 [Internet]. 2015. Available from: https://www.gov.uk/government/publications/code-of-practice-mental-health-act-1983
6. Dimond MB. *Legal aspects of nursing*, 7th edition. Harlow: Pearson; 2015.
7. Department of Health, Concordat signatories. Mental Health Crisis Care Concordat [Internet]. 2014. Available from: https://www.gov.uk/government/publications/mental-health-crisis-care-agreement
8. Katona C, Cooper C, Robertson M. *Psychiatry at a glance*, 6th edition. Chichester: Wiley-Blackwell; 2015.
9. Gunderson JG. Borderline personality disorder. *New England Journal of Medicine*, 2011 May 25;364(21):2037–42.
10. Royal Society of Psychiatrists. Self-harm, suicide and risk: helping people who self-harm [Internet]. 2010. Available from: https://www.rcpsych.ac.uk/docs/default-source/improving-care/better-mh-policy/college-reports/college-report-cr158.pdf?sfvrsn=fcf95b93_2
11. Warden S, Spiwak R, Sareen J, Bolton JM. The SAD PERSONS scale for suicide risk assessment: a systematic review. *Archives of Suicide Research*, 2014 Oct 2;18(4):313–326.
12. Joint Royal Colleges Ambulance Liaison Committee, Association of Ambulance Chief Executives. JRCALC Clinical Guidelines. Cited from JRCALC Plus (Version 1.2.13) [Mobile application software]. Bridgwater: Class Publishing Ltd; 2021.
13. National Poisons Information Service. TOXBASE – poisons information database for clinical toxicology advice [Internet]. 2021. Available from: https://www.toxbase.org/
14. Morris J, editor. *ABC of eating disorders*. Oxford: Wiley-Blackwell/BMJ Books, Blackwell Pub; 2008. (ABC series).
15. Hay P, Chinn D, Forbes D, Madden S, Newton R, Sugenor L, et al. Royal Australian and New Zealand College of Psychiatrists clinical practice guidelines for the treatment of eating disorders. *Australian and New Zealand Journal of Psychiatry*, 2014 Nov 1;48(11):977–1008.
16. American Psychiatric Association. *Diagnostic and statistical manual of mental disorders*, 5th edition (DSM-5®). American Psychiatric Pub; 2013. 1629 p.
17. Mitchison D, Hay PJ. The epidemiology of eating disorders: genetic, environmental, and societal factors. *Clinical Epidemiology*, 2014 Feb 17;6:89–97.
18. Campbell IC, Mill J, Uher R, Schmidt U. Eating disorders, gene–environment interactions and epigenetics. *Neuroscience & Biobehavioral Reviews*, 2011 Jan;35(3):784–793.
19. Zipfel S, Löwe B, Reas DL, Deter H-C, Herzog W. Long-term prognosis in anorexia nervosa: lessons from a 21-year follow-up study. *The Lancet*, 2000 Feb 26;355(9205):721–722.
20. Smink FRE, van Hoeken D, Hoek HW. Epidemiology, course, and outcome of eating disorders. Current Opinion in Psychiatry, 2013 Nov;26(6):543–548.
21. Blythin SPM, Nicholson HL, Macintyre VG, Dickson JM, Fox JRE, Taylor PJ. Experiences of shame and guilt in anorexia and bulimia nervosa: a systematic review. *Psychology and Psychotherapy: Theory, Research and Practice*, 2020;93(1):134–59.
22. National Institute for Mental Health. Eating disorders: about more than food [Internet]. 2018. Available from: https://www.nimh.nih.gov/health/publications/eating-disorders/
23. National Institute for Health and Care Excellence. Eating disorders: recognition and treatment [Internet]. NICE; 2020. Available from: https://www.nice.org.uk/guidance/NG69

24. Morgan JF, Reid F, Lacey JH. The SCOFF questionnaire: assessment of a new screening tool for eating disorders. *British Medical Journal*, 1999 Dec 4;319(7223):1467–1468.
25. Trent SA, Moreira ME, Colwell CB, Mehler PS. ED management of patients with eating disorders. *American Journal of Emergency Medicine*, 2013 May;31(5):859–865.
26. Simon C. *Oxford Handbook of General Practice*, 5th edition. Oxford: Oxford University Press; 2020. 1155 p. (Oxford handbooks).

10 Older People

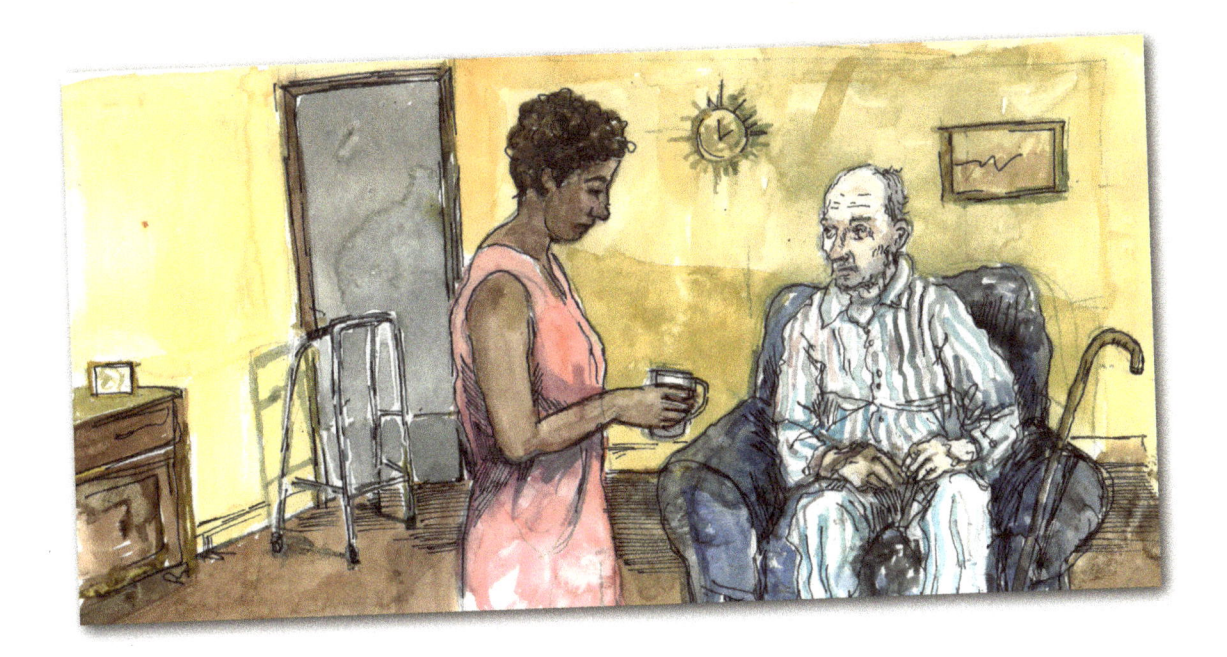

Frailty

By Dolly McPherson

You are watching the clock tick over the final minute of your meal break when you hear the familiar sound of a job coming through to your radio. After mobilising and getting the vehicle's wheels in motion, you and your crewmate get a look at the job. It is an 88-year-old male 'stuck in his chair'. You note thankfully that the job hasn't been in very long and hope your poor patient hasn't waited too long to call.

On arrival you find a waifish male sitting in a deep low chair; a walking stick is hung over the armrest and there's a walking frame tucked away in the corner. His carer welcomes you in and says the dreaded phrase, "I'm only new and don't know Mr Brown very well." You take an inward sigh and ask her what has been happening. She states that when she arrived Mr Brown was sitting in his chair and was unable to get out of it when she prompted him to.

When she met Mr Brown for the first time a week ago he was able to do so, but with some effort. She has not seen him again until today. You turn your attention to Mr Brown and apologise for talking about him prior to introducing yourself. When you ask what he would like to be called he says, "Bill," and

Chapter 10 Older People

he proceeds to tell you that over the last few days he has felt weaker on his legs and has taken to sleeping in his chair. He thinks he has been out of his chair today but can't be sure. Your initial impression reassures you that this patient doesn't need any time-critical interventions, so you ask your colleague if she wouldn't mind getting an initial set of observations and a pain score while you go in search of some good collateral history.

After some hunting through the kitchen you manage to get hold of the patient's care notes, a district nurse's folder from one month ago and a phone number for the patient's son. You ring the son, who informs you that in addition to his worsening mobility, his father has also seemed slightly more confused than normal and he wonders if his father has a 'water infection' again. You return to the lounge room to collate your findings.

Supporting history and pertinent negatives

Bill reports no chest pain, no falls in the last week, no coughs, colds, dysuria or frequency. There is an increase in confusion as reported by the carers and Bill's son, and Bill sometimes feels dizzy on standing. He hasn't had a bowel movement today but is unsure about his last bowel opening, but the care notes show patient is eating and drinking normally.

Previous medical history

Early stage dementia
Recurrent urinary tract infections (UTIs)
Hypertension
Falls
Myocardial infarction (MI) 10 years ago
Atrial fibrillation (AF)
Benign prostatic hypertrophy

Medications

Furosemide
Bisoprolol
Amiodarone
Ramipril
Donepezil
Apixaban
Tamsulosin
Laxido sachets

Social history

Carers twice a day with good family support
Walks with a stick in his right hand (has a frame from a previous hospitalisation but hasn't needed to use it recently)
Lives in a bungalow
Only leaves the house if his son takes him in the car for lunch
Has a keysafe and pendant alarm

Allergies

Penicillin – but no one knows what effect it has on him

Airway

Clear
Self-maintained
No upper airway noises

Breathing

Respiratory rate: 16 breaths per minute
SpO_2: 97% on air
Chest clear
No respiratory distress
Equal bilateral chest expansion
Resonant throughout to percussion

Circulation

Heart rate: 76–89 beats/min, irregular
Blood pressure: 168/87 sitting, 140/73 standing (asymptomatic)

Heart sounds: S1+S2+0
Strong bilateral radial pulses
Abdomen soft with mild diffuse tenderness plus dullness to percussion over the descending colon

Disability

GCS score: 15/15
Abbreviated Mental Test 4 (AMT4) score: (Age, Date of birth, Place, Year) = 3 (doesn't know the year)
No evidence of head injury

Environment/Everything else

Temperature: 36.1°C
Care notes confirm patient had been out of the chair this morning (3 hours earlier) but did seem less stable on his feet
You think you can smell urine when you move closer to the patient
After helping the patient out of his very low chair he is able to walk with his stick but appears unsteady. When you introduce his frame, he appears much safer when using it
Rockwood Clinical Frailty Score: 6
You calculate Bill's National Early Warning Score (NEWS2) as a 3

> What do you do now: **Take the patient to hospital** for further investigation and management (read on), **Request treatment for a UTI** (skip the next paragraph), OR **Contact your local frailty unit** (skip the next two paragraphs)?

Take the patient to hospital

You know that older frail people can present with relatively simple symptoms despite serious underlying illnesses and you want to be sure that this doesn't get missed. You advise Bill that he needs to go to hospital. You drop him off with a comprehensive handover and hope that he will be home soon. Six hours later when you are bringing your last patient into hospital you see Bill still lying on an emergency department (ED) trolley looking uncomfortable and tired. You ask one of the nursing staff what the plan is, and they state that he will be admitted for the night as it is too late to send him home. Hopefully he will be out first thing in the morning. You follow up on Bill a few weeks later and find out that he developed a pressure sore in the ED, resulting in a delay in discharging him while district nurses were arranged to treat the sore. It subsequently became infected, leading to a 2-week stay in hospital. Bill was discharged to a dementia nursing home as he was no longer strong enough to live independently with carers and the stress of admission had exacerbated his dementia. You know that this is not a good outcome for your patient.

Request treatment for a UTI

Given Bill's recent increase in confusion and the smell of urine, you are confident that this is just a UTI and he is 'off-legs' as a result. You decide to ring the GP for antibiotics, thereby demonstrating your Sherlock Holmes-like diagnostic deductive skills. It will be an easy referral as this patient has had multiple doses of antibiotics for a UTI in the past and the GP simply sends the prescription to the local pharmacy to be collected by the patient's son. You feel happy with your plan. However, you then remember listening to a podcast on frailty where you heard that many older patients are incorrectly diagnosed with UTIs based on confusion alone. This leads to antibiotic resistance and deterioration from the true source of confusion. You wonder if maybe you've been too quick to diagnose

Chapter 10 Older People

Bill, and perhaps it would be a good idea to contact the local frailty unit (read on).

Contact your local frailty unit

The more you think about it, the more you are not fully convinced that this is a UTI, so you decide to contact your local frailty unit. You speak to a very pleasant charge nurse who agrees that Bill sounds perfect for the service. You follow up on Bill the following shift and find out he was diagnosed with constipation and discharged back to his own home the following morning. He received a comprehensive geriatric assessment (CGA) and was given laxatives with good effect. He was taken off his furosemide temporarily due to a postural blood pressure drop and has a GP and district nurse review in 1–2 weeks. He was also seen and assessed by an occupational therapist who noted your concerns about his low chair and organised an urgent home visit to assess and correct this.

The scale of the problem

Frailty is defined as a vulnerability to stressors that would not stress the non-frail person.[1,2] These stressors are not limited to disease processes and can include bereavement and depression. In the clinical context this translates into a multisystem loss of reserves leading to increased physiological vulnerability. It is estimated that around 14% of people aged 60 and over are frail and this increases with age. For example, while 6.5% of people aged 60–69 are frail, in the over 90 age group, this jumps to 65%.[3]

Historically, frailty has been defined under two different models. These are the 'frailty phenotype model' and the 'cumulative deficit model'.[1] The frailty phenotype grades patients across five domains: unintentional weight loss, low energy expenditure, weak grip, self-reported exhaustion and slow gait speed. The cumulative deficit model uses tools such as the frailty index or the comprehensive geriatric assessment to identify individual patient deficits, with the understanding that the more deficits a person has, the more likely they are to be frail.[2]

While frailty increases with, and is worsened by age, it is important to recognise that advancing age does not equal frailty. This is the same for patients with disability and/or multiple co-morbidities.[1] The process of pattern recognition can mean that only patients who 'appear' frail with low body weight are identified as such; however, it is important to remember that frailty exists in bariatric patients as well.[4]

Terms

In the field of frailty there are several terms that have been used in the past but that no longer have a place in clinical practice. Not only do these terms belittle the seriousness of frailty, they will also earn you a wry and possibly condescending look from any geriatric-sensitive clinician. Some of these terms are:[5,6]

- Acopia: This term is all too often used as a diagnosis by those unable to unpick the clinical complexities of the frail older person. It suggests lazy assessment and places the blame of decline onto the patient – for example, 'they just can't cope because they are old and frail', not 'they have [insert diagnosis here] that is overwhelming for their circumstances'.
- Off legs: Very similar to the above. Diagnosing your patient with 'Acopia' and/or 'Off legs' can be very dangerous.[9] Labelling your patient with social terms can result in bias leading to missed important medical diagnoses.[7] As paramedics, we can be the start of this

bias through our handovers – don't underestimate your power!
- Mechanical fall: Once again, 'Fall' is not a diagnosis, it is a presenting complaint – the diagnosis is the underlying cause of the fall and/or any injuries sustained during that fall. If you must use a term, try using 'Fall ?cause', which will at least make you and anyone reading your notes consider what the contributing factors were to cause the fall in the first place.
- Failed discharge: This term implies that a system or the patient failed, thus creating a negative experience for all involved. These are high-risk patients who are likely to re-present to all healthcare settings.[6] Instead of saying 'failed discharge' in your handover, simply state the fact that they were discharged recently from hospital.

Geriatric giants

In 1965, a geriatrician named Bernard Isaacs coined the term 'geriatric giants' to highlight the key chronic disabilities that afflicted the older person: immobility, instability, incontinence and impaired intellect/memory.[8] More recently, these have been refined into the four 'new' syndromes of frailty, sarcopenia (progressive loss of skeletal muscle mass), the anorexia of ageing and cognitive impairment.[9]

Assessment

Your challenge is to operationalise the assessment of management of frailty while still being mindful of the 'geriatric giants'. A suggested approach is to utilise the Geriatric 5Ms (Table 10.1). While originally conceived to assist clinicians determine when input from geriatrician specialist clinicians would be beneficial to patients, they can also help you to focus in on specific areas that adversely affect the older person if not well managed.[10]

Table 10.1 The geriatric 5Ms.

Geriatric 5M	Description
Mind	Mentation Dementia Delirium Depression
Mobility	Impaired gait and balance Fall injury prevention
Medications	Polypharmacy Optimal prescribing/deprescribing Adverse medication effects and medication burden
Multicomplexity	Multimorbidity Complex biopsychosocial situations
Matters most	Each individual's own meaningful health outcome goals and care preferences

Source: Molnar and Frank, 2019.

A thorough clinical assessment is vital and should include a complete physical assessment including respiratory, cardiovascular, neurological, gastrointestinal and genitourinary as appropriate to identify underlying causes.[11] Remember to expose your patient to examine them but do be cognisant of maintaining dignity. Changes to skin colour and texture, peripheral oedema, rashes, scars, distention and deformity can all inform your clinical decision-making.[12] While you are likely to record physiological observations and calculate the patient's National Early Warning Score (NEWS2), there are two further tools that can assist you in the assessment of frailty: the Clinical Frailty Score and the AMT4.

Chapter 10 Older People

Rockwood Clinical Frailty Scale

There are several ways to score frailty but perhaps the simplest version is the Rockwood Clinical Frailty Scale (Figure 10.1).[13] This scale is increasingly being used in practice and offers a quick reference for scoring frailty, although is designed to reflect the person's frailty in times of health, not during acute illness. It can be determined using collateral history, if the patient is unable to provide the information required. In addition, consider scoring the patient twice: once to reflect their baseline at times of normal health; and a second time to reflect their needs at the point of assessment.

AMT4 score

While the Abbreviated Mental Test Score (AMTS) is a more thorough test of cognition than the Abbreviated Mental Test 4 (AMT4) score, it is longer and does not always suit the time constraints of the emergency care environment. Instead, a shortened tool, the AMT4, has been created and validated to evaluate fluctuating cognition in your patient.[14,15] The AMT4 score asks only four questions:

- Age
- Date of birth
- Place
- Year.

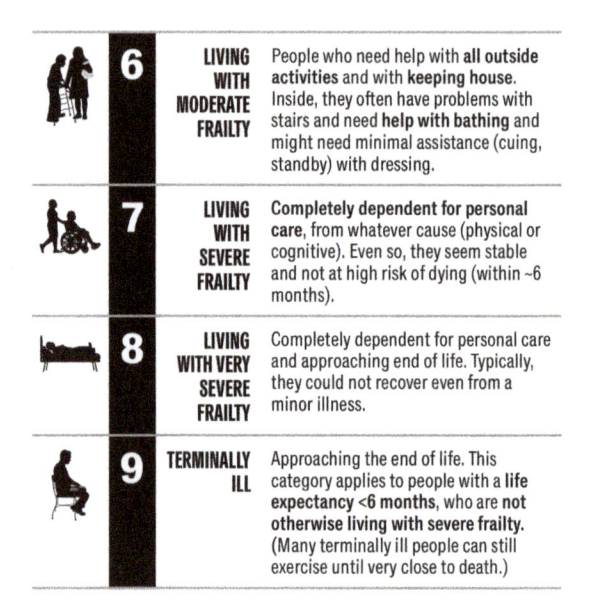

CLINICAL FRAILTY SCALE

	1	VERY FIT	People who are robust, active, energetic and motivated. They tend to exercise regularly and are among the fittest for their age.
	2	FIT	People who have **no active disease symptoms** but are less fit than category 1. Often, they exercise or are very **active occasionally**, e.g., seasonally.
	3	MANAGING WELL	People whose **medical problems are well controlled**, even if occasionally symptomatic, but often are **not regularly active** beyond routine walking.
	4	LIVING WITH VERY MILD FRAILTY	Previously "vulnerable," this category marks early transition from complete independence. While **not dependent** on others for daily help, often **symptoms limit activities**. A common complaint is being "slowed up" and/or being tired during the day.
	5	LIVING WITH MILD FRAILTY	People who often have **more evident slowing**, and need help with **high order instrumental activities of daily living** (finances, transportation, heavy housework). Typically, mild frailty progressively impairs shopping and walking outside alone, meal preparation, medications and begins to restrict light housework.
	6	LIVING WITH MODERATE FRAILTY	People who need help with **all outside activities** and with **keeping house**. Inside, they often have problems with stairs and need **help with bathing** and might need minimal assistance (cuing, standby) with dressing.
	7	LIVING WITH SEVERE FRAILTY	**Completely dependent for personal care**, from whatever cause (physical or cognitive). Even so, they seem stable and not at high risk of dying (within ~6 months).
	8	LIVING WITH VERY SEVERE FRAILTY	Completely dependent for personal care and approaching end of life. Typically, they could not recover even from a minor illness.
	9	TERMINALLY ILL	Approaching the end of life. This category applies to people with a **life expectancy <6 months**, who are not otherwise living with severe frailty. (Many terminally ill people can still exercise until very close to death.)

SCORING FRAILTY IN PEOPLE WITH DEMENTIA

The degree of frailty generally corresponds to the degree of dementia. Common **symptoms in mild dementia** include forgetting the details of a recent event, though still remembering the event itself, repeating the same question/story and social withdrawal.

In **moderate dementia**, recent memory is very impaired, even though they seemingly can remember their past life events well. They can do personal care with prompting.

In **severe dementia**, they cannot do personal care without help.

In **very severe dementia** they are often bedfast. Many are virtually mute.

DALHOUSIE UNIVERSITY

Clinical Frailty Scale ©2005–2020 Rockwood, Version 2.0 (EN). All rights reserved. For permission: www.geriatricmedicineresearch.ca
Rockwood K et al. A global clinical measure of fitness and frailty in elderly people. CMAJ 2005;173:489–495.

Figure 10.1 Rockwood Clinical Frailty Scale.
Source: Rockwood et al., 2005. Clinical Frailty Scale © 2005–2020 Rockwood, Version 2.0 (EN). All rights reserved. Reproduced with permission.

Urine dipstick testing/urinalysis

Become a 'Urosceptic': urinalysis has extremely poor specificity for identification of urinary tract infection (UTI) and will most likely diagnose an asymptomatic bacteraemia.[16] It should not be used to routinely investigate patients presenting with frailty as it can lead to over-prescription of antibiotics and delayed treatment for the true underlying cause. The diagnosis of UTI is made on the history of specific signs and symptoms, but be aware that confusion is not a sufficient symptom in isolation – constipation is a more common cause of confusion than UTI in this patient group.[17]

Management

One of the most significant decisions you are going to have to make with respect to managing the frail patient is whether to take them to hospital. Hospital admission for the frail older person can have a long-term and sometimes irreversible detrimental effect on functionality and physical health.[17] A week-long admission for a frail older person can result in deconditioning of muscles by up to 10%! Not only does a stay in hospital result in poor outcomes for these patients, transport to the ED even without onward admission can result in adverse events such as pressure sores and missed or late administration of medication.[18,19]

Community pathways include social services, rapid access clinic for the older person, emergency medical unit, community hospitals, GP home visits, hospital at home, specialist community services such as community respiratory or heart failure teams, older persons mental health teams, charitable societies and many more. If you are unsure what is available in your area, some good people to approach for information are the acute medical team, the geriatrics team/medicine for the older person, the occupational health team at your local hospital or some of your local GPs.

If you are making a referral to community services, it is important to be clear about what you are hoping to achieve. Using the SBAR (Situation, Background, Assessment and Recommendations) mnemonic is helpful and recognisable to all clinicians and can help you to arrange your thoughts as these patients rarely have a straightforward clinical story to tell. Explain your reasons for considering a community pathway (especially if the patient has a higher acuity) and don't be afraid to make recommendations from your findings, such as medication review, bloods to identify biochemical or haematological causes of Acute Frailty Syndromes, antibiotics, laxatives, and so on.

If your patient does require transport to ED, it is worth considering their discharge planning early. This can be done by documenting the patient's home situation along with social support, lining up family to collect the patient or to be at home for discharge, having a keysafe code documented, packing the patient's clothes to help prevent 'pyjama paralysis' and bringing key medications with the patient so that they don't have to wait for the hospital pharmacy prior to departure.

Conclusion

The assessment, management and referral of the patient living with frailty can be a challenge for even the most experienced geriatrician. These patients require a careful balancing act of providing treatment and maintaining independence. Using a thorough and conscientious approach aiming to avoid acute admission when clinically possible will usually be sufficient to ensure high-quality care.

Chapter 10 Older People

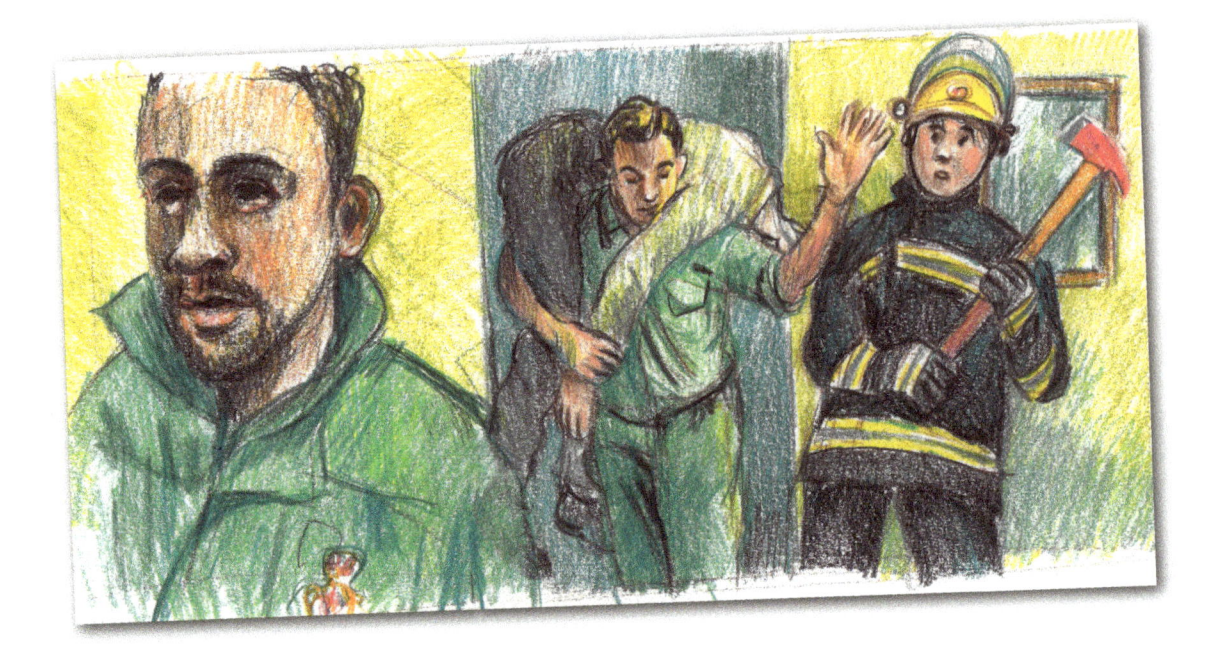

Dementia

You are on standby having a laugh and joke with your colleague, who is recounting a hilarious (and potentially perilous) tale involving a boat, a numb leg and a ship called the Pride of Normandy, when you are passed details of an elderly woman who has fallen. Your colleague's tale ends just as you turn into the street, giving you just enough time to focus on finding the address. As you suspected, it is a block of flats housing elderly residents.

You press the entry buzzer and are greeted by a much younger voice than the 93-year-old patient and take this to be a relative. After ascending two flights of stairs, you arrive at a scene of devastation. It turns out that the son-in-law had to take a sledgehammer to the door as he could not gain entry. This was all the more frustrating since there is a perfectly good key safe just adjacent to the front door, but that was of no use since the patient had left her key in the door lock.

The son-in-law and daughter show you into the bedroom, where Elisabeth, the patient, is seated. You introduce yourself and establish that the patient likes to be called Liz. Thanks to her dementia, she cannot remember much about what has happened, but is happy to defer to her daughter to tell the story. Apparently, Liz had fallen, but luckily was wearing an alarm pendant around her neck and pushed it straight away. The alarm company had dutifully called the family rather than the ambulance service (which makes a change). The daughter and her husband, once they had destroyed the door, found Liz on the floor next to the bed. She appeared uninjured and they had assisted her back onto the bed. They are quite correct: after a thorough check, you cannot find anything wrong with her either and the main problem seems to be Liz forgetting to use her walking frame.

What are you going to do: **Leave** (read on) or **Investigate further** (skip the next paragraph)?

Leave

"Marvellous, we'll leave it with you then," you find yourself saying. The daughter's face drops. "Aren't you going to check her blood pressure or record an ECG?" she asks. Either she watches lots of those fly-on-the-wall emergency department documentaries, or she is a healthcare professional. You decide to obtain some observations before leaving.

Investigate further

Despite Liz's protestations that she is fine and does not want to go to hospital, she is happy for you to examine her in the flat once you remind her of your name, again. You set about gaining a set of observations, including a lying and standing blood pressure:

Airway

Patent

Breathing

Respiratory rate: 16 breaths/min
SpO_2: 96% on air
Bilateral air entry on auscultation

Circulation

Pulse: 84 beats/min and regular
Blood pressure:
  Lying: 180/90 mmHg
  Standing: 140/85 mmHg
Capillary refill time: 2 seconds

Disability

GCS score: 14/15
Pupils: Equal, round and reacting to light
Blood sugar: 6.6 mmol/l

Exposure/Environment

Temperature: 36.7°C
No rashes

Having reviewed the observations, what are you going to do now: **Leave** (read on) or **Do something else** (skip the next paragraph)?

Leave

After loudly commenting that these observations are better than yours, the daughter frowns as she surveys her mother's blood pressure. "She has a postural drop of more than 20 mmHg systolic," she says, pointing at the two blood pressures. You have another look and see that the daughter is quite right. She must be a healthcare professional: this is not the sort of knowledge you get from watching TV documentaries. You decide to do something else.

Do something else

With a postural drop in systolic blood pressure of more than 20 mmHg, Liz really needs to go to hospital. However, on broaching the subject of taking a ride in your ambulance, she gives you a scowl and makes it clear that she is not going. The daughter explains that she has had bad experiences in the past and gets very disorientated in hospital. She asks if there is anything else you can do. You consider how this is going to look if your clinical record is randomly selected for audit and can't think of a way to make a 40 mmHg postural drop look good on paper. However, while recording the standing blood pressure, Liz did remain on her feet for a full 3 minutes, and had no symptoms of chest pain, shortness of breath or dizziness. You give the out-of-hours GP a ring to discuss things further. Luckily, you get through to a very pleasant and helpful doctor who understands your predicament, but thinks if

Chapter 10 Older People

the patient feels strongly that she wants to stay at home and the family are prepared to stay with her, then the risk is reasonable and the patient should see her own GP in the morning. Liz and her family are very pleased with the news and you complete your documentation appropriately.

You are just completing the non-conveyance form when you hear the building fire-alarm going off. After this continues for a minute, with no apparent sign of stopping, you decide that you are going to have to evacuate. You assist Liz from the flat and decide that if she can manage two flights of stairs, then she is definitely safe to remain at home, assuming that it is not consumed by fire. As you descend, your colleague looks at the floor above, which appears to be filling with smoke. Without a word, he shoots upstairs, only to return a moment later to borrow the son-in-law's sledgehammer. As he disappears into the smoke, you pause for a moment, and then continue down the stairs with the family.

It transpires that one of the residents on the third floor had awoken to find his utility room alight thanks to an electrical fault. Luckily, he had let himself out, but in the process, filled the corridor with smoke. Your colleague has assisted two of the residents on the smoke-filled floor downstairs, and by the time the fire and rescue service arrived to put the fire out, he had already triumphantly emerged.

You request a second crew to take one of the residents exposed to smoke, while you take the other. On the basis that 'no good deed goes unpunished', the doctor at the emergency department decides that your colleague needs a blood gas and sends a medical student in to stab his radial artery … three times.

Scale of the problem

Dementia is a set of behaviours or 'symptoms' which suggest difficulties with cognitive function. The most common symptoms include:[20]

- Memory loss
- Confusion
- Mood and personality changes
- Problems with planning
- Problems with doing tasks in the right order.

Dementia is diagnosed when the symptoms cause such problems with the everyday tasks of daily life that the person affected can no longer carry on living independently, without care.

It is an 'organic' disorder, meaning there is an associated physical deterioration of the brain tissue, which can be seen via a brain scan or, after death, at autopsy. Dementia is progressive – the damage and symptoms get worse over time. It is therefore not a normal result of ageing, but rather is the result of a disease.[20]

There are over 100 types of dementia, with Alzheimer's disease being the most common single cause in the UK, making up around 66% of cases, with vascular dementia coming in second (17%). However, multiple disease processes also occur, with Alzheimer's disease and vascular dementia and Alzheimer's disease and Lewy body dementia common combinations.[21] It is estimated that 7.1% of people over 65 have dementia in the UK.[22]

Types of dementia

Alzheimer's disease (AD)

This is the most common type of dementia and also the most well-understood. AD occurs due to the formation of beta-amyloid containing plaques. In healthy cells, amyloid is removed, but in patients with AD, it forms plaques around the neurons, interrupting the neuronal signalling system that cells use to communicate. In addition, another protein, tau, is abnormal in patients with AD. Tau is an important part of the internal cellular network, and helps to transport nutrients around the cell. However, in AD an abnormal form of tau is produced, which forms clumps (or neurofibrillary tangles, NFT), disrupting the cell structure and causing cell death.[23]

AD is often split into three subtypes:

- Typical
- Posterior cortical atrophy
- Logopenic aphasia.

Typical

This mostly affects older people, particularly those in their late 70–80s. There is a gradual worsening of memory, most notably with new learning, but recall of long-term memory also becomes problematic. Typically, attention and concentration are preserved in the early stages. The onset of disease starts medially in the brain, but gradually spreads throughout the cortex, with the exception of the occipital lobe, which is often spared. Language impairment and amnesia are usually subtle to start with, but as the disease progresses, they become increasingly obvious and are associated with difficulty recalling words and names (anomia) and the grammatical complexity of conversation declines. In severe disease, basic understanding and communication are severely impaired and physical function is also affected, with decreasing mobility, poor swallowing and incontinence. Together, they make a patient vulnerable to life-limiting infections and poor nutrition.[24]

Posterior cortical atrophy

As the name implies, this form of AD predominantly affects the occipital lobe, with visual recognition and visual spatial skills adversely affected. The spatial skills are particularly important, as without the ability to think in three dimensions, practical skills such as dressing become difficult. This form of AD is more common in younger patients, and in the early stages it spares other parts of the brain, leading to patients performing well in basic cognitive tests, which can delay diagnosis.

Logopenic aphasia

This form of AD is a progressive aphasia, manifesting early on with alterations in speech fluency, gradually progressing to resemble typical AD.

Vascular dementia

Ischaemic damage of the brain can also cause dementia. There are a variety of mechanisms, including small vessel disease and vasculitis, as well as the larger infarcts caused by strokes, that lead to lacunar infarction.[25] Unsurprisingly, the greater the cell volume loss, the more impairment that will result, although the location is also important, with bilateral thalamic infarcts causing amnesia, for example.

The presentation of vascular dementia is classically described as a stepwise deterioration with a plateauing of symptoms in between ischaemic strokes. In reality, patients rarely suffer from a pure infarct, but typically have mixed pathophysiology (such as vascular dementia with AD), meaning that this pattern does not emerge so clearly.[24]

Dementia vs delirium

If dementia can be thought of as chronic brain failure, then delirium is acute brain failure.[26] It is a common and serious condition that is characterised by disruptions in thinking, consciousness, attention, cognition and perception. Unlike dementia, it has a short onset (typically hours to days). To complicate matters, patients with dementia can also develop delirium: a combination that has been associated with serious complications and poor outcome, including death.[27]

Chapter 10 Older People

Differentiating between delirium and dementia can be difficult, so if in doubt, it is safer to assume delirium and ensure patients receive prompt medical attention.[28] However, there are a number of features that can assist with the diagnosis of delirium in the out-of-hospital setting.[29]

- Onset: This is usually abrupt in delirium, although initial loss of mental clarity can be subtle.
- Duration: Dementia is a slow, progressive disease and does not 'get better'. Delirium on the other hand tends to last hours to days (although it can be prolonged in some cases).
- Attention: Patients with delirium have a reduced ability to focus, sustain, or shift attention. This is absent in dementia, except in severe cases.
- Consciousness: This fluctuates in delirium so repeated assessment is important. However, patients will typically exhibit a reduced level of consciousness and impaired orientation.
- Cause: Delirium is caused by an underlying medical condition, substance intoxication or a side effect of prescription medication. Dementia on the other hand is causes by an underlying neurological process (for example, amyloid beta-plaque accumulation in Alzheimer's disease).

Delirium is often divided into three variants:[28]

- Hyperactive: Characterised by anxiety, restlessness, irritability, anger and frustration. Patients may be easily startled and distracted, and unable to sit still. Speech can be loud, but incoherent with frequent topic hopping.
- Hypoactive: Patients with hypoactive delirium are typically lethargic, apathetic, slow in movement, withdrawn, drowsy and difficult to wake.
- Mixed: A combination of the two other variants, with patients fluctuating between hyperactive and hypoactive delirium throughout the day.

Causes of delirium

Delirium can be the result of virtually any medical condition or drug treatment as well as a number of other causes, including:[28]

- Infection: Examples include urinary tract infections, pneumonia, or fever from a viral infection
- Medication: Such as anticholinergics, analgesics and corticosteroids. Polypharmacy
- Serious medical illnesses: For example diseases of the liver, kidney, lungs and heart
- Sudden alcohol and/or drug withdrawal
- Major surgery
- Acute stress
- Epilepsy
- Brain injury or infection
- Terminal illness
- Constipation
- Urinary catheters
- Immobility.

Assessment of delirium

If you suspect that a patient is suffering from delirium, you can use the 4AT assessment screening tool (Table 10.2). This four-part screening tool takes less than 2 minutes to complete and incorporates the AMT4 (covered earlier in the chapter).[30] A score of 4 or more indicated possible delirium with/without cognitive impairment. A score of 1–3 indicates possible cognitive impairment.

Communication

Although you are well versed in the art of communication, there are some additional points to consider when you are caring for a patient with dementia:[31]

Table 10.2 The 4AT test.

Alertness	
This includes patients who may be markedly drowsy (for example, difficult to rouse and/or obviously sleepy during assessment) or agitated/ hyperactive. Observe the patient. If asleep, attempt to wake with speech or gentle touch on shoulder. **Ask the patient to state their name and address to assist rating.**	
Normal (fully alert, but not agitated, throughout assessment)	0
Mild sleepiness for <10 seconds after waking, then normal	0
Clearly abnormal	4
AMT4	
Age, date of birth, place (name of the hospital or building), current year.	
No mistakes	0
1 mistake	1
2 or more mistakes/untestable	2
Attention	
Ask the patient: **"Please tell me the months of the year in backwards order, starting at December."** To assist initial understanding, one prompt of **"What is the month before December?"** is permitted.	
Achieves 7 months or more correctly	0
Starts but scores < 7 months / refuses to start	1
Untestable (cannot start because unwell, drowsy, inattentive)	2
Acute change or fluctuating course	
Evidence of significant change or fluctuation in: alertness, cognition, other mental function (for example, paranoia, hallucinations) arising over the last 2 weeks and still evident in the last 24 hours.	
No	0
Yes	4

- Get their attention: Approach the patient from the front so they can see you coming. Try to make eye contact and ensure they can see your face and body movements.
- Use their name: Using their name can help them understand that you are not a stranger (although this may not be true), which can be reassuring.
- Frequently remind them who you are: This can reduce anxiety and avoid the patient becoming alarmed at being treated by a stranger.
- Keep ambient noise and activity to a minimum: Reducing distractions, activity and noise will help a patient with dementia (indeed most patients) to concentrate on what you are saying.
- Don't rush: Take your time. Slowing your rate of speech can help, but increase the time spent speaking AND listening. It may help if you silently count to seven between

short sentences, and then give the patient the same time to answer.
- Keep calm: Adopt a calm tone and manner to reduce distress and make the patient feel more comfortable with you. Patients with dementia maintain the ability to determine your body language even after their ability to understand speech has been lost.
- Keep things simple: Avoid jargon and speak in short and simple to understand sentences. When giving instructions, break down the task into simple stages. Give clear instructions, for example rather than saying "sit there" you could try saying "sit in this blue chair, please."
- Use the patient's preferred method of communication: Establish this early from the patient and others who know them. This includes speaking to the patient in their first language or using communication aids such as pictures or talking mats.

Challenging behaviour

Many patients with dementia are placid and sweet-tempered, but over 90% will exhibit some form of challenging behaviour. This includes:[26]

- Sleeplessness
- Wandering
- Agitation
- Pacing
- Aggression (including spitting)
- Disinhibition
- Jealousy (especially sexual jealousy).

Challenging behaviour needs to be seen as the result of an unmet need, which the patient may not be able to express, such as boredom, frustration and/or annoyance.

Managing challenging behaviour

It is important to appreciate that each patient will be slightly different, so the best way of managing challenging behaviour will need to be tailored to them. Advice from carers and/or relatives may help, but general principles include:[31]

- Trying to find out what is the cause of the behaviour
- Reducing the stress and/or demands placed on the patient
- Explaining what is happening using the patient's name and saying who you are. You are likely to have to repeat this process often
- Giving patients time to respond to your requests or questions
- Trying not to show criticism or irritation and avoiding confrontation with patients
- Watching for warning signs that they are becoming more anxious or agitated. Get help if the situation does not calm down quickly
- Including carers and/or relatives who know the patient and who will have experience in managing the patient's challenging behaviour
- Not making sudden movements or using a sharp tone. Instead, remain calm and keep your voice low.

Assessment of pain in dementia

The Abbey pain scale is currently included in the *JRCALC Clinical Guidelines* (Figure 10.2).[32] However, it requires a score sheet and is recommended to be conducted during patient movement, which might make it impractical for use in some acute pre-hospital situations. In addition, with the lack of recent studies into its use, other pain scores for patients with severe cognitive impairment have been advocated instead.[33] One example, is the Pain in Advanced. Dementia (PAINAD) score,[34] which has been favourably evaluated in one paramedic study.[35] The takeaway point here is that pain scoring using alternative methods in patients with dementia is important if these patients are not to be left in pain.

The Abbey Pain Scale

For measurement of pain in people with dementia who cannot verbalise.

How to use scale: While observing the resident, score questions 1 to 6.

Name of resident:...

Name and designation of person completing the scale:..

Date:.. Time:..

Latest pain relief given was.. at.....................hrs.

Q1. Vocalisation
eg whimpering, groaning, crying
Absent 0   Mild 1   Moderate 2   Severe 3

Q1 [ ]

Q2. Facial expression
eg looking tense, frowning, grimacing, looking frightened
Absent 0   Mild 1   Moderate 2   Severe 3

Q2 [ ]

Q3. Change in body language
eg fidgeting, rocking, guarding part of body, withdrawn
Absent 0   Mild 1   Moderate 2   Severe 3

Q3 [ ]

Q4. Behavioural change
eg increased confusion, refusing to eat, alteration in usual patterns
Absent 0   Mild 1   Moderate 2   Severe 3

Q4 [ ]

Q5. Physiological change
eg temperature, pulse or blood pressure outside normal limits, perspiring, flushing of pallor
Absent 0   Mild 1   Moderate 2   Severe 3

Q5 [ ]

Q6. Physical changes
eg skin tears, pressure areas, arthritis, contractures, previous injuries
Absent 0   Mild 1   Moderate 2   Severe 3

Q6 [ ]

Add scores for Q1 to Q6 and record here ➔ Total pain score [ ]

Now tick the box that matches the Total Pain Score ➔

0–2 No pain	3–7 Mild	8–13 Moderate	14+ Severe

Finally, tick the box which matches the type of pain ➔

Chronic	Acute	Acute on chronic

Abbey J, De Bellis A, Piller N, Esterman A, Gilles L, Parker D, Lowcay B. The Abbey Pain Scale. Funded by the JH & JD Gunn Medical Research Foundation 1998–2002.
(This document may be reproduced with this reference retained.)

Figure 10.2 The Abbey pain score.

Chapter 10 Older People

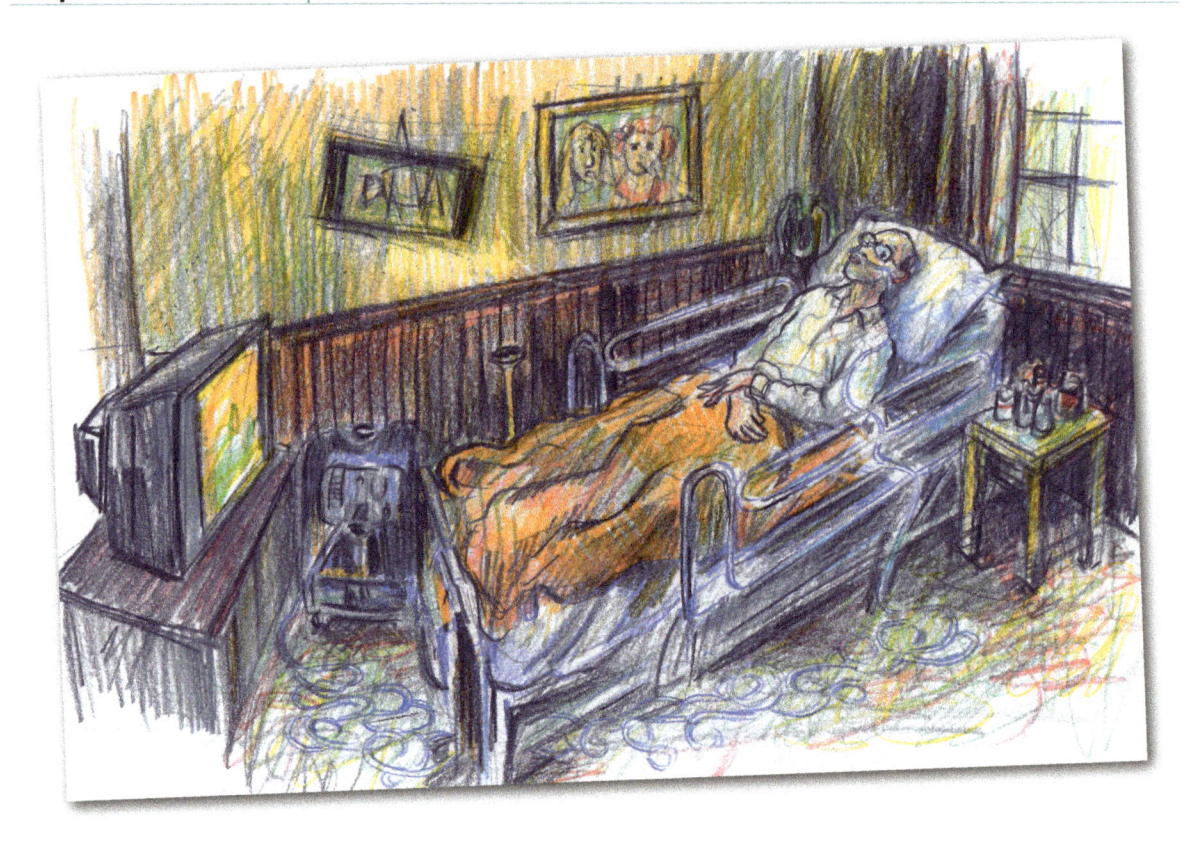

End-of-Life Care

You are on standby with just over an hour of the shift left. Your colleague is getting increasingly fidgety as the final 45 minutes of the shift approaches, since the new standby policy demands that you are returned to station after this time. As the clock changes to exactly 45 minutes until shift end, your colleague reaches for the radio to contact the emergency operations centre (EOC). However, he is beaten by the MDT, which passes you details of a 70-year-old male who has fallen. "They must have cameras in here," says your colleague, who starts looking suspiciously around the cab. Still, he is hopeful that with the incident location and the hospital close by, you'll be able to pop the patient in the back of the ambulance, get to the emergency department (ED) and only be 20 minutes off late. You press mobile and head towards the patient's address, which is only 5 minutes from your current location.

As you pull up outside the address, you can't help thinking that you have been here before, although it must be over three years ago. The nicotine-stained walls clinch it and you remember that the patient suffers with COPD and is on home oxygen (see Chapter 1).

His wife, Jean, shows you into the living room, which has not changed apart from the hospital bed that has replaced the comfy chair whose arms were peppered with holes caused by hot ash falling from the patient's cigarettes, and a newer TV.

End-of-Life Care

The oxygen concentrator is chugging away in the corner of the room and is attached to the patient by the longest piece of oxygen tubing you have ever seen. About a metre of this tubing is currently wrapped tightly around the patient's legs, which probably explains why he has fallen onto the floor. Jean explains that her husband, Eric, had been trying to use a urine bottle, but had become tangled in his oxygen tubing and lost his balance. Jean had helped him slump to the floor, which ensured that he did not get hurt, but could not save him. "I'm no spring chicken myself," she cackles, "even if he is my toy boy!"

Your colleague is trying to talk to Eric but is not having much luck, despite speaking increasingly slower and louder. Unsurprisingly, this is not proving to be an effective communication strategy. "It's no good," your colleague says dejectedly, "I'll get a collar and board." Before you can respond, he is off out of the door.

> What are you going to do: **Maintain cervical-spine immobilisation** (read on) or **Assess the patient** (skip the next paragraph)?

Maintain cervical-spine immobilisation

You attempt to take hold of Eric's head, but he does not like that at all and tries to peel your hands off his head. He is clearly confused and you cannot rationalise with him about the need for immobilisation. As he gets more agitated, Jean becomes upset and as you try to explain to her why you need to hold Eric's head, she retorts with "But he only slid to the floor. I made sure he didn't go with a bang." She has a point, the mechanism sounds benign. Just then, your colleague returns with the spinal board, headblocks, collars and what looks like a pelvic binder. You make the decision that immobilisation is not appropriate, and your colleague turns back to the front door, grumbling all the way to the ambulance.

Assess the patient

From the history, you determine that the mechanism of injury (MOI) is benign and the risk of injury, low. Instead, you focus your energy on performing a patient assessment and checking for injuries. You call back your colleague and ask him to record some baseline observations:

Appearance

Patient looks cachexic

Airway

Patent.

Breathing

Laboured, with a prolonged expiratory phase
Nasal prongs in situ with oxygen running at 2 l/min
Poor air entry generally, with a mixture of wheeze and crackles everywhere
Respiratory rate: 26 breaths/min
SpO_2: 84% on oxygen
Peripheral cyanosis and finger clubbing present.

Circulation

Weak radial pulse at a rate of 96 beats per minute
Blood pressure: 86/51 mmHg
Skin pale and non-diaphoretic

Disability

Disorientated and confused
Unable to follow commands
Blood sugar: 9.2 mmol/l

Chapter 10   Older People

Exposure/Environment

Temperature: 35.8°C.

A head-to-toe examination does not reveal any injuries so you gently lift the patient back into bed.

You ask Jean about Eric's medical history and she tells you that he has COPD, lung cancer and recurrent urinary tract infections (UTIs), which cause him to think he needs to pass urine, although it sounds as if he has not passed much in the last few days. Eric has also spent a week at a local hospice recently.

> Eric is clearly very unwell and respiratory failure is approaching. What are you going to do: **Take Eric to hospital** (read on) or **Find out more** (skip the next paragraph)?

Take Eric to hospital

You suggest taking Eric to hospital and both Jean and your colleague shout "NO!" in unison. You turn first to your colleague who is trying, unsuccessfully, to subtly show you his watch, intimating that there is only 15 minutes of the shift left and a referral to an advanced practitioner or GP might still lead to a reasonable finish time. You turn your attention to Jean, who has tears welling up in her eyes, and you enquire what the matter is (read on).

Find out more

"He's come home to die," she sniffs quietly. "He went to the hospice and the staff were lovely, even offered him a bed, until ... the end, but he wanted to come home." Eric's lung cancer is terminal and has infiltrated his lymph nodes, and a number of other organs. His condition has been deteriorating over the past week and the Macmillan nurse and GP have been preparing the family for the inevitable. Jean tells you that Eric has an advance care plan (ACP), but when you ask to see it, she cannot find it, despite bustling around the living room, seemingly glad to have something to do. After 10 minutes, she admits defeat. "I can't understand it, the district nurses were looking at it only this morning." You do find a box of anticipatory medication, complete with a prescription and clear guidance on when it should be administered. Some of these look useful, but midazolam for restlessness and breathlessness is not the indication provided in the *JRCALC Clinical Guidelines*. The rattle from the secretions in his airway would also benefit from the hyoscine, but that is not in the guidelines at all.

> What are you going to do: **Stick to the guidelines** (read on) or **Administer the drugs** (skip the next paragraph)?

Stick to the guidelines

You'll get into trouble if you give these drugs, you're sure of it. Instead, you administer a salbutamol nebuliser, which makes little difference to the patient's conditions, but at least you feel better for doing something. Jean still cannot locate the ACP, but does produce a phone number for the hospice. Perhaps it is worth giving it a ring (read on)?

Administer the drugs

The anticipatory drugs are prescribed for the patient and there are clear instructions on how and when they should be administered. As a healthcare professional, you know that you can administer the drugs in this instance. However, you have little experience of the drugs in the box, and since Jean has located a phone number for the hospice, you elect to give them a ring.

After briefly speaking to the hospice nurse, the palliative care consultant comes onto the phone. She listens to your description of events and the patient's clinical signs, and enquires about the presence of anticipatory medication. You reel off the list in the box and she advises that you administer both the midazolam and hyoscine subcutaneously. In addition, she enquires about whether family members are present and suggests that they are contacted now and their presence requested.

Feeling reassured, you pass the phone to Jean and the consultant has a chat with her. You administer the midazolam and hyoscine as instructed, and after 10 minutes the patient is visibly more relaxed and settled. It takes nearly an hour for family members to turn up at the door, but they are in time to say their goodbyes and hold a vigil for Eric, who slips into respiratory, and then cardiorespiratory, arrest.

You contact the patient's GP who confirms that he has seen the patient recently and is happy to certify to cause of death, which means that the police are not required. One of the daughters recalls the contact details of the undertakers and, sensing that your presence is no longer required, you gently say your goodbyes. Jean gives you and your colleague a hug and thanks you for being there. It's very moving and even your battle-hardened colleague's eyes start to water. You close the door on the way out and return to station in silence.

Scale of the problem

Every year in England and Wales, 500,000 people die; almost half of these in hospital.[36] In most cases, death is expected, providing an opportunity for end-of-life care planning, including the location of death. While there is some debate about whether most patients actually want to die at home,[37] it is clear that a significant proportion of patients do not die in their preferred location. The reasons for this are multi-factorial, but include a lack of anticipatory care planning, lack of communication between healthcare agencies and insufficient community resources.[38,39]

Physiology of dying

Normal body function involves highly complex and interactive processes to maintain homeostasis. As death approaches, homeostasis is disrupted, which leads to multi-organ failure. This will typically manifest as one or more of the following:[40]

- Acidosis
- Uraemia
- Electrolyte imbalances
- Hypoxaemia
- Hypoalbuminaemia.

Acidosis

This is caused by a number of factors including excess fat catabolism, which causes cachexia; intestinal obstruction, which causes a reduction in bicarbonate due to diarrhoea and vomiting; and an accumulation of carbon dioxide due to inadequate ventilation.

Uraemia

Acute kidney failure usually occurs in the days approaching death, and as the kidneys begin to fail, they stop excreting urea in the urine, leading to a rapid increase in blood levels of urea.

Electrolyte imbalances

These are also a consequence of kidney failure, with signs and symptoms depending on the electrolytes. For example, high levels of phosphate in the blood leads to tetany and muscle twitching, hyperkalaemia causes cardiac arrhythmias, and low levels of sodium are responsible for weakness, confusion, convulsions and coma.

Chapter 10 Older People

Hypoxaemia

This is probably the one that you are most familiar with, and is caused by inadequate oxygenation of the tissues, due to hypoventilation and/or insufficient numbers of red blood cells.

Hypoalbuminaemia

This is usually caused by a failing liver, which is responsible for the synthesis of proteins (of which albumin is one). In addition, the excess catabolism that leads to cachexia also causes excessive protein breakdown. Since albumin is required to maintain oncotic pressure inside the vessels, its reduction leads to water moving out of the general circulation and into the tissues, causing central and peripheral oedema.[41]

As organs are damaged, they begin to fail and there is a cascade of liver, kidney and respiratory failure, hypercalcaemia and intestinal obstruction. This is responsible for the signs and symptoms that precede death, which include the following:[42]

- Abdominal ascites
- Cheyne-Stokes respirations
- Cool peripheries with mottling and/or cyanosis
- Decreased oral intake
- Delirium
- Difficulty swallowing medication
- Drowsiness
- Global weakness
- Incontinence
- Jaundice
- Noisy moist breathing (due to inability to clear secretions), sometimes called the death rattle
- Respiratory distress.

Advance care planning

In terminal conditions, death can often be anticipated, which provides patients with the opportunity to consider their wishes and preferences about future care, particularly as they are likely to be unable to do so when close to death. Unfortunately, only 5% of people put these wishes and preferences in writing by means of an advance care plan (ACP, sometimes also called a preferred priorities for care document) or Recommended Summary Plan for Emergency Care and Treatment (ReSPECT) document.[43] The contents of an ACP are not legally binding, but any best interests decision about patients must take into account the patient's wishes and preferences.[42]

Advanced decisions to refuse treatment (ADRT)

ADRTs (also known as living wills) are documents that outline specific aspects of care that the patient does not wish to receive. This is then typically referred to when the patient is unable to make these wishes clear. Examples of the interventions that a patient may refuse include being ventilated, tube fed, receiving antibiotics and not being admitted to hospital unless they are suffering from a complaint with a treatable cause.

Unlike the ACP, this is a legal document and, as long as the phrase "even if life is at risk" is present, and the document is signed, dated and witnessed, the contents must be respected by healthcare staff. Note that treatment can only be declined and not requested and the ADRT only comes into effect once the patient loses mental capacity.[44]

Do not attempt cardiopulmonary resuscitation (DNACPR) decisions

DNACPR decisions are made by a senior clinician, usually with involvement from the patient's clinical team. This will normally be a consultant, GP or suitably experienced nurse. There are four broad situations when a DNACPR decision will be made:[45]

- A mentally competent patient refuses resuscitative treatment

End-of-Life Care

- A valid advanced directive clearly states that the patient does not want CPR
- CPR is unlikely to be successful
- Successful CPR is possible, but the length and quality of life following resuscitation is not in the patient's best interests.

Ideally, this is written and agreed ahead of time and documentary evidence of the decision will be presented to you before you commence resuscitation. However, even if there is no formal DNACPR in place, you can still elect not to start or continue resuscitation if the patient is in the final stages of a terminal illness and you think that CPR would not be successful. Ultimately, if you are unsure about the validity of previously made decisions, then commencing resuscitation is appropriate while you obtain further information to guide your decision-making.[45]

Anticipatory medication

Anticipatory (sometimes called just-in-case) medications are drugs that are prescribed before symptoms occur on the assumption that they will be required prior to death. They are typically given subcutaneously, which, although having a slower onset time than the intravenous route, is generally safer and the effects of administration are likely to be seen within a few minutes (up to 15 minutes). Dosages vary and may need to be increased if the patient is already having the same drug administered via a syringe driver.[40]

Symptoms that anticipatory medications are intended to manage include:[42]

- Pain
- Shortness of breath
- Cough
- Nausea and vomiting
- Agitation and restlessness
- Secretions.

Typical types of drugs used to manage these symptoms are opioids, benzodiazepines, dopamine antagonists and anticholinergics (Table 10.3). Drugs are selected so that any combination (and all) of the drugs can be administered together, safely.

Table 10.3 Typical anticipatory medication.

Drug	Drug type	Symptoms managed	Side effects
Diamorphine	Opioid	Pain Breathlessness Cough	Nausea and vomiting Constipation Urinary retention Dry mouth and sweats
Midazolam	Benzodiazepine	Restlessness Breathlessness Cough Muscle twitching Convulsions Muscle pain/spasm	Drowsiness Respiratory depression Addiction and tolerance
Haloperidol	Dopamine receptor antagonist	Nausea and vomiting Agitation Sedation	Secretions Colic Urinary spasm
Hyoscine butylbromide	Anticholinergic	Secretions (particularly death rattle) Colic Urinary spasm	Dry mouth Constipation Urinary retention

Adapted from: Watson, 2019.

Chapter 10   Older People

Subcutaneous injections

As previously mentioned, the subcutaneous (SC) route is most commonly used for anticipatory medication. It has the benefit of providing slower absorption of the drug, due to lower blood flow in the subcutaneous tissues. It is also relatively pain free if small needles and low volumes are used, for example 0.5–2 ml. A good technique is important to avoid inadvertent intramuscular administration of the drug (Table 10.4).

Site

Suitable sites for SC administration are the upper arm, thighs and peri-umbilical area of the abdomen. When choosing a site, consider avoiding previously used sites as irritation, scarring and hardening of the tissues can occur with repeated injections. Also avoid sites where there is evidence of inflammation or wounds.[46]

Table 10.4   Technique for administering a subcutaneous injection.

Action	Rationale
Check prescription and patient notes	Ensure right drug, dose, route and time Avoid duplication of administration
Explain procedure to patient and double check drug allergies	Enables patient to give informed consent Maintains safety
Wash hands or clean with antibacterial hand rub Put on gloves	Reduces risk of cross-infection/contamination
Make a space for your kit Collect and visually inspect items Check drug including expiry date with colleague	Minimises risk of infection Prevents disruption to procedure Maintains patient safety
Choose site, considering need for rotation of injection sites Check it is clean. Wash with soap and water if necessary	Maximises drug absorption NOTE: swabbing with an alcohol wipe does not reduce incidence of infection and repeated use of wipes leads to hardening of skin
If the syringe is not prefilled, draw up drug and then exchange needle for injection needle	Ensures needle is clean, sharp and the correct length
Using your non-dominant hand, pinch skin between thumb and index finger to make a fold	Lifts tissue away from muscle to ensure insertion into SC tissue and not muscle
Insert needle into skin about 6 mm deep at an angle of 90° If the patient is cachexic or the needle is large, insert at an angle of 45° Administer drug (there is no need to pull back on syringe)	Ensures correct administration and minimises discomfort Chance of inadvertent vessel injection is very small
Keep hold of skin fold until needle removed Withdraw needle and place in sharps bin	Prevent needlestick injuries
Document administration	Legal requirement

Source: Hunter 2008.

Emergencies in end-of-life care (EOLC)

Although much of the focus of EOLC is preparation for death, there are still emergencies that require prompt medical intervention. These are mainly due to complications of cancer and include:[42]

- Sepsis in the neutropenic patient
- Metastatic spinal cord compression
- Superior vena cava occlusion
- Haemorrhage
- Convulsions.

Sepsis in the neutropenic patient

Any patient on anti-cancer treatment who becomes unwell should be suspected of suffering from neutropenic sepsis. Early signs include flu-like symptoms, but watch for other signs of sepsis and/or a temperature above 38°C. These patients need intravenous antibiotics as soon as possible.[47]

Metastatic spinal cord compression

This occurs in up to 6% of patients with cancer and the most common sign is back pain. The patient may also complain of weakness and altered sensation in both legs and difficulty in passing urine. High-dose steroids and prompt decompression, if appropriate, are the best ways to avoid the patient becoming paraplegic.

Superior vena cava occlusion

This can be caused by external compression, a thrombus forming inside the vein, or direct invasion by a cancer. It is most commonly caused by cancer of the bronchus. Clinical signs and symptoms include Horner's syndrome, breathlessness, headache and swelling of the face, neck and arms. Without treatment, these patients usually die within a few days.[42]

Haemorrhage

Haemorrhage can be caused directly, by erosion of a cancer into a vessel, or indirectly by medication such as steroids and non-steroidal anti-inflammatory drugs, that cause gastric and duodenal erosion. Erosion of a major artery can rapidly lead to death, which will be very distressing for the patient and relatives. In some cases, the palliative care team may provide anticipatory medication to sedate an acutely bleeding patient.

Convulsions

This is probably the condition you are most comfortable with. Most convulsions are self-limiting and will only require supportive care. In the case of prolonged convulsions, anticipatory medication may be available, or diazepam can be administered from the vehicle supply.

Chapter 10 Older People

References

1. British Geriatrics Society. Introduction to Frailty [Internet]. British Geriatrics Society. 2014. Available from: https://www.bgs.org.uk/resources/introduction-to-frailty
2. Clegg A, Young J, Iliffe S, Rikkert MO, Rockwood K. Frailty in elderly people. *Lancet (London, England)*, 2013 Mar 2;381(9868):752–762.
3. Gale CR, Cooper C, Aihie Sayer A. Prevalence of frailty and disability: findings from the English Longitudinal Study of Ageing. *Age and Ageing*, 2015 Jan 1;44(1):162–165.
4. University of York Centre for Reviews and Dissemination. Effectiveness Matters: Recognising and managing frailty in primary care [Internet]. 2017. Available from: https://www.york.ac.uk/media/crd/effectiveness-matters-may-2017-frailty.pdf
5. Oliver D. 'Acopia' and 'social admission' are not diagnoses: why older people deserve better. Journal of the Royal Society of Medicine, 2008 Apr 1;101(4):168–174.
6. Oliver D. The Geriatrics "Profanisaurus." Words and phrases we should ban? [Internet]. British Geriatrics Society. 2013. Available from: https://www.bgs.org.uk/blog/the-geriatrics-%E2%80%9Cprofanisaurus%E2%80%9D-words-and-phrases-we-should-ban
7. Kee Y-YK, Rippingale C. The prevalence and characteristic of patients with 'acopia'. *Age and Ageing*, 2009 Jan;38(1):103–105.
8. Hughes L. The Geriatric 5Ms - have the 'giants' changed [Internet]. GM. 2018. Available from: https://www.gmjournal.co.uk/the-geriatric-5ms-an-important-new-construct-in-geriatric-medicine
9. Morley JE. The new geriatric giants. *Clinics in Geriatric Medicine*, 2017 Aug 1;33(3):xi–xii.
10. Molnar F, Frank CC. Optimizing geriatric care with the GERIATRIC 5Ms. *Canadian Family Physician*, 2019 Jan;65(1):39.
11. British Geriatrics Society. Recognising frailty [Internet]. British Geriatrics Society. 2014. Available from: https://www.bgs.org.uk/resources/recognising-frailty
12. Innes JA, Dover AR, Fairhurst K, Britton R, Danielson E. *Macleod's clinical examination*, 14th edition. Edinburgh: Elsevier; 2018.
13. Rockwood K, Song X, MacKnight C, Bergman H, Hogan DB, McDowell I, et al. A global clinical measure of fitness and frailty in elderly people. *Canadian Medical Association Journal*, 2005 Aug 30;173(5):489–495.
14. Locke T, Keat S, Tate M, Bown A, Hart A, Ghosh R. Assessing the performance of the four question abbreviated mental test in the acute geriatric setting. *Acute Medicine*, 2013;12(1):13–17.
15. Swain DG, Nightingale PG. Evaluation of a shortened version of the Abbreviated Mental Test in a series of elderly patients. Clinical Rehabilitation, 1997 Aug;11(3):243–248.
16. National Institute for Health and Care Excellence. Urinary tract infections in adults [Internet]. NICE; 2015. Available from: https://www.nice.org.uk/guidance/qs90
17. Abbott C, Dykes L. Geriatric Medicine: A selection of top tips to get you started [Internet]. DrLindaDykes. 2017. Available from: https://docs.wixstatic.com/ugd/bbd630_9068591ed32045ef9e10c04cdf3086a2.pdf?index=true
18. Royal College of Emergency Medicine. Early to bed [Internet]. 2018. Available from: https://www.rcem.ac.uk/docs/Safety/RCEM%20Safety%20Alert%20-%20Pressure%20Ulcers%20FINAL.pdf
19. Royal College of Emergency Medicine. Time critical medicines [Internet]. 2017. Available from: https://www.rcem.ac.uk/docs/Safety%20Resources%20+%20Guidance/Time%20critical%20meds%20-%20Nov%202017%20.pdf
20. Social Care Institute for Excellence, National Institute for Health and Clinical Excellence. Dementia – Supporting people with dementia and their carers in health and social care [Internet]. 2006. Available from: https://www.scie.org.uk/publications/misc/dementia/
21. Neuropathology Group of the Medical Research Council Cognitive Function and Ageing Study. Pathological correlates of late-onset dementia in a multicentre, community-based population in England and Wales. Neuropathology Group of the Medical Research Council Cognitive Function and Ageing Study (MRC CFAS). *The Lancet*, 2001 Jan 20;357(9251):169–175.

References

22. Ray S, Davidson S. *Dementia and cognitive decline: a review of the evidence*. London: Age UK; 2014.
23. Ross J, Horton-Szar D. *Crash course nervous system*, 4th edition. Smith C, editor. London: Mosby; 2015.
24. Richards FA, Coope B, editors. *ABC of dementia*, 2nd edition. Hoboken: John Wiley & Sons; 2020. (ABC series).
25. Loeb C, Gandolfo C, Croce R, Conti M. Dementia associated with lacunar infarction. *Stroke*, 1992 Sep 1;23(9):1225–1229.
26. Barrett E, Burns A. Dementia revealed: what primary care needs to know [Internet]. 2015. Available from: https://dementiapartnerships.com/resource/dementia-the-view-from-primary-care/
27. Morandi A, Davis D, Bellelli G, Arora RC, Caplan GA, Kamholz B, et al. The diagnosis of delirium superimposed on dementia: an emerging challenge. *Journal of the American Medical Directors Association*, 2017 Jan 1;18(1):12–18.
28. Scottish Ambulance Service. Dementia Learning Resource [Internet]. 2014. Available from: https://www.nes.scot.nhs.uk/media/nlqdz3fn/scottish_ambulance_service.pdf
29. Fong TG, Davis D, Growdon ME, Albuquerque A, Inouye SK. The interface between delirium and dementia in elderly adults. *The Lancet Neurology*, 2015 Aug 1;14(8):823–832.
30. Tieges Z, Maclullich AMJ, Anand A, Brookes C, Cassarino M, O'connor M, et al. Diagnostic accuracy of the 4AT for delirium detection in older adults: systematic review and meta-analysis. *Age and Ageing*, 2021 May 1;50(3):733–743.
31. Yorkshire Ambulance Service NHS Trust. Dementia Learning Resource for Ambulance Staff [Internet]. 2014. Available from: https://dementiapartnerships.com/wp-content/uploads/sites/2/DementiaLearningResourceforAmbulanceStaff.pdf
32. Joint Royal Colleges Ambulance Liaison Committee, Association of Ambulance Chief Executives. JRCALC Clinical Guidelines. Cited from JRCALC Plus (Version 1.2.13) [Mobile application software]. Bridgwater: Class Publishing Ltd; 2021.
33. Schofield P. The assessment of pain in older people: UK national guidelines. *Age and Ageing*, 2018 Mar 1;47(suppl_1):i1–22.
34. Warden V, Hurley AC, Volicer L. Development and psychometric evaluation of the Pain Assessment in Advanced Dementia (PAINAD) scale. *Journal of the American Medical Directors Association*, 2003 Feb;4(1):9–15.
35. Lucas PV, Mason R, Annear M, Harris W, McCall M, Robinson A, et al. Pain assessment in older adults with dementia: an exploratory pilot study of paramedic students' perceptions of the utility of two validated assessment tools. Australasian Journal of Paramedicine, [Internet]. 2016 Jul 31;13(3). Available from: https://ajp.paramedics.org/index.php/ajp/article/view/481
36. Health Quality Improvement Partnership. National Audit of Care at the End of Life [Internet]. NHS Benchmarking Network. 2020. Available from: https://www.nhsbenchmarking.nhs.uk/nacel-audit-outputs
37. Hoare S, Morris ZS, Kelly MP, Kuhn I, Barclay S. Do patients want to die at home? A systematic review of the UK literature, focused on missing preferences for Place of Death. PLOS ONE. 2015 Nov 10;10(11):e0142723.
38. Collis E, Al-Qurainy R. Care of the dying patient in the community. *British Medical Journal*, 2013 Jul 3;347(jul03 1):f4085–f4085.
39. Hoare S, Kelly MP, Prothero L, Barclay S. Ambulance staff and end-of-life hospital admissions: a qualitative interview study. *Palliative Medicine*, 2018 Oct 1;32(9):1465–1473.
40. Kirkwood Hospice. *Going, going, gone. Key issues in palliative and end of life care*. Huddersfield: Kirkwood Hospice; 2014.
41. Marieb E, Hoehn K. Human anatomy & physiology, 11th edition. Pearson; 2019.
42. Watson MS, Campbell R, Vallath N, Ward S, Wells J. *Oxford handbook of palliative care*, 3rd edition. Oxford: Oxford University Press; 2019. (Oxford handbooks).
43. NatCen Social Research. British social attitudes research for dying matters [Internet]. 2013. Available from: http://www.dyingmatters.org/sites/default/files/BSA30_Full_Report.pdf

Chapter 10   Older People

44. NHS Improving Quality. Capacity, care planning and advance care planning in life limiting illness [Internet]. 2014. Available from: https://www.england.nhs.uk/improvement-hub/wp-content/uploads/sites/44/2017/11/ACP_Booklet_2014.pdf
45. Resuscitation Council (UK). Decisions relating to cardiopulmonary resuscitation [Internet]. 2017. Available from: https://www.resus.org.uk/library/publications/publication-decisions-relating-cardiopulmonary
46. Hunter J. Subcutaneous injection technique. *Nursing Standard*, 2008 Jan 29;22(21):41–44.
47. Blackmore T. *Palliative and end of life care for paramedics*. Bridgwater: Class Professional Publishing; 2020.

Assessment

Airway and Breathing

Severe airway contamination in cardiac arrest

1. The normal pressure of the lower oesophageal sphincter is:
   a. 30 cmH$_2$O
   b. 20 cmH$_2$O
   c. 10 cmH$_2$O
   d. 5 cmH$_2$O

2. Which of the following is NOT true about gastric distention?
   a. Increases risk of regurgitation
   b. Decreases lung movement
   c. Decreases respiratory system compliance
   d. Lowers the diaphragm

3. The upper oesophageal sphincter is formed by ____ parts of the inferior pharyngeal constrictor muscle.
   a. 5
   b. 4
   c. 3
   d. 2

4. The pharyngeal reflex is also known as the ____ reflex:
   a. Gip
   b. Gag
   c. Cough
   d. Splutter

5. Which conditions put patients at increased risk of aspiration?
   a. Obesity
   b. Pregnancy
   c. Chronic lung disease
   d. All of the above

6. Which of the following airway management techniques is NOT routinely recommended in cardiac arrest?
   a. Patient positioning
   b. Cricoid pressure
   c. Suction
   d. None of the above

7. The 'L' in SALAD stands for:
   a. Laryngoscopy
   b. Larynx
   c. Laryngeal
   d. Large

8. _____ is an alternative technique to cricoid pressure.
   a. Right paratracheal compression
   b. Right parasternal compression
   c. Left paratracheal compression
   d. Left parasternal compression

9. When performing the SALAD technique, you insert the index finger of the right hand into the right-hand side of the oropharynx to create a 'channel' for tracheal tube. This is known as the SALAD:
   a. Poke
   b. Point
   c. Prod
   d. Pick

10. Blind insertion of a tracheal tube usually results with the tube in the patient's:
    a. Eyeball
    b. Nostril
    c. Larynx
    d. Oesophagus

Answers: Q1: b, Q2: d, Q3: d, Q4: b, Q5: d, Q6: b, Q7: a, Q8: c, Q9: a, Q10: d.

Assessment

Tracheostomies

1. What is the most important difference between a laryngectomy and tracheostomy?
   a. Laryngectomy patients have a potentially patent upper airway
   b. Minimising of anatomical dead space
   c. Laryngectomy patients have no patent upper airway
   d. None of the above

2. Tracheostomy patients have a reduction in anatomical dead space of up to ____%:
   a. 20
   b. 30
   c. 40
   d. 50

3. Which tracheostomy tube is best for positive pressure ventilation?
   a. Uncuffed, fenestrated
   b. Cuffed, unfenestrated
   c. Uncuffed, double-cannula
   d. Any of the above

4. Patients with cuffed tracheostomy tubes should not be able to:
   a. Eat
   b. Breathe
   c. Speak
   d. Sleep

5. Respiratory distress in a tracheostomy patient can be observed clinically by the presence of:
   a. Accessory muscle use
   b. Increased respiratory rate
   c. Increased airway pressures
   d. All of the above

6. What type of red flag symptom is pain at the tracheostomy site?
   a. Airway
   b. Breathing
   c. Specific tracheostomy
   d. General

7. When assessing the breathing of a patient with a tracheostomy, you should look, listen and feel:
   a. At the mouth only
   b. At the tracheostomy site only
   c. At the face and tracheostomy site
   d. At the face only

8. What item is used to assist insertion of a tracheostomy tube?
   a. Decannulation cap
   b. Speaking valve
   c. Swedish nose
   d. Obturator

9. Speaking valves should NEVER be fitted to:
   a. Fenestrated tubes
   b. Double-cannula tubes
   c. Cuffed tubes
   d. None of the above

10. What can you use to ventilate a patient with a laryngectomy?
    a. Paediatric face-mask
    b. Laryngeal mask airway
    c. Endotracheal tube
    d. Any of the above

Answers: Q1: c, Q2: d, Q3: b, Q4: c, Q5: d, Q6: a, Q7: c, Q8: d, Q9: c, Q10: d.

Pneumothorax

1. The inner layer of the pleural membrane is known as the _____ pleura.
   a. Visceral
   b. Parietal
   c. Diaphragmatic
   d. None of the above

2. Boyle's Law states that as the volume of a gas increases, the pressure:
   a. Increases
   b. Stays the same
   c. Decreases
   d. Is too much to bear

3. Many patients with PSP have small blisters on their lungs called:
   a. Plebs
   b. Blebs
   c. Pleura
   d. Viscera

4. Patients with SSP typically have underlying lung disease such as:
   a. COPD
   b. Cystic fibrosis
   c. Tuberculosis
   d. All of the above

5. Which type of pneumothorax only affects women?
   a. Primary
   b. Secondary
   c. Iatrogenic
   d. Catamenial

6. Which type of pneumothorax is commonly caused by transthoracic needle aspiration?
   a. Primary
   b. Secondary
   c. Iatrogenic
   d. Catamenial

7. Patients at increased risk of pneumothorax include:
   a. Non-smokers
   b. Tall, thin males
   c. Short, obese females
   d. All of the above

8. Tension pneumothorax most often occurs in:
   a. Ventilated patients in intensive care
   b. Trauma
   c. Cardiac arrest
   d. All of the above

9. Which of the following is a reliable and early sign of tension pneumothorax in the awake patient?
   a. Decreasing respiratory rate
   b. Hypotension
   c. Agitation
   d. Distended neck veins

10. The typical length of a 14 gauge cannula is:
    a. 25 mm
    b. 35 mm
    c. 45 mm
    d. 55 mm

Answers: Q1: a, Q2: c, Q3: b, Q4: d, Q5: d, Q6: c, Q7: b, Q8: d, Q9: c, Q10: c.

Assessment

Chronic obstructive pulmonary disease

1. Risk factors for COPD include:
   a. Smoking
   b. Dust exposure
   c. Alpha-1 antitrypsin deficiency
   d. All of the above

2. Which of the following shifts the oxyhaemoglobin dissociation curve to the right?
   a. Decreased acidity
   b. Increased PaO_2
   c. Decreased $PaCO_2$
   d. Increased 2,3 DPG

3. How much CO_2 is typically dissolved in blood plasma?
   a. 1.5%
   b. 9%
   c. 27%
   d. 64%

4. How much ipratropium would you administer to a patient with COPD?
   a. 5 mg
   b. 5 mcg
   c. 500 mcg
   d. 500 ml

5. What do the following arterial blood gas results show?
   pH: 7.3
   PaO_2: 12 kPa
   $PaCO_2$: 7 kPa
   HCO_{3-}: 24 mmol/l
   a. Metabolic acidosis
   b. Respiratory acidosis
   c. Metabolic alkalosis
   d. Respiratory Alka-Seltzer

6. Pulmonary arterioles are different to systemic capillaries because they:
   a. Dilate when PAO_2 is low
   b. Constrict when PAO_2 is low
   c. Dilate when $PACO_2$ is high
   d. Constrict when HCO_{3-} is low

7. Hyperoxia can cause hypercapnic respiratory failure due to:
   a. The Bohr Effect
   b. The Haldane Effect
   c. Dalton's Law
   d. All of the above

8. An ABG from an 'acute on chronic' exacerbation of COPD would show which of these results?
   a. Increased pH
   b. Increased HCO_{3-}
   c. Decreased $PaCO_2$
   d. All of the above

9. Above __ breaths/min, the flow rate for a Venturi mask should be increased to __% above the recommended flow rate.
   a. 10, 30
   b. 20, 40
   c. 30, 50
   d. 40, 60

10. You should suspect that your patient has COPD if they have a history of chronic breathlessness on minor exertion and:
    a. Are over 50 years of age
    b. Are long-term smokers
    c. Have no known cause of breathlessness
    d. All of the above

Answers: Q1: d, Q2: d, Q3: b, Q4: c, Q5: b, Q6: b, Q7: b, Q8: b, Q9: c, Q10: d.

Circulation

Chest pain

1. Contra-indications for aspirin include administration of the drug to children less than 16 years of age because it may rarely lead to _____ syndrome
   a. Cushing's
   b. Reye's
   c. Exploding head
   d. Cauda equina

2. An example of a drug used to treat erectile dysfunction is:
   a. Simvastatin
   b. Ramipril
   c. Frusemide
   d. Sildenafil

3. What is the mortality rate of patients who have right ventricular involvement in inferior wall MIs?
   a. 2–9%
   b. 25–30%
   c. 30–50%
   d. 50–60%

4. Left dominance refers to the fact that the posterior descending artery branches from which artery?
   a. Acute marginal
   b. Left coronary
   c. Circumflex
   d. Sinoatrial nodal

5. From which arteries do diagonal branches originate?
   a. LCA and RCA
   b. RCA and PDA
   c. RCA and Cx
   d. RCA and LAD

6. Proximal RCA occlusions may result in which arrhythmia?
   a. SVT
   b. Sinus tachycardia
   c. Atrial fibrillation
   d. VT

7. The Frank-Starling law of the heart states that increased stretching of the ventricles causes:
   a. Increased contractility
   b. Decreased contractility
   c. Increased heart rate
   d. Decreased stroke volume

8. Which non-standard leads can increase the chances of identifying right ventricular involvement in an inferior wall MI?
   a. V_7 and V_8
   b. MCL and MCR
   c. III and V_1
   d. V_3R and V_4R

9. JVD with clear lung fields suggests which diagnosis?
   a. Pulmonary embolism
   b. Cardiac tamponade
   c. Right ventricular infarction
   d. All of the above

10. If a shocked patient with a right ventricular infarction responds to a fluid bolus, which drug should you use with caution?
    a. Aspirin
    b. Oxygen
    c. GTN
    d. Morphine

Answers: Q1: b, Q2: d, Q3: a, Q4: c, Q5: d, Q6: c, Q7: a, Q8: d, Q9: d, Q10: d.

Assessment

Pacemakers and ICDs

1. Modern electrophysiology stems back to Luigi Galvani's experiments on:
   a. Cats
   b. Dogs
   c. Frogs
   d. Rats

2. What type of batteries power pacemakers?
   a. Alkaline
   b. Nickel cadmium
   c. Rechargeable
   d. Lithium iodide

3. What is the most common type of pacing lead fixator?
   a. Tines
   b. Screws
   c. Superglue
   d. Sutures

4. What does the 3rd letter position of the NBG code signify?
   a. Chamber(s) paced
   b. Response to sensing
   c. Rate modulation
   d. Chamber(s) sensed

5. Which chamber is sensed when the pacemaker mode is set to VVI?
   a. Atrium
   b. Ventricle
   c. Both atrium and ventricle
   d. None of the above

6. A CRT pacemaker is most commonly used to treat:
   a. Sinus pauses of over 6s
   b. Severe heart failure
   c. Recurrent sustained VT
   d. Bundle branch block

7. The key difference between a CRT pacemaker and other types is that they pace the:
   a. Right ventricle
   b. Left ventricle
   c. Right atrium
   d. Left atrium

8. Superior vena cava syndrome is an example of what type of complication?
   a. Implant-related
   b. Pacemaker malfunction
   c. A shocking ICD
   d. All of the above

9. Pacemaker leads can become twisted and coiled because of a patient intervention known as:
   a. Twiddler's syndrome
   b. Fiddler's syndrome
   c. Fettler's syndrome
   d. None of the above

10. Placing a magnet over a CIED will normally:
    a. Stop it pacing
    b. Cause it to pace at a fixed rate
    c. Make it deliver a shock
    d. All of the above

Answers: Q1: c, Q2: d, Q3: a, Q4: b, Q5: b, Q6: b, Q7: b, Q8: a, Q9: a, Q10: b.

Sickle cell disease

1. Complications of sickle cell disease that are common to both adults and children do NOT include:
   a. Dactylitis
   b. Stroke
   c. Chronic anaemia
   d. Vaso-occlusive crisis

2. If there are multiple forms of a gene that code for the same trait and that are found in the same position within a homologous chromosome, they are known as:
   a. Homologues
   b. Alleles
   c. Genotypes
   d. Heterozygous

3. Each red blood cell contains approximately _____ million haemoglobin.
   a. 80
   b. 160
   c. 280
   d. 4.8

4. The typical lifespan of a red blood cell is:
   a. 30 days
   b. 60 days
   c. 90 days
   d. 120 days

5. Homozygous sickle-cell anaemia is denoted as:
   a. HbA
   b. HbS
   c. HbAS
   d. HbSS

6. Sickle red blood cells are fragile, with a reduced lifespan of _____ days.
   a. 10–20
   b. 20–30
   c. 30–60
   d. 60–90

7. The generation of reactive oxygen species in response to haemolysis interferes with _____ signalling.
   a. CO
   b. NO
   c. O_2
   d. CO_2

8. The most common cause of admission for patients with SCD is:
   a. Splenic sequestration
   b. Vaso-occlusive crisis
   c. Acute chest syndrome
   d. Bacterial sepsis

9. Which of the following signs or symptoms in a patient with SCD warrant urgent referral to hospital?
   a. New neurological symptoms
   b. Haematuria
   c. Severe sepsis
   d. All of the above

10. Which drug has been proven to reduce the incidence of painful crisis in patients with SCD?
    a. Morphine
    b. Aspirin
    c. Hydroxyurea
    d. Blood

Answers: Q1: a, Q2: b, Q3: c, Q4: d, Q5: d, Q6: d, Q7: a, Q8: b, Q9: b, Q10: c.

Assessment

Tachyarrhythmias

1. Which of the following is NOT a tachyarrhythmia?
   a. Atrial fibrillation
   b. Atrial flutter
   c. AV-nodal re-entry tachycardia
   d. Sinus tachycardia

2. Which tachyarrhythmia is a PSVT?
   a. AVNRT
   b. AVRT
   c. Atrial tachycardia
   d. All of the above

3. Which tachyarrhythmia would lead to the appearance of F waves?
   a. Atrial fibrillation
   b. Atrial flutter
   c. AV-nodal re-entry tachycardia
   d. Sinus tachycardia

4. Which structures border the triangle of Koch?
   a. Coronary sinus ostium
   b. Tendon of Todaro
   c. Septal leaflet of tricuspid valve
   d. All of the above

5. The most common type of AVNRT is:
   a. Fast-slow
   b. Slow-fast
   c. Slow-slow
   d. Quick-quick-slow

6. In which tachyarrhythmia would you expect to see delta waves?
   a. AVNRT
   b. Ventricular tachycardia
   c. Atrial flutter
   d. Wolff–Parkinson–White

7. The most common form of AVRT is:
   a. Orthodromic
   b. Antidromic
   c. Retrograde
   d. Antegrade

8. Ventricular tachycardias that last for more than 30 seconds are called:
   a. Long
   b. Prolonged
   c. Sustained
   d. Delayed

9. When assessing tachyarrhythmias, adverse signs include:
   a. Shock
   b. Syncope
   c. Myocardial ischaemia
   d. All of the above

10. Irregular broad complex tachycardias are mostly likely to be caused by:
    a. Ventricular fibrillation
    b. Atrial fibrillation with a bundle branch block
    c. Atrial flutter
    d. A letter from the HCPC

Answers: Q1: d, Q2: d, Q3: b, Q4: d, Q5: b, Q6: d, Q7: a, Q8: c, Q9: d, Q10: b.

Disability

Brain attack

1. What is the rhythm of the ECG in Figure 3.1 (p. 77)?
   a. Atrial fibrillation
   b. Sinus arrhythmia
   c. Normal sinus rhythm
   d. Supraventricular tachycardia

2. Stroke is typified by disturbances in cerebral function which last longer than:
   a. 12 hours
   b. 24 hours
   c. 48 hours
   d. 72 hours

3. Two pairs of arteries serve the brain. What are they?
   a. External carotid and subclavian
   b. Internal and external carotid
   c. Basilar and vertebral
   d. Vertebral and internal carotid

4. Which of the following is not a modifiable risk factor for stroke?
   a. Hypertension
   b. Smoking
   c. Atrial fibrillation
   d. Age

5. Why is it important to exclude hypoglycaemia when you suspect an acute stroke?
   a. It can mimic the signs of a stroke
   b. Diabetics can have a stroke
   c. Stroke patients survive longer with a high blood sugar
   d. Hypoglycaemic patients can be violent

6. Which age category below could suffer from a stroke?
   a. Adults
   b. Children
   c. Babies
   d. All of the above

7. One problem with the FAST tool is that it does not recognise:
   a. Facial palsy
   b. Unilateral arm weakness
   c. Speech disturbance
   d. Unilateral leg weakness

8. Why do most stroke signs occur on the opposite side to the affected hemisphere?
   a. Hemispheric dominance
   b. Decussation of nerve fibres
   c. Left-right confusion
   d. Cranial nerve palsies

9. Which artery is likely to be responsible for dysphasia?
   a. Anterior cerebral
   b. Middle cerebral
   c. Posterior cerebral
   d. Basilar

10. Which drug should not be routinely administered to patients suffering from a stroke?
    a. Ketamine
    b. Oxygen
    c. Amiodarone
    d. All of the above

Answers: Q1: a, Q2: b, Q3: d, Q4: d, Q5: a, Q6: d, Q7: d, Q8: b, Q9: b, Q10: b.

Assessment

Transient loss of consciousness

1. Approximately what percentage of the UK population will suffer from TLoC at some point in their lives?
   a. 10%
   b. 30%
   c. 50%
   d. 70%

2. What is the most common type of syncopal TLoC?
   a. Reflex syncope
   b. Syncope due to orthostatic hypotension
   c. Cardiac syncope
   d. Psychogenic pseudo-TLoC

3. Classic orthostatic hypotension is defined as a systolic blood pressure drop of at least _____ mmHg within 3 minutes of standing:
   a. 10
   b. 20
   c. 30
   d. 40

4. Causes of cardiac syncope include:
   a. Cardiomyopathy
   b. Long QT syndrome
   c. Valvular disease
   d. All of the above

5. The key difference between epilepsy and TLoC is:
   a. The short duration
   b. It's self-limiting
   c. Loss of consciousness
   d. The pathophysiology

6. POTS is a type of _____ TLoC.
   a. Syncopal
   b. Non-syncopal
   c. Apparent
   d. None of the above

7. Drugs administered to psychiatric patients that cause drug-induced orthostatic hypotension include:
   a. Phenothiazines
   b. Tricyclic anti-depressants
   c. Mono-amine oxidase inhibitors
   d. All of the above

8. Which of the following is NOT a prodromal symptom?
   a. Feeling hot/warm
   b. Nausea
   c. Dizziness
   d. None of the above

9. Which type of movement would not necessarily suggest an epileptic seizure?
   a. Myoclonic
   b. Tonic
   c. Clonic
   d. None of the above

10. Which of the following is a red flag sign on a 12-lead ECG?
    a. Brugada syndrome
    b. Abnormal T-wave inversion
    c. Left ventricular hypertrophy
    d. All of the above

Answers: Q1: c, Q2: a, Q3: b, Q4: d, Q5: d, Q6: a, Q7: d, Q8: d, Q9: a, Q10: d.

Headache

1. Migraine and cluster headaches are classified as:
   a. Primary headaches
   b. Secondary headaches
   c. Tertiary headaches
   d. None of the above

2. Migraines are divided into two types, based on whether they are associated with:
   a. Head pain
   b. An aura
   c. Nausea
   d. Loss of vision

3. Prodromal symptoms can occur up to _____ hours before a migraine starts.
   a. 1–2
   b. 4–12
   c. 12–24
   d. 24–48

4. The pain of a cluster headache is always severe and:
   a. Generalised
   b. Frontal
   c. Unilateral
   d. All of the above

5. The most common type of secondary headache is:
   a. Subarachnoid haemorrhage
   b. Medication-overuse
   c. Intracranial tumour
   d. Meningitis

6. Which of the serious causes of secondary headaches is typically worse when lying down?
   a. Meningitis
   b. Subarachnoid haemorrhage
   c. Giant cell arteritis
   d. Intracranial tumour

7. Thunderclap headaches are classically associated with:
   a. Cluster headaches
   b. Subarachnoid haemorrhage
   c. Carbon monoxide poisoning
   d. Meningitis

8. Jaw claudication is considered a diagnostic sign of:
   a. Meningitis
   b. Intracranial tumours
   c. Giant cell arteritis
   d. None of the above

9. Recurrent episodes of early morning headaches could be a sign of:
   a. Hangover or a raised ICP
   b. Meningitis or GCA
   c. Subarachnoid haemorrhage
   d. Extradural or subdural haemorrahge

10. Although not advocated by the *JRCALC Clinical Guidelines*, oxygen is useful in _____ headaches.
    a. Primary
    b. Secondary
    c. Frontal
    d. Generalised

Answers: Q1: a, Q2: b, Q3: d, Q4: c, Q5: b, Q6: d, Q7: b, Q8: c, Q9: a, Q10: a.

Assessment

Autonomic dysreflexia

1. The most common cause of a spinal cord injury is a:
   a. Fall
   b. RTC
   c. Sporting injury
   d. Stabbing

2. Autonomic dysreflexia typically affects those with an injury at _____ or above:
   a. C6
   b. T6
   c. L6
   d. M6

3. The sympathetic nervous system helps to control:
   a. Blood pressure
   b. Thermoregulation
   c. Urogenital function
   d. All of the above

4. Which arm of the autonomic nervous system connects with a chain of ganglia outside the CNS, but close to either side of the vertebral column?
   a. Enteric
   b. Parasympathetic
   c. Sympathetic
   d. None of the above

5. Which cranial nerves are utilised by the parasympathetic nervous system?
   a. I, II and XII
   b. II, V and VI
   c. III, VII and IX
   d. VIII, XI and XII

6. Complications of neuroplasticity include all of the following EXCEPT:
   a. Muscle spasticity
   b. Poikilothermia
   c. Autonomic dysreflexia
   d. Neuropathic pain

7. Neurogenic shock can last for _____ following injury.
   a. Days to weeks
   b. Hours to days
   c. Minutes to hours
   d. Seconds to minutes

8. Common causes of autonomic dysreflexia include:
   a. Pressure sores
   b. Bladder and bowel irritation
   c. Kidney stones
   d. All of the above

9. Signs and symptoms of autonomic dysreflexia do NOT include:
   a. Chest pain
   b. Pounding headache
   c. Severe hypertension
   d. Nasal congestion

10. A patient may be prescribed which drug to take during an episode of autonomic dysreflexia, if their blood pressure stays above 150 mmHg despite non-pharmacological intervention?
    a. Nifedipine
    b. GTN
    c. Nitrates
    d. All of the above

Answers: Q1: a, Q2: b, Q3: d, Q4: c, Q5: c, Q6: b, Q7: a, Q8: d, Q9: a, Q10: d.

Exposure

Drowning

1. A victim who has suffered a primary respiratory impairment from submersion in a liquid but survives has:
   a. Drowned
   b. Near-drowned
   c. Almost drowned
   d. Fatally drowned

2. Most drowning incidents are:
   a. Accidental
   b. Suicide
   c. Criminal in intent
   d. Due to natural causes

3. Laryngospasm:
   a. Is responsible for dry-drowning
   b. Causes hypoxic cardiac arrest
   c. Is rapidly terminated by cerebral hypoxia
   d. Leaves you speechless when nervous

4. The cold shock response can be reduced by all of the following EXCEPT:
   a. Clothing
   b. Habituation
   c. Orientation on immersion
   d. Holding your breath

5. The diving response is caused by stimulation of which nerve?
   a. Trigeminal
   b. Olfactory
   c. Trochlear
   d. Optic

6. Simultaneous stimulation of both sympathetic and parasympathetic pathways in drowning can lead to:
   a. Automatic dysreflexia
   b. Autonomic conflict
   c. A cold shock response
   d. All of the above

7. Clinical signs of aspirated water include:
   a. Blood-stained pulmonary oedema
   b. Bronchospasm
   c. Widespread atelectasis
   d. All of the above

8. When rescuing a drowning victim, you should remember to:
   a. Stop, drop and roll
   b. Hop, step and jump and fall
   c. Call, reach, throw, wade and row
   d. None of the above

9. After rescuing an adult drowning victim and finding that they are in cardiac arrest, you should:
   a. Start chest compressions
   b. Attach a defibrillator
   c. Ventilate
   d. Recognise death

10. In water above 6°C, survival for more than _____ minutes of submersion is unlikely
    a. 15
    b. 30
    c. 60
    d. 90

Answers: Q1: a, Q2: a, Q3: c, Q4: d, Q5: a, Q6: b, Q7: d, Q8: c, Q9: c, Q10: b.

Assessment

Heat-related illness

1. Although there is no definition of a 'heatwave', excess deaths are known to occur when ambient temperatures exceed:
   a. 20°C
   b. 24.5°C
   c. 30°C
   d. 34.5°C

2. Groups at higher risk of heat-related illness include patients who are:
   a. Over 75 years
   b. Female
   c. Living on their own
   d. All of the above

3. Which of the following is not a method of heat exchange?
   a. Conduction
   b. Convection
   c. Complexion
   d. Radiation

4. A mild form of heat-related illness is called:
   a. Heat stroke
   b. Heat exhaustion
   c. Heat syncope
   d. Heat stress

5. An example of an environmental risk factor for heat illness would be:
   a. Lack of heat acclimatisation
   b. Lack of shelter
   c. Poor physical fitness
   d. Malignant hyperthermia

6. What rise in blood temperature is sufficient to activate sympathetic mediated peripheral vasodilation?
   a. <1°C
   b. <2°C
   c. <3°C
   d. <4°C

7. Endotoxins leaving the porous gut are detected by:
   a. HSPs
   b. TLRs
   c. EMTs
   d. CWIs

8. Elevating the extremities is an effective treatment for:
   a. Heat cramps
   b. Heat stroke
   c. Heat oedema
   d. All of the above

9. The most serious type of heat-related illness is:
   a. Heat stroke
   b. Heat exhaustion
   c. Heat syncope
   d. Heat stress

10. Which of the following areas of the body are glabrous?
    a. Palms of the hands
    b. Forearms
    c. Groin
    d. Legs

Answer: Q1: b, Q2: d, Q3: c, Q4: d, Q5: b, Q6: a, Q7: b, Q8: c, Q9: a, Q10: a.

Carbon monoxide poisoning

1. Sources of CO poisoning include:
   a. Portable burner
   b. Barbecues in confined spaces
   c. Shisha
   d. All of the above

2. The most common location for CO poisoning is the:
   a. Pub
   b. Home
   c. Caravan
   d. Tent

3. At physiological levels, CO is thought to control:
   a. Inflammation
   b. Apoptosis
   c. Cell proliferation
   d. All of the above

4. How much CO binds with haemoglobin after being inhaled?
   a. 10–20%
   b. 20–40%
   c. 40–80%
   d. 80–90%

5. What CO concentration in air is required to produce a COHb of 14%?
   a. 10 ppm
   b. 50 ppm
   c. 100 ppm
   d. 500 ppm

6. Which factor is neuro- and cardioprotective at low levels of CO?
   a. Hypoxia-inducible
   b. Krypton
   c. Immune
   d. Coma

7. What does the C in the mnemonic COMA stand for?
   a. Chest pain
   b. Cardiac arrest
   c. Confusion
   d. Cohabitees

8. The most commonly reported symptom of CO poisoning is:
   a. Nausea
   b. Weakness
   c. Headache
   d. Vertigo

9. Baseline COHb in pregnant women can be as high as:
   a. 0.5%
   b. 1%
   c. 3%
   d. 5%

10. The half-life of COHb is approximately 320 minutes, which can be reduced to around _____ minutes if high-flow oxygen is administered.
    a. 204
    b. 104
    c. 74
    d. 34

Answers: Q1: d, Q2: b, Q3: d, Q4: d, Q5: c, Q6: a, Q7: d, Q8: c, Q9: d, Q10: c.

Assessment

Medical Emergencies

Anaphylaxis

1. Anaphylaxis by envenomation typically causes cardiac arrest within:
   a. 1 minute
   b. 5 minutes
   c. 10 minutes
   d. 15 minutes

2. Which of the following is a non-immunological trigger for anaphylaxis?
   a. Exercise
   b. Complement system
   c. Latex
   d. Insect sting

3. Which preformed mediator(s) cause bronchoconstriction?
   a. Prostaglandin D2
   b. Leukotrienes
   c. Platelet Activating Factor
   d. All of the above

4. Which cells are responsible for the chain of events leading to anaphylaxis?
   a. Red blood cells and basophils
   b. Basophils and mast cells
   c. Mast cells and leukotrienes
   d. Mast cells and white blood cells

5. The general order of anaphylaxis management in the hypotensive patient consists of:
   a. Oxygen, adrenaline, IV fluids
   b. Adrenaline, oxygen, IV fluids
   c. Chlorphenamine, oxygen, hydrocortisone
   d. IV fluids, oxygen, chlorphenamine

6. Rapidly progressing skin changes are present in around _____% of anaphylaxis cases.
   a. 10%
   b. 20%
   c. 80%
   d. 100%

7. Common differential diagnoses for anaphylaxis include all of the following EXCEPT:
   a. Acute asthma
   b. Neurological events
   c. Scombroidosis
   d. Acute generalised urticaria

8. The preferred route for administration of adrenaline in anaphylaxis is:
   a. Anterolateral thigh
   b. Deltoid
   c. Largest vein possible
   d. By mouth

9. The correct dose of IV fluids in hypotensive children with anaphylaxis is:
   a. 5 ml/kg
   b. 10 ml/kg
   c. 20 ml/kg
   d. 40 ml/kg

10. Signs of anaphylaxis include:
    a. Urticaria
    b. Angioedema
    c. Respiratory compromise
    d. All of the above

Answers: Q1: d, Q2: a, Q3: d, Q4: b, Q5: b, Q6: c, Q7: c, Q8: a, Q9: b, Q10: d.

Hypoglycaemia

1. Which cells in the islets of Langerhans secrete glucagon?
   a. Alpha
   b. Bravo
   c. Charlie
   d. Delta

2. Which organ consumes over 50% of the body's glucose?
   a. Heart
   b. Brain
   c. Liver
   d. Pancreas

3. What can cause hypoglycaemia associated autonomic failure?
   a. Sleep
   b. Previous hypoglycaemia
   c. Strenuous exercise
   d. All of the above

4. The glucose counter-regulatory process consists of two defences:
   a. Alpha and beta
   b. Endocrine and exocrine
   c. Physiological and behavioural
   d. Type 1 and 2

5. 10g of glucose is found in all of the following EXCEPT:
   a. 100ml Diet Coca-Cola
   b. 3–4 teaspoons of sugar
   c. 1–2 tubes of 40% glucose gel
   d. 5–7 Dextrosol tablets

6. The *JRCALC Clinical Guidelines* recommend the administration of IV glucose in which concentration?
   a. 5%
   b. 10%
   c. 20%
   d. 50%

7. Diabetic patients who have been successfully treated for hypoglycaemia should still be encouraged to attend hospital if:
   a. They have been treated with glucagon
   b. They are taking sulphonylureas
   c. There are signs of illness/infection
   d. All of the above

8. Neuroglycopaenic signs and symptoms include:
   a. Hunger
   b. Malaise
   c. Confusion
   d. None of the above

9. Which of the following cells does insulin target?
   a. Fat
   b. Liver
   c. Muscle
   d. All of the above

10. Which hormone has similar effects on the liver as glucagon?
    a. Insulin
    b. Adrenaline
    c. Somatostatin
    d. Raging teenage

Answers: Q1: a, Q2: b, Q3: d, Q4: c, Q5: a, Q6: b, Q7: d, Q8: c, Q9: d, Q10: b.

Assessment

Pulmonary embolism

1. An embolus can consist of?
   a. Air
   b. Fat
   c. Amniotic fluid
   d. All of the above

2. The most common cause of a pulmonary embolism is:
   a. Deep vein thrombosis
   b. Pregnancy
   c. Air travel
   d. Pleurisy

3. Virchow's triad does NOT include:
   a. Hypercoagulopathy
   b. Stasis
   c. Hypothermia
   d. Intimal injury

4. High risk factors for VTE include:
   a. Spinal cord injury
   b. Air travel
   c. Obesity
   d. All of the above

5. A deep vein thrombosis can grow to lengths of:
   a. 5cm
   b. 10cm
   c. 50cm
   d. 1m

6. What is the Wells score for the patient in the case study?
   a. 0–1
   b. 2–5
   c. 6–9
   d. 10 or more

7. What is the Revised Geneva Score for the patient in the case study?
   a. 0–5
   b. 6–10
   c. 11–20
   d. More than 20

8. Signs of right ventricular strain on a 12-lead ECG include:
   a. Right bundle branch block
   b. T-wave inversion in anterior leads
   c. S1Q3T3
   d. All of the above

9. If thrombolytics are administered in cardiac arrest in an attempt to treat a suspected PE, CPR should be continued for:
   a. 20–40 minutes
   b. 40–60 minutes
   c. 60–90 minutes
   d. 90–120 minutes

10. Pulmonary embolism can present in all of the following ways EXCEPT:
    a. Circulatory collapse
    b. Shortness of breath only
    c. Tender, hot and swollen calf
    d. Pulmonary haemorrhage

Answers: Q1: d, Q2: a, Q3: c, Q4: d, Q5: a, Q6: c, Q7: b Q8: d, Q9: c, Q10: c.

Addison's disease

1. Which zone of the adrenal glands secretes mineralocorticoids?
   a. Zona fasciculata
   b. Zona glomerulosa
   c. Zona reticularis
   d. Zona fabricartis

2. Aldosterone helps to regulate:
   a. Sodium and calcium
   b. Potassium and calcium
   c. Potassium and sodium
   d. Sodium and chloride

3. Cortisol has a number of functions including:
   a. Glucose formation
   b. Breaking down proteins
   c. Depressing the immune response
   d. All of the above

4. Raised plasma levels of _____ act on the zona glomerulosa leading to a release of aldosterone.
   a. Sodium
   b. Calcium
   c. Cortisol
   d. Potassium

5. What type of drug is lisinopril?
   a. Anti-platelet
   b. ACE inhibitor
   c. Diuretic
   d. None of the above

6. Which organ is mostly responsible for the conversion of angiotensin I to II?
   a. Heart
   b. Liver
   c. Brain
   d. Lungs

7. The hypothalamus receives input from:
   a. Limbic system
   b. Cerebral cortex
   c. Thalamus
   d. All of the above

8. The most common form of Addison's disease in developed countries is:
   a. Autoimmune
   b. Infective
   c. Genetic
   d. None of the above

9. The most common cause of adrenal crisis is:
   a. Injury
   b. Flu-like illness
   c. Diarrhoea and vomiting
   d. Anxiety

10. Signs and symptoms of Addison's disease include:
    a. Inexplicable weight loss
    b. Fatigue/tiredness
    c. Skin colour changes
    d. All of the above

Answers: Q1: b, Q2: c, Q3: d, Q4: d, Q5: b, Q6: d, Q7: d, Q8: a, Q9: c, Q10: d.

Assessment

Trauma

Thermal burns

1. What is the most common burn type causing injury to children?
   a. Contact
   b. Flame
   c. Scalds
   d. Acid

2. Keratinocytes are found in which layer of the skin?
   a. Epidermis
   b. Dermis
   c. Hypodermis
   d. Reticular region

3. Which of the following is NOT a function of the skin?
   a. Protection
   b. Sensory perception
   c. Synthesis of vitamin B
   d. Excretion

4. The correct term for 1st degree burns is:
   a. Superficial
   b. Mid-dermal
   c. Full thickness
   d. Epidermal

5. Loss of sensation in burns usually occurs at which depth?
   a. Epidermal
   b. Deep dermal
   c. Mid-dermal
   d. Superficial dermal

6. The zone of stasis is:
   a. The point of maximal injury
   b. Characterised by reduced perfusion
   c. Characterised by increased perfusion
   d. None of the above

7. Which gas binds to haemoglobin with 250 times the affinity of oxygen?
   a. Carbon monoxide
   b. Carbon dioxide
   c. Cyanide
   d. Hydrogen chloride

8. Using the rule of nines, what %TBSA does an adult patient with deep dermal circumferential burns to both legs have?
   a. 9
   b. 18
   c. 27
   d. 36

9. Signs of inhalation injury do NOT include:
   a. Singed nasal hair
   b. Green sputum
   c. Cyanosis
   d. Hoarseness

10. Burns of greater than _____% in children may require IV fluids.
    a. 5
    b. 10
    c. 20
    d. 30

Answer: Q1: c, Q2: a, Q3: c, Q4: d, Q5: b, Q6: b, Q7: a, Q8: d, Q9: b, Q10: b.

Conducted electrical devices

1. A Taser is held against the subject's body and the trigger is pulled with no probes being fired. This is referred to as:
   a. Red dot
   b. Fired
   c. Drive stun
   d. Drawn

2. Although a Taser can generate 50,000 volts, a subject is likely to be exposed to:
   a. 500 volts
   b. 800 volts
   c. 1,000 volts
   d. 1,200 volts

3. Alpha-motor neurons are important in innervating _____ muscle fibres.
   a. Extrafusal
   b. Intrafusal
   c. Cardiac
   d. Bladder

4. The average age of a person who is 'Tasered' is:
   a. 20 years
   b. 30 years
   c. 40 years
   d. 50 years

5. People who are at increased risk of injury during a fall following incapacitation with a Taser include those with:
   a. Osteoporosis
   b. Clotting disorders
   c. Anti-coagulant medication
   d. All of the above

6. Reported injuries following CED exposure include:
   a. Fractures
   b. Miscarriage
   c. Burns
   d. All of the above

7. If you are asked to remove Taser barbs, you should first:
   a. Ask the patient for consent to remove the barbs
   b. Ask the officer to remove the cartridge from the Taser
   c. Ask the officer if they need to keep the barbs for evidential purposes
   d. None of the above

8. Transport to hospital is recommended for patients who have been incapacitated by a Taser if they:
   a. Show signs of ABD
   b. Have a significant cardiac history
   c. Have a vagal nerve stimulator
   d. All of the above

9. Taser barbs should not be removed from the:
   a. Back
   b. Leg
   c. Genitalia
   d. Buttocks

10. A 12-lead ECG should be recorded following Taser incapacitation for:
    a. All patients
    b. Patients with a CIED
    c. No patients
    d. None of the above

Answers: Q1: c, Q2: d, Q3: a, Q4: b, Q5: d, Q6: d, Q7: b, Q8: d, Q9: c, Q10: b.

Assessment

Ankle injuries

1. The ankle joint cannot perform which of the following movements?
   a. Inversion
   b. Eversion
   c. Adduction
   d. Dorsiflexion

2. Which bones form the ankle joint?
   a. Tibia
   b. Fibula
   c. Talus
   d. All of the above

3. The distal end of which bone forms the medial malleolus?
   a. Tibia
   b. Fibula
   c. Talus
   d. Calcaneus

4. The lateral ligamentous complex comprises the anterior and posterior talofibular ligaments and the:
   a. Tibiofibular ligament
   b. Syndesmotic ligament
   c. Calcaneofibular ligament
   d. None of the above

5. Which ligament is most commonly damaged in an ankle injury?
   a. Tibiotalar ligament
   b. Calcaneofibular
   c. Anterior tibiofibular
   d. Anterior talofibular

6. Which grade of sprain would indicate a complete rupture of part of the ligament complex?
   a. 1
   b. 2
   c. 3
   d. None of the above

7. When considering the mechanism of injury, it is useful to form a mental image of the:
   a. Duration of the force
   b. Magnitude of the force
   c. Direction of the force
   d. All of the above

8. What is the correct order to examine the ankle joint?
   a. Joint above, move, feel, look
   b. Look, feel, move, joint above
   c. Joint above, look, feel, move
   d. Joint above, feel, look, move

9. When using the Ottawa ankle rules, you should check for bony tenderness in which two areas of the midfoot zone?
   a. Navicular and base of 5th metatarsal
   b. Lateral and medial malleolus
   c. Calcaneus and navicular
   d. Scaphoid and base of 5th metacarpal

10. The mnemonic PRICE stands for:
    a. Party, rest, ice cream, cake and eat it
    b. Protect, rest, ice, compression, elevation
    c. Pronate, raise injury, compress and elevate
    d. None of the above

Answers: Q1: c, Q2: d, Q3: a, Q4: c, Q5: d, Q6: b, Q7: d, Q8: c, Q9: a, Q10: b.

Pelvic trauma

1. The pelvic ring is made up of:
   a. two pelvic bones and the sacrum
   b. Ilium, ischium and pubis
   c. Symphysis pubis and sacroiliac joints
   d. All of the above

2. Anterior pelvic ring stability is provided by which ligament?
   a. Sacroiliac
   b. Iliolumbar
   c. Symphysis pubis
   d. None of the above

3. The most common type of pelvic ring fracture using the Young-Burgess system is:
   a. Combined mechanical
   b. Vertical shear
   c. Anterior-posterior
   d. Lateral compression

4. Vertical shear fractures typically occur with:
   a. Frontal impact RTC
   b. Lateral impact RTC
   c. Falls from height
   d. Vehicle rollover

5. A Tile type B pelvic fracture is:
   a. Rotationally and vertically unstable
   b. Rotationally unstable only
   c. Stable
   d. Rotationally stable

6. Bleeding from pelvic fractures originates from:
   a. Cancellous, fractured bone
   b. Retroperitoneal veins
   c. Internal iliac arteries
   d. All of the above

7. Compared with adults, pelvic ring fractures in children are:
   a. More common
   b. Less common
   c. Just as common
   d. More unstable

8. A clinical examination of a suspected fractured pelvis does NOT involve:
   a. Looking for deformity
   b. Noting if one leg is shorter than the other
   c. Springing the pelvis
   d. Identifying bleeding from the rectum

9. Concerns have been expressed about the use of commercial pelvic binders on which Tile type fractures?
   a. B1
   b. C
   c. A
   d. B3

10. The correct placement of a pelvic binder is usually over the:
    a. Iliac crests
    b. Pubic rami
    c. Greater trochanters
    d. Femurs

Answers: Q1: a, Q2: c, Q3: d, Q4: c, Q5: b, Q6: d, Q7: b, Q8: c, Q9: d, Q10: c.

Assessment

Obstetrics and Gynaecology

Care of the newborn

1. The APGAR score should be assessed at:
   a. Birth and 1 minute
   b. 1 and 5 minutes
   c. 2 and 8 minutes
   d. 5 and 10 minutes

2. The amount of baby's blood in the cord and placenta at birth can be up to:
   a. 300 ml
   b. 30 ml
   c. 10 ml
   d. 150 ml

3. The baby should pink up and cry:
   a. At the point of birth
   b. Within 90 seconds
   c. Within an hour
   d. It doesn't matter when

4. The umbilical cord should be cut:
   a. Immediately at birth
   b. After 3 hours
   c. At the child's graduation
   d. When it has stopped pulsating

5. Skin-to-skin is not an effective way to keep babies warm:
   a. False, it is effective as long as the head is covered and the baby has at least 2 towels or blankets covering them to ensure warmth
   b. True, they will always get cold
   c. Agree, midwives don't do it
   d. Agree, it will teach the baby bad habits

6. The infant's lungs in utero are filled with:
   a. Air
   b. Helium
   c. Fluid
   d. Nothing – they are in a collapsed state

7. The 'G' component of the APGAR score stands for:
   a. Growl
   b. Groan
   c. Greatness
   d. Grimace

8. SpO_2 probes should be placed on the:
   a. Left hand
   b. Right hand
   c. Left foot
   d. Right foot

9. At 2 minutes after birth the SpO_2 level should be:
   a. 80%
   b. 65%
   c. 100%
   d. 40%

10. The newborn's heart rate should be:
    a. 100–140 bpm
    b. 110–140 bpm
    c. 100–160 bpm
    d. 110–160 bpm

Answers: Q1: b, Q2: d, Q3: b, Q4: d, Q5: a, Q6: c, Q7: d, Q8: d, Q9: b, Q10: d.

Childbirth complications

1. Shoulder dystocia has an annual incidence of:
   a. 0.10–0.65%
   b. 0.58–0.70%
   c. 3–4%
   d. 5–7%

2. The second stage of labour starts when:
   a. The cervix is fully dilated
   b. The woman requests an epidural
   c. The baby is delivered
   d. Regular contractions commence

3. How long does the first stage of labour typically last in a woman's first pregnancy?
   a. 6–10 hours
   b. 16–20 hours
   c. 12–14 hours
   d. Up to 30 minutes

4. If a loop of umbilical cord lies beside the presenting part it is known as:
   a. Cord presentation
   b. Cord prolapse
   c. Occult presentation
   d. None of the above

5. The most practical position for a woman with a cord prolapse on an ambulance trolley is:
   a. Knees to chest
   b. Supine
   c. McRoberts'
   d. Right lateral with hips raised

6. Shoulder dystocia is difficult to predict with ____% of cases having no risk factors and in babies of normal weight.
   a. 10
   b. 20
   c. 30
   d. 50

7. Once you recognise shoulder dystocia, place the mother in the _____ position.
   a. Knees to chest
   b. Supine
   c. McRoberts'
   d. Left lateral with hips raised

8. The most common breech presentation is:
   a. Frank
   b. Betty
   c. Complete
   d. Footling

9. In a breech birth, the baby should be born within _____ minutes of the umbilicus becoming visible
   a. 1–2
   b. 2–3
   c. 3–5
   d. 5–10

10. Inserting a urinary catheter to fill the bladder with 500 ml of normal saline is undertaken by midwives to manage:
    a. Shoulder dystocia
    b. Cord prolapse
    c. Breech presentation
    d. All of the above

Answers: Q1: b, Q2: a, Q3: c, Q4: c, Q5: d, Q6: d, Q7: c, Q8: a, Q9: c, Q10: b.

Postpartum haemorrhage

1. The amount of blood that has to be lost to be classed as a PPH is:
   a. >200 ml
   b. >400 ml
   c. >500 ml
   d. >800 ml

2. The most common cause of PPH is:
   a. Tone
   b. Tissue
   c. Thrombin
   d. Trauma

3. The 'living ligatures' in the placental bed occlude which arteries in the uterine tissue?
   a. Broad
   b. Spiral
   c. Ovarian
   d. Femoral

4. If the uterus is well contracted and the placenta complete, which is the cause of PPH?
   a. Trauma
   b. Tissue
   c. Thrombin
   d. Tone

5. Syntometrine is a synthetic version of the hormone oxytocin combined with:
   a. Progesterone
   b. Ergometrine
   c. Testosterone
   d. Misoprostol

6. Leaving the umbilical cord intact to stop pulsating:
   a. Increases iron levels
   b. Increases blood volume
   c. Provides antibodies
   d. All of the above

7. The physiological changes of pregnancy allow for a blood volume loss of up to ____% before any changes in vital signs are noted.
   a. 20
   b. 30
   c. 40
   d. 50

8. After delivery, the placenta should be:
   a. Thrown away
   b. Inspected for completeness
   c. Cooked up and eaten
   d. None of the above

9. Trauma to the genital tract occurs in ____% of childbirths.
   a. 20
   b. 50
   c. 75
   d. 85

10. Contraindications to the administration of Syntometrine include:
    a. Hypertension
    b. Severe renal disease
    c. Multiple/concealed pregnancy
    d. All of the above

Answers: Q1: c, Q2: a, Q3: b, Q4: a, Q5: b, Q6: d, Q7: d, Q8: b, Q9: d, Q10: d.

Female genital mutilation

1. Which type of FGM includes narrowing of the vaginal opening through the creation of a covering seal?
   a. 1
   b. 2
   c. 3
   d. 4

2. What percentage of women who give birth in England and Wales have FGM?
   a. 1.5
   b. 2.5
   c. 5
   d. 10

3. FGM is typically carried out on girls aged between:
   a. Birth and 1 year
   b. 5 and 10 years
   c. 10 and 14 years
   d. 14 and 16 years

4. What are the benefits of carrying out FGM?
   a. Less painful childbirth
   b. Increased fertility
   c. There are no benefits
   d. Better protection for husbands during sex

5. Long-term effects of FGM include:
   a. Recurrent UTIs
   b. Fistula formation
   c. Chronic pelvic pain
   d. All of the above

6. Which type of FGM is associated with increased maternal and newborn mortality?
   a. 1
   b. 2
   c. 3
   d. 4

7. How many specialist centres are there in the UK that receive women with FGM?
   a. 5
   b. 10
   c. 15
   d. 20

8. FGM has been illegal in the UK since:
   a. 2004
   b. 2008
   c. 2014
   d. 2015

9. Women with type 3 FGM will often require a corrective procedure called:
   a. Episiotomy
   b. De-infibulation
   c. Infibulation
   d. Caesarean section

10. The fold of skin surrounding the clitoris is known as the:
    a. Prepuce
    b. Labia majora
    c. Labia minora
    d. Urethra

Answers: Q1: c, Q2: a, Q3: c, Q4: c, Q5: d, Q6: c, Q7: c, Q8: a, Q9: b, Q10: a.

Assessment

Paediatrics

Croup

1. What effect does 1 mm of oedema have on the diameter of an infant's airway?
   a. Increases diameter by 200%
   b. Decreases diameter by 40%
   c. Increases diameter by 25%
   d. Decreases diameter by 44%

2. The narrowest portion of a child's airway is at the level of the:
   a. Tongue
   b. Epiglottis
   c. Cricoid ring
   d. Vocal cords

3. Croup can be divided into two types, acute laryngotracheitis and _____.
   a. Spastic croup
   b. Spasmodic croup
   c. Nocturnal croup
   d. Gloopy croup

4. 95% of the cases of croup are caused by:
   a. Respiratory syncytial virus
   b. Parainfluenza virus
   c. Metapneumovirus
   d. None of the above

5. What is the Westley croup score of a child who when agitated has moderate chest wall recession, stridor, cyanosis, mildly decreased air entry but a normal level of consciousness?
   a. 4
   b. 8
   c. 12
   d. 16

6. The majority of cases of croup occur in the:
   a. Spring
   b. Summer
   c. Autumn
   d. Winter

7. Classic signs and symptoms of croup include:
   a. Barking cough
   b. Stridor
   c. Hoarse voice
   d. All of the above

8. Differential diagnoses for croup include all of the following EXCEPT:
   a. Coryza
   b. Epiglottitis
   c. Diptheria
   d. Retropharyngeal abscess

9. What is the modified Taussig score of a child who has stridor and intercostal recession when crying?
   a. 0
   b. 2
   c. 4
   d. 6

10. The dose of oral dexamethasone advocated by the *JRCALC Clinical Guidelines* is:
    a. 0.15 mg/kg
    b. 2.5 mg/kg
    c. 3.1 mg/kg
    d. 1.4 mg/kg

Answers: Q1: d, Q2: c, Q3: b, Q4: b, Q5: b, Q6: c, Q7: d, Q8: a, Q9: b, Q10: a.

Feverish illness

1. A temperature of _____°C or higher in a 3-month-old is classed as high risk according to the NICE traffic light system.
   a. 37
   b. 38
   c. 39
   d. 40

2. Fever is perceived in which of the following ways by parents and healthcare professionals?
   a. As a disease
   b. As a diagnostic sign
   c. As a symptom
   d. All of the above

3. Non-infectious illnesses that can cause fever include:
   a. Myocardial infarction
   b. Pulmonary embolism
   c. Cancer
   d. All of the above

4. What type of pyrogens do not cross the blood–brain barrier, but instead bind to toll-like receptors?
   a. Endogenous
   b. Exogenous
   c. Cytokine
   d. None of the above

5. Anti-pyretic drugs such as ibuprofen reduce fever by inhibiting:
   a. PGE2
   b. COX-2
   c. cAMP
   d. TLR

6. With every 1°C increase in body temperature, the body's metabolic rate increases by about:
   a. 1%
   b. 5%
   c. 10%
   d. 20%

7. A respiratory rate of more than ____ breaths/min in children is an intermediate risk factor of serious illness in a feverish child.
   a. 20
   b. 30
   c. 40
   d. 50

8. Red traffic light signs for the feverish child include:
   a. Decreased activity
   b. Crackles on auscultation
   c. Fever for 5 or more days
   d. None of the above

9. Dry, cracked mucous membranes, bilateral conjunctival injection and a strawberry-coloured tongue are signs of:
   a. Meningococcal disease
   b. Septic arthritis
   c. Herpes simplex encephalitis
   d. Kawasaki disease

10. What age group are forehead thermometers suitable for?
    a. Children under 5 years
    b. Infants under 4 weeks
    c. Infants over 4 weeks
    d. None of the above

Answers: Q1: b, Q2: d, Q3: d, Q4: b, Q5: b, Q6: c, Q7: c, Q8: d, Q9: d, Q10: d.

Assessment

Meningococcal disease

1. Meningococcal disease is most common in which age group?
   a. Infants
   b. Children
   c. Teenagers
   d. The elderly

2. The most common serogroup of meningococcus in the UK is:
   a. A
   b. B
   c. C
   d. WD40

3. Which of the following are proinflammatory cytokines?
   a. Tumour necrosis factor alpha
   b. Interleukin 1
   c. Interleukin 8
   d. All of the above

4. Circulating antithrombin III is activated by:
   a. Factor X
   b. Tissue plasminogen activator
   c. Heparan
   d. von Willebrand factor

5. When stimulated by endotoxins and cytokines, endothelial cells:
   a. Release tPa
   b. Release PAI-1
   c. Gain surface heparans
   d. All of the above

6. The extrinsic pathway of the clotting cascade is activated by:
   a. Tissue factor
   b. The X factor
   c. Factor V
   d. Damaged endothelium

7. Infants with meningitis are less likely to display which sign/symptom?
   a. Bulging fontanelle
   b. Neck stiffness
   c. Paradoxical irritability
   d. None of the above

8. When should you administer benzylpenicillin to a sick child with suspected meningococcal disease?
   a. If there is a non-blanching rash
   b. After correcting A and B problems
   c. En route to hospital
   d. All of the above

9. Hypoglycaemia should be corrected with the administration of ____ ml/kg of ____% glucose.
   a. 5, 5
   b. 5, 10
   c. 10, 5
   d. 10, 10

10. Fluid administration over ____ ml/kg will lead to pulmonary oedema.
    a. 5
    b. 10
    c. 20
    d. 40

Answers: Q1: a, Q2: b, Q3: d, Q4: c, Q5: b, Q6: a, Q7: b, Q8: d, Q9: b, Q10: b.

Mental Health

Mental disorders and the mental health act

1. An AMHP is usually which type of healthcare professional?
   a. Social worker
   b. Paramedic
   c. Psychiatrist
   d. Psychologist

2. Which person is top of the nearest relative hierarchy?
   a. Relative who usually lives with the patient
   b. The child of the patient
   c. The sister of the patient
   d. The patient's best friend

3. Under Section 2 of the MHA, a patient can be detained in hospital for up to _____.
   a. 72 hours
   b. 14 days
   c. 28 days
   d. 6 months

4. An application for Section _____ of the MHA can be overridden by the nearest relative.
   a. 2
   b. 3
   c. 4
   d. 136

5. Section _____ of the MHA is rarely used as it is seen as an incomplete Section _____.
   a. 4, 2 or 3
   b. 2, 4 or 3
   c. 1, 3
   d. 135, 136

6. Which Section of the MHA allows a police officer to gain entry to a property and remove the patient to a place of safety?
   a. 1
   b. 135
   c. 136
   d. All of the above

7. Under Section 137, as an authorised person, you have the same powers, authorities, protection and privileges of:
   a. An AMHP
   b. A paramedic
   c. Section 12 doctor
   d. A police officer

8. Making seemingly random connections between verbal statements in conversation is known as:
   a. Derailment
   b. Neologisms
   c. Concrete thinking
   d. None of the above

9. Using words in a special way or making up words is known as:
   a. Creating a word salad
   b. Concrete thinking
   c. Creating neologisms
   d. Derailment

10. Which mental disorder is characterised by the presence of a maladaptive and rigid coping mechanism?
    a. Schizophrenia
    b. Personality disorder
    c. Bi-polar affective disorder
    d. Deliberate self-harm

Answers: Q1: a, Q2: a, Q3: c, Q4: b, Q5: a, Q6: b, Q7: d, Q8: a, Q9: c, Q10: b.

Assessment

Eating disorders

1. 'Recurrent inappropriate compensatory behaviours in order to prevent weight gain' is a characteristic of:
   a. Anorexia
   b. Bulimia
   c. Binge-eating disorder
   d. All of the above

2. Patients with which eating disorder are typically underweight?
   a. Anorexia
   b. Bulimia
   c. Binge-eating disorder
   d. All of the above

3. The prevalence of eating disorders in the UK is highest for girls aged:
   a. 1–5 years
   b. 5–10 years
   c. 10–15 years
   d. 15–19 years

4. Around a third of all deaths in anorexia are due to:
   a. Infection
   b. Falls
   c. Bingeing
   d. None of the above

5. Amenorrhoea is common in women once their BMI is below:
   a. 20
   b. 17.5
   c. 15
   d. 12.5

6. The most serious complication of purging by vomiting or laxative/diuretic abuse is:
   a. Electrolyte abnormalities
   b. Losing weight
   c. Obesity
   d. Decreased gut motility

7. Russell's sign is caused by:
   a. Not eating
   b. Bingeing
   c. Laxative abuse
   d. Inducing vomiting

8. On a patient's ECG, _____ prolongation is common at low weights.
   a. P wave
   a. PR
   c. T wave
   d. QT

9. Which questionnaire can be helpful to determine the risk of an eating disorder being present?
   a. CAGE
   b. SCOFF
   c. MUNCH
   d. BINGE

10. The second 'F' in SCOFF stands for:
    a. Fat
    b. Flab
    c. Flatus
    d. Food

Answers: Q1: b, Q2: a, Q3: d, Q4: a, Q5: b, Q6: a, Q7: d, Q8: d, Q9: b, Q10: d.

Older People

Frailty

1. Which terms have NO place in clinical practice when referring to frailty?
   a. Acopia
   b. Off legs
   c. Failed discharge
   d. All of the above

2. Which of the following is NOT one of the geriatric 5Ms?
   a. Mind
   b. Mobility
   c. Management
   d. Matters most

3. A patient with a Rockwood clinical frailty score of 4 is:
   a. Fit
   b. Living with very mild frailty
   c. Living with mild frailty
   d. Living with moderate frailty

4. How might you verify abnormal findings as normal for the patient in front of you?
   a. Talk to family
   b. Find old discharge notes
   c. Discuss with their GP
   d. All of the above

5. What are the four questions of the AMT4 score?
   a. Age, Date of birth, Place, Year
   b. Age, Month, Year, Place
   c. Time, Place, Events, Year
   d. End of World War 2, current monarch, recognise 2 people, remember an address

6. Which scores are helpful when assessing a patient with frailty?
   a. NEWS2
   b. Rockwood Clinical Frailty Score
   c. AMT4 score
   d. All of the above

7. Which test should not be routinely used to investigate patients presenting with frailty?
   a. Urinalysis
   b. GCS
   c. NEWS2
   d. Blood pressure

8. A week-long admission for a frail older person can result in deconditioning of muscles by up to:
   a. 1%
   b. 2%
   c. 5%
   d. 10%

9. Who would be a good person to talk to regarding community referrals for the person living with frailty?
   a. GP
   b. Occupational therapist
   c. Acute medical team/medicine for the older person team
   d. All of the above

10. Which of these is the most important consideration if transporting someone to hospital?
    a. Patient's toothbrush
    b. Discharge plans: keysafe code, lifts home, etc.
    c. Which route to take to hospital
    d. The location of the vomit bowls

Answers: Q1: d, Q2: c, Q3: b, Q4: d, Q5: a, Q6: d, Q7: a, Q8: d, Q9: d, Q10: b.

Assessment

Dementia

1. Dementia is a set of 'symptoms' that includes which of the following?
   a. Memory loss
   b. Confusion
   c. Mood changes
   d. All of the above

2. What type of dementia makes up around 66% of cases?
   a. Alzheimer's disease
   b. Vascular dementia
   c. Lewy body dementia
   d. None of the above

3. Approximately, what percentage of people over 65 are thought to have dementia?
   a. 5%
   b. 7%
   c. 10%
   d. 15%

4. What type of Alzheimer's disease is a progressive aphasia?
   a. Typical
   b. Posterior cortical atrophy
   c. Logopenic aphasia
   d. Pogo-stick atrophy

5. Which of the following is NOT a sign of delirium?
   a. Sudden onset
   b. Disruptions in thinking
   c. Reduced ability to focus
   d. Hallucinations

6. Which of the following can be a cause of delirium?
   a. Infection
   b. Medication
   c. Constipation
   d. All of the above

7. The 4AT test incorporates which other scoring system?
   a. GCS
   b. AMT4
   c. ABCD2
   d. Abbey

8. Challenging behaviour displayed by patients with dementia can include:
   a. Wandering
   b. Pacing
   c. Sexual jealousy
   d. All of the above

9. Which of the following is NOT helpful when managing challenging behaviour?
   a. Involving relatives
   b. Repeatedly saying who you are
   c. Using a sharp tone of voice
   d. Finding the cause of the behaviour

10. In order to avoid patients with dementia being left in pain, you should:
    a. Always give IV morphine
    b. Score pain using alternative methods
    c. Always use the numerical pain rating scale
    d. Give every patient with dementia two paracetamol

Answers: Q1: d, Q2: a, Q3: b, Q4: c, Q5: c, Q6: d, Q7: b, Q8: d, Q9: c, Q10: b.

End-of-life care

1. What percentage of deaths occur in UK hospitals?
   a. Over 80%
   b. Over 70%
   c. Over 60%
   d. Over 50%

2. Multi-organ failure typically manifests as:
   a. Acidosis
   b. Uraemia
   c. Electrolyte imbalances
   d. All of the above

3. Tetany and muscle twitching are caused by high blood levels of:
   a. Phosphate
   b. Bicarbonate
   c. Potassium
   d. Urea

4. Which of the following is NOT a sign or symptom that precedes death?
   a. Abdominal ascites
   b. Delirium
   c. Respiratory distress
   d. Warm peripheries

5. When is a DNACPR decision likely to be made?
   a. When a mentally incompetent patient refuses CPR
   b. There is a valid ADRT stating the patient does not want CPR
   c. CPR is likely to be successful
   d. All of the above

6. Which drug might be used to treat the death rattle?
   a. Diamorphine
   b. Midazolam
   c. Haloperidol
   d. Hyoscine

7. Which anticipatory drug does NOT cause urinary retention or spasm?
   a. Diamorphine
   b. Midazolam
   c. Haloperidol
   d. Hyoscine

8. Suitable sites for subcutaneous injection include:
   a. Upper arms
   b. Thighs
   c. Peri-umbilical area
   d. All of the above

9. Which end-of-life emergency causes headache, breathlessness and facial swelling?
   a. Sepsis in the neutropenic patient
   b. Spinal cord compression
   c. Superior vena cava occlusion
   d. Convulsions

10. With a 6mm needle, what angle should you use to give a subcutaneous injection assuming the patient is NOT cachexic?
    a. 30°
    b. 45°
    c. 90°
    d. 180°

Answers: Q1: d, Q2: d, Q3: a, Q4: d, Q5: b, Q6: d, Q7: b, Q8: d, Q9: c, Q10: c.

Index

A
Abbey pain score, 295
Abbreviated Mental Test Score (AMTS), 286
Absorption atelectasis, 32
Acute asthma symptoms, 140
Acute chest syndrome, 60
Acute pulmonary embolism, 152
Acute smoke inhalation injury, 172
Addison's disease, 155–163
    causes of, 161
    signs and symptoms, 162
Adrenal cortex, 158–159
Adrenal crisis, 161–162
    management of, 162–163
    precipitating factors for, 162
Adrenal glands, 157, 158
Adrenaline, 137
Adrenocorticotrophic hormone (ACTH), 160, 161
Advance care plan (ACP), 298
Advanced decisions to refuse treatment (ADRT), 300
Airway and breathing
    carbon monoxide poisoning, 131
    chronic obstructive pulmonary disease (COPD), 25–32
        absorption atelectasis, 32
        blood gases, 30–31
        carbon dioxide transport, 30
        gases, 28
        Haldane effect, 32
        hydrogen ion transport, 30
        management of, 32
        oxygen physiology, 28–29
        oxygen transport, 29–30, 30
        pathophysiology of, 31–32
        risk factors for, 28
        ventilatory drive, 31–32
        V/Q mismatch, 31
    pneumothorax, 17–24
        assessment of, 23–24
        management of, 24
        pathophysiology, 21–23
        physiology, 19–21
        spontaneous, 19
        traumatic, 19
    severe airway contamination in cardiac arrest, 1–8
        anatomy and physiology, 4–5
        management of, 6–8
        pathophysiology, 4–5
        risk factors, 5
    tracheostomies, 9–16
        cuffed/uncuffed tubes, 12–13
        fenestrated tubes, 13
        indications for, 12
        inner cannulas, 13
        management of, 14–16
        patient assessment, 13–14
        physiological changes with, 12
Alveoli, 30
Amiodarone, 70
Anaphylaxis, 135–140
    causes of, 137
    differential diagnoses, 139–140
    management, 140
    mediators., actions of, 139
    pathophysiology, 137–139
Ankle injuries, 181–187
    examination, 185–186
    foot, anatomy and physiology, 183–185
    history of, 185
    management of, 186–187
    Ottawa ankle rules, 186, 187
    pathophysiology, 185
Anorectal injuries, 193
Anterior cerebral arteries, 79
Anterior-posterior compression (APC) fractures, 190, 192
Antihistamines, 140
Antithrombin III (ATIII), 255
Aplastic crisis, 60
Approved mental health professional (AMHP), 264
Arterial oxygen tension, 28
Assessment of, delirium, 292
Associated abdominal injuries, 193
Atrial fibrillation (AF), 65, 67
Atrial flutter, 66
Atrial tachycardia, 66
Autonomic dysreflexia, 99–106
    anatomy and physiology, 101–103
    causes of, 105–106
    management of, 106
        non-pharmacological interventions, 106
        pharmacological interventions, 106
    parasympathetic division, 103, 104
    pathophysiology, 103, 105
    signs and symptoms of, 106
AV junction, electrophysiology of, 67
AV-nodal re-entry tachycardia (AVNRT), 66, 67–68, 68
AV node, 67
AV re-entry tachycardia (AVRT), 66, 68–69

Index

B

Bacterial sepsis, 60
Bag-valve-mask (BVM), 240
Basophils, 137
Beta-thalassaemia, 58
Bilateral bundle branch block (BBB), 51
Bipolar pacing, 49–50
Blood gases, 30–31
Bohr effect, 30
Boyle's Law, 20
Brain attack, 75–82
    anatomy and physiology, 77–79
    causes and pathophysiology of, 80–81
    management, 82
    modifiable risk factors for, 80
    non-modifiable risk factors for, 79–80
    signs and symptoms of, 82
Breech presentation
    cephalic presentation, 214
    factors, 216
    frank breech position, 217
    head-down birth, 219
    stages of, 215–216
    tum to bum position, 217
Broad complex tachycardias (BCTs), 63, 71
Bronchodilators, 140
Bundle branch block (BBB), 51
Burn injury, 167–174
    assessment, 173
    classification, 170, 171
    history of, 173
    management, 173–174
        analgesia, 174
        cooling, 173–174
        covering/dressing, 174
        fluid, 174
        safety, 173
        stopping burning process, 173
        transport, 174
    pathophysiology of, 170–173
        acute smoke inhalation injury, 172
        local response, 171–172
        systemic response, 172

C

Carbon dioxide transport, 30
Carbon monoxide (CO) poisoning, 96, 126–132
    management, 131–132
        airway and breathing, 131
        circulation, 131
        scene safety, 131
    pathophysiology, 128–129
    signs and symptoms of, 131
Cardiac arrest, severe airway contamination in, 1–8
    anatomy and physiology, 4–5
    management of, 6–8
    pathophysiology, 4–5
    risk factors, 5
Cardiac output, 43
Cardiac resynchronisation therapy (CRT), 51–52
    types of, 52
Cardiac syncope, 87
Cardiopulmonary resuscitation (CPR), 1
Cardiovascular compromise, 152
Cardiovascular implanted electronic devices (CIEDs), 52, 178
Cardioversion, 70
Carotid sinus syncope, 85
Catamenial pneumothoraces, 19, 21
Causes of, delirium, 292
Chest pain, 23, 37–44
    fluid bolus, 44
    management of, 43
    pathophysiology, 41–43
    recognition, 43
Childbirth complications
    breech presentation, 214–219
    cord prolapse, 210–211
    knees to chest position, 211
    mother's position, 209
    scale of the problem, 210
    shoulder dystocia, 211–214
    stages of labour, 210
Chlorphenamine, 140
Chronic lung disease, 5
Chronic obstructive pulmonary disease (COPD), 17, 25–32
    absorption atelectasis, 32
    blood gases, 30–31
    carbon dioxide transport, 30
    gases, 28
    Haldane effect, 32
    hydrogen ion transport, 30
    management of, 32
    oxygen physiology, 28–29
    oxygen transport, 29–30, 30
    pathophysiology of, 31–32
    risk factors for, 28
    ventilatory drive, 31–32
    V/Q mismatch, 31
Circulation
    carbon monoxide poisoning, 131
    chest pain, 37–44
    implantable cardioverter defibrillators, 45–53
        complications, 52
        implantation of, 51
        management of, 53
        shocking, 53
    pacemakers, 45–53
        anatomy of, 49–50

cardiac resynchronisation therapy, 51–52
codes, 50–51
implantation of, 51
indications for, 51
malfunctions, 53
pacing leads, 49–50
sickle cell disease, 54–61
assessment of, 60–61
complications of, 56
management of, 61
paracetamol, 55
pathophysiology of, 58–60
quick primer in genetics, 57
scale of problem, 56–57
signs and symptoms, 60
tachyarrhythmias, 62–71
assessment and management, 69–71
atrial fibrillation, 67
atrial flutter, 66
AV node, 67
AV re-entry tachycardia, 68–69
re-entry tachycardias, 66
ventricular tachycardias, 69
Circumflex artery (Cx), 41
Classical orthostatic hypotension, 86–87
Cluster headaches, 95
Cold shock, 114
Cold-water immersion (CWI), 119, 125
Combined mechanical (CM) fractures, 192
Comprehensive geriatric assessment (CGA), 284
Conducted electrical device (CED), 175–180
management for, 179–180
pathophysiology of, 179
Conducted electrical weapon (CEW). *See* Conducted electrical device (CED)
Conduction, 121
Convection, 121
Coronary artery anatomy, 39, 40
left coronary artery (LCA), 41
right coronary artery (RCA), 40–41
Cortisol, 158
Cricoid pressure, 6
Croup
airway resistance, 241
anatomy, 240–241
disability, 239
management of, 243
Modified Taussig score, 243
pathophysiology, 241–242
SMS assess, 238
SpO_2 probe, 239
symptoms, 242
Westley scoring system, 243
Cuffed/uncuffed tubes, 12–13

Cyanide poisoning, 174
Cyclic-adenosine monophosphate (cAMP), 248

D
Deep vein thrombosis (DVT), 149, 150
pathophysiology, 150
Delayed (progressive) orthostatic hypotension, 87
Deltoid ligamentous complex, 184
Dementia
assessment of, 294–295
challenging behaviour, 294
communication, 292–294
vs. delirium, 291–292
observations, 289
scale of problem, 290
types of
Alzheimer's disease (AD), 290–291
vascular dementia, 291
Dermis, 170
Direct contact burns, 171
Disability
autonomic dysreflexia, 99–106
anatomy and physiology, 101–103
causes of, 105–106
management, of, 106
parasympathetic division, 103, 104
pathophysiology, 103, 105
signs and symptoms of, 106
sympathetic division, 101–103
brain attack, 75–82
anatomy and physiology, 77–79
causes and pathophysiology of, 80–81
management, 82
modifiable risk factors for, 80
non-modifiable risk factors for, 79–80
signs and symptoms of, 82
headache, 91–98
assessment, 96–97
differential diagnosis of, 98
primary, 93–95
secondary, 93–96
signs and symptoms, 97
treatment, 97–98
transient loss of consciousness (TLoC), 83–90
assessment for, 88–90
management, 90
non-syncopal, epileptic seizures, 87
onset of, 89
psychogenic, 88
rare causes, 88
syncopal, 85–87
Distributive shock, 140
Do not attempt cardiopulmonary resuscitation (DNACPR) decisions, 300–301
Double-cannula tubes, 13

Index

Double-lumen tubes, 13
Drowning, 5, 111–117
   autonomic conflict, 115
   management of, 116–117
   pathophysiology of, 114
Dyspnoea, 23

E

Eating disorders
   administer IV drugs, 274
   anorexia nervosa, 275
   assessment and management, 278
   binge-eating disorder, 275–276
   bingeing, 277–278
   bulimia nervosa, 275
   causes of, 276
   chronic fasting and starvation, 276–277
   comparison of, 274–275
   observations, 273
   scale of problem, 274
   weight control strategy, 277
Edinburgh Hypoglycaemia Scale, 146
Electromagnetic interference (EMI). *See* Cardiovascular implanted electronic devices (CIEDs)
Emergencies in end-of-life care (EOLC), 303
Emergency operations centre (EOC), 212, 263, 296
Emphysema-like changes, 21
End-of-life care
   advance care planning
      advanced decisions to refuse treatment (ADRT), 300
      DNACPR decisions, 300–301
   anticipatory medication, 301
   assessment of, 297–298
   cervical-spine immobilisation, 297
   drugs, 298–299
   emergencies in end-of-life care (EOLC), 303
   physiology of
      acidosis, 299
      electrolyte imbalance, 299
      hypoalbuminaemia, 300
      hypoxaemia, 300
      uraemia, 299
   scale of problem, 299
   subcutaneous injection, 302
Entonox, 44, 55, 56, 61
Epidermis, 169–170
Epileptic seizures, 87
Erythrocytes, anatomy and physiology of, 57
Estimated time of arrival (ETA), 223
Evaporation, 121–122
Exposure
   carbon monoxide poisoning, 126–132
      management, 131–132
      pathophysiology, 128–129
      signs and symptoms of, 131
   drowning, 111–117
      autonomic conflict, 115
      management of, 116–117
      pathophysiology of, 114
   heat-related illness, 118–125
      cold-water immersion, 119
      evaporative cooling, 120
      heat exchange, 121–122
      management, 123–125
      pathophysiology, 122–123
      physiology, 121
      risk factors for, 122–123
Extrafusal muscle fibres, 178

F

Female genital mutilation (FGM)
   childbirth management, 234
   culture of, 233–234
   safeguarding, 234
   stages of labour, 230
   types, 231–233
Fenestrated tubes, 13
Fenestrations, 21
Feverish in children
   assessment of, 245
   NICE traffic light system, 249
   paediatric assessment, 248
   patient anti-pyretics, 251
   physiology of, 246–248
   safety netting, 251
   scale of problem, 246
   symptoms and signs, 250
   thermometers, 251
   transport *vs.* safety netting, 251
Fight-or-flight division. *See* Sympathetic division
Fluid bolus, 44
4AT assessment, 293
Frailty
   AMT4 score, 286
   Clinical Frailty Scale, 286
   geriatric giants, 285
   history of, 282–283
   local frailty unit, 284
   scale of problem, 284
   terms, 284–285
   urine dipstick testing/urinalysis, 287
   UTI, 283–284
Frank-Starling law, 42

G

General practitioner (GP), 252
Geriatric 5Ms, 285
Giant cell arteritis (GCA), 96
Glasgow Coma Scale (GCS), 127

Index

Glucagon, 142, 144
Glucocorticoids, 160–161
Glucose counter-regulation, 144
Glucose oral gel, 142
Glyceryl trinitrate (GTN), 38
Glycosaminoglycan (GAG), 255
Graves' disease, 161
Greater trochanters, 190

H
Haemoglobin, 57–58
Haemolysis, 60
Haemolytic anaemia, 60
Haemophilus influenzae type b (HiB), 242
Haemorrhage, 192
Haldane effect, 32
Headache, 91–98
    assessment, 96–97
    differential diagnosis of, 98
    primary, 93–95
    secondary, 93–96
    signs and symptoms, 97
    treatment, 97–98
Heart failure, severe, 69
Heat exchange, 121–122
Heat exhaustion, 122, 125
Heat-related illness, 118–125
    cold-water immersion, 119
    evaporative cooling, 120
    heat exchange, 121–122
    management, 123–125
    pathophysiology, 122–123
    physiology, 121
    risk factors for, 122–123
Heat-shock proteins (HSPs), 123
Heat stress, 122
Heat stroke, 122–124, 125
Histamine poisoning, 140
Homozygous sickle-cell anaemia (HbSS), 58
Hydrocortisone, 157, 158, 163
Hydrogen ion transport, 30
Hydroxycarbamide (hydroxyurea), 61
Hyper acute stroke unit, 76–77
Hypercapnia, 32
Hypodermis, 169, 170
Hypoglycaemia, 76, 141–147, 142, 143
    management of, 146–147
    pancreas, anatomy of, 143, 145
    pathophysiology, 146
    physiology, 143–145
    signs and symptoms of, 147
Hyponatraemia, 162
Hypothermia, 116, 174
Hypoxaemia, 152
Hypoxic pulmonary vasoconstriction (HPV), 31

I
Iatrogenic pneumothoraces, 19, 21
Iliac crests, 190
Implantable cardioverter defibrillators (ICDs), 52
    complications, 52
    implantation of, 51
    management of, 53
    shocking, 53
Inferior vena cava (IVC), 201
Inner cannulas, 13
Intentional oesophageal intubation, 6
Interleukin 6 (IL-6), 257
Internal cardio-defibrillator (ICD), 48, 178
Internal carotid arteries, 79
Intracranial tumours, 95–96
IPAP suicide risk assessment, 269–270
Ischaemic penumbra, 81
Ischaemic stroke, 80, 82
IV access, 169
IV infusion, 157

J
Jugular venous distension (JVD), 43

K
Kendrick Traction Device, 194
Keratin, 170
Keratinocytes, 169
Kidneys, 158

L
Laryngeal reflexes, 5
Laryngectomy, 11, 12
    management of, 16
    physiological changes with, 12
Lateral compression (LC) fractures, 190
Lateral ligamentous complex, 184
Lead infection, 52
Left bundle branch block (LBBB), 52
Left coronary artery (LCA), 41
Life-threatening endocrine disease, 156–157
Lipopolysaccharide binding protein (LBP), 254
Los Angeles Prehospital Stroke Scale, 81
Lower oesophageal sphincter (LOS), 4
Lungs, 20

M
Major trauma centre (MTC), 169
Mast cells, 138
Mechanism of injury (MOI), 297
Medial ligamentous complex, 184
Medical emergencies
    Addison's disease, 155–163
        causes of, 161
        signs and symptoms, 162
    anaphylaxis, 135–140
        causes of, 137

Index

  differential diagnoses, 139–140
  management, 140
  mediators., actions of, 139
  pathophysiology, 137–139
 hypoglycaemia, 141–147
  management of, 146–147
  pancreas, anatomy of, 143, 145
  pathophysiology, 146
  physiology, 143–145
  signs and symptoms of, 147
 pulmonary embolism, 148–154
  high risk factors for, 150
  low risk factors for, 150–151
  management of, 154
  moderate risk factors for, 150
  pathophysiology, 150–153
  signs and symptoms of, 153–154
Medication overuse headache (MOH), 93, 95
Meningitis, 96
Meningococcal disease
 benzylpenicillin, 253
 clotting cascade, 255–256
 complement cascade, 254–255
 definition, 254
 general practitioner, 252
 management of, 259
 meningococcal meningitis, 258
 myocardial dysfunction, 257–258
 pathophysiology of, sepsis, 257
 signs and symptoms
  fever, 258
  meningism, 259
  rash, 258
  sepsis and shock, 258
 vascular endothelium, 255
Mental disorders
 bi-polar affective disorder, 269
 personality disorder (PD), 268
 principles, 266–267
 psychosis, 268
 scale of problem, 265
 schizophrenia, 269
 transport, 267–268
Mental health
 eating disorders
  administer IV drugs, 274
  anorexia nervosa, 275
  assessment and management, 278
  binge-eating disorder, 275–276
  bingeing, 277–278
  bulimia nervosa, 275
  causes of, 276
  chronic fasting and starvation, 276–277
  comparison of, 274–275
  observations, 273

  scale of problem, 274
  weight control strategy, 277
 mental disorders
  bi-polar affective disorder, 269
  personality disorder (PD), 268
  principles, 266–267
  psychosis, 268
  scale of problem, 265
  schizophrenia, 269
  transport, 267–268
The Mental Health Act 1983, 265
 AMHP, 266
 risk of, 269
 roles, 266
 suicide and deliberate self-harm, 269–270
 tips, 270–271
Metabolic alkalosis, 27
Migraines, 94–95
Minor heat-related illness, 123, 125
Misoprostol, 226–227
Morphine, 43
Myocardial capture, 178–179
Myocardial infarction (MI), 39
Myocardial ischaemia, 69

N
Narrow complex tachycardia (NCT), 63–64, 70
Naso-oropharygeal and mucosal burns, 172
NASPE/BPEG generic (NBG) code, 50
National Early Warning Score (NEWS), 119, 285
National Institute for Health and Care Excellence (NICE), 246
Neurogenic shock, 105
Neuroplasticity, 105
Newborn care
 APGAR score, 204
 blood glucose, 205
 fetal circulation, 201, 202
 oxygen saturation, 204, 205
 respiratory and heart rate, 204–205
 resuscitation, 206
 skin-to-skin contact, 205
 SpO_2 values, 205
 transition, 202, 203
 unclamped cord, 205, 206
Newcastle Face Arm Speech Test (FAST), 81
Non-iatrogenic pneumothoraces, 19, 21
Non-steroidal anti-inflammatory drugs (NSAIDs), 93, 97, 248

O
Obesity, 5
Obsessive compulsive disorder (OCD), 265
Obstetrics and gynaecology
 childbirth complications
  breech presentation, 214–219

Index

cord prolapse, 210–211
knees to chest position, 211
mother's position, 209
scale of the problem, 210
shoulder dystocia, 211–214
stages of labour, 210
female genital mutilation (FGM)
 childbirth management, 234
 culture of, 233–234
 safeguarding, 234
 stages of labour, 230
 types, 231–233
newborn care
 APGAR score, 204
 blood glucose, 205
 fetal circulation, 201, 202
 oxygen saturation, 204, 205
 respiratory and heart rate, 204–205
 resuscitation, 206
 skin-to-skin contact, 205
 SpO$_2$ values, 205
 transition, 202, 203
 unclamped cord, 205, 206
postpartum haemorrhage
 anatomy and physiology, 224
 benefits, 221
 carry chair, 222–223
 Patricia's observations, 221–222
 pre-hospital management, 224–228
 risk factors, 224
 scale of the problem, 223–224
 walk, 222
Older people
 dementia
  assessment of, 294–295
  challenging behaviour, 294
  communication, 292–294
  vs. delirium, 291–292
  observations, 289
  scale of problem, 290
  types of, 290–291
 end-of-life care
  advance care planning, 300–301
  anticipatory medication, 301
  assessment of, 297–298
  cervical-spine immobilisation, 297
  drugs, 298–299
  emergencies in end-of-life care (EOLC), 303
  physiology of, 299–300
  scale of problem, 299
  subcutaneous injection, 302
 frailty
  AMT4 score, 286
  Clinical Frailty Scale, 286
  geriatric giants, 285
  history of, 282–283
  local frailty unit, 284
  scale of problem, 284
  terms, 284–285
  urine dipstick testing/urinalysis, 287
  UTI, 283–284
Open book injury, 192
Opiates, 92
Oropharyngeal airway (OPA), 10, 240
Orthodromic AVRT, 69
Orthopaedic (scoop) stretcher, 189
Orthostatic hypotension, 85–87
Ottawa ankle rules, 186, 187
Oxygen physiology, 28–29
Oxygen transport, 29–30
Oxyhaemoglobin dissociation curve, 29

P

Pacemaker-mediated tachycardia, 53
Pacemakers, 45–53
 anatomy of, 49–50
 cardiac resynchronisation therapy, 51–52
 codes, 50–51
 implantation of, 51
 indications for, 51
 malfunctions, 53
 pacing leads, 49–50
Paediatric intensive care unit (PICU), 240
Paediatrics
 croup
  airway resistance, 241
  anatomy, 240–241
  disability, 239
  management of, 243
  Modified Taussig score, 243
  pathophysiology, 241–242
  SMS assess, 238
  SpO$_2$ probe, 239
  symptoms, 242
  Westley scoring system, 243
 feverish in children
  assessment of, 245
  NICE traffic light system, 249
  paediatric assessment, 248
  patient anti-pyretics, 251
  physiology of, 246–248
  safety netting, 251
  scale of problem, 246
  symptoms and signs, 250
  thermometers, 251
  transport *vs.* safety netting, 251
 meningococcal disease
  benzylpenicillin, 253
  clotting cascade, 255–256
  complement cascade, 254–255

Index

definition, 254
general practitioner, 252
management of, 259
meningococcal meningitis, 258
myocardial dysfunction, 257–258
pathophysiology of, sepsis, 257
signs and symptoms, 258–259
vascular endothelium, 255
Pain in Advanced. Dementia (PAINAD) score, 294
Pancreatic cells, 144
Paracetamol, 55
Paroxysmal supraventricular tachycardias (PSVT), 66
Partial pressure of oxygen (PaO$_2$), 28, 29
Pelvic binders, 194
Pelvic ring fractures, 191, 192
Pelvic trauma, 188–194
associated abdominal injuries, 193
haemorrhage, 192
management of, 193–194
mechanism of, 190, 192
pelvis, anatomy of, 190, 191
Tile's classification, 192
Pericardial effusion, 52
Plasminogen activator inhibitor (PAI-1), 255
Pleura, 20
Pneumothorax, 17–24, 52
assessment of, 23–24
management of, 24
pathophysiology, 21–23
physiology, 19–21
spontaneous, 19
traumatic, 19
Pocket haematoma, 52
Pocket infection, 52
Pollen-food allergy syndrome, 140
Postganglionic neurons, 101
Post-synaptic neurons, 101
Post-traumatic stress disorder (PTSD), 233
Postural orthostatic tachycardia syndrome (POTS), 87
Potassium
regulation of, 159
Pregnancy, 5
Pre-hospital management
causes, 224
drug therapy
Misoprostol, 226–227
Syntometrine, 226–227
Tranexamic acid (TXA), 227–228
extreme cases, 226
fundal massage, 226
thrombin, 226
tissue, 226
tone, 225
trauma, 226
Premature atrial complex (PAC), 67

Primary adrenal insufficiency, 157
Primary headaches, 93–95
migraines, 94–95
Primary percutaneous coronary intervention (PPCI), 43
Primary postpartum haemorrhage (PPH), 223
Primary spontaneous pneumothorax (PSP), 21
Prostaglandin E2 (PGE2), 248
Psychogenic non-epileptic seizures (PNES), 88
Psychogenic pseudo-syncope (PPS), 88
Psychogenic transient loss of consciousness (TLoC), 88
Pulmonary embolism, 148–154
high risk factors for, 150
low risk factors for, 150–151
management of, 154
moderate risk factors for, 150
pathophysiology, 150–153
signs and symptoms of, 153–154

R

Radiation, 122
Rapid response vehicle (RRV), 220
Re-entry tachycardias, 66
Reflex syncope, 85–86
Regurgitation, 4
Renin-angiotensin-aldosterone pathway, 159, 160
Respiratory acidosis, 27–28
Respiratory syncytial virus (RSV), 240
Right coronary artery (RCA), 40–41
Right ventricular infarction (RVI), 43
Russell's sign, 278

S

SALAD poke, 7, 8
SALAD technique, 6–8
Salbutamol, 136–137
Secondary headaches
carbon monoxide (CO) poisoning, 96
giant cell arteritis (GCA), 96
intracranial tumours, 95–96
medication overuse headache (MOH), 95
meningitis, 96
subarachnoid haemorrhage (SAH), 96
Secondary spontaneous pneumothorax, 19, 21
Severe airway contamination in cardiac arrest, 1–8
anatomy and physiology, 4–5
management of, 6–8
pathophysiology, 4–5
risk factors, 5
Shock, 69
Shoulder dystocia
applying suprapubic pressure, 213
axial traction, 212
documentation, 214
Sickle cell crisis, 60, 61
Sickle cell disease, 54–61
assessment of, 60–61

Index

complications of, 56
management of, 61
paracetamol, 55
pathophysiology of, 58–60
quick primer in genetics, 57
scale of problem, 56–57
signs and symptoms, 60
Sickle-cell trait, 58
Sickle haemoglobin, 58
Simmons test, 186
Skin
    anatomy, 169–170
    physiology, 170
Sodium, 159
    regulation of, 159
Spinal cord injury (SCI), 100–101, 105
Spinal shock, 105
Splenic sequestration, 60
Spontaneous pneumothorax, 19
    pathophysiology, 21
Stroke, 75–82, 77, 142
    anatomy and physiology, 77–79
    causes and pathophysiology of, 80–81
    management, 82
    modifiable risk factors for, 80
    non-modifiable risk factors for, 79–80
    signs and symptoms of, 82
Subarachnoid haemorrhage (SAH), 88, 96
Subclavian steal syndrome, 88
Suicide and deliberate self-harm (DSH), 269–270
Superficial fascia. *See* Hypodermis
Superior vena cava syndrome, 52, 201
Supraventricular tachycardia (SVT), 62
Sympathetic division, 101–103
Syncope, 69
Syndesmotic ligamentous complex, 184
Syntometrine, 226–227
Systemic inflammatory response syndrome (SIRS), 123
Systemic toxins, 172

T

Tachyarrhythmias, 62–71
    assessment and management, 69–71
    atrial fibrillation, 67
    atrial flutter, 66
    AV node, 67
    re-entry tachycardias, 66, 68–69
    ventricular tachycardias, 69
Tachycardia, pacemaker-mediated, 53
Taser
    mechanism of action, 177–179
    types, 177
Tension pneumothorax, 22–23
    assessment of, 23–24
Tension-type headache (TTH), 93, 95

Thermal burns, 167–174. *See also* Burn injury
Tile's classification, 192
Tissue plasminogen activator (tPA), 255
Toll-like receptors (TLRs), 123
Total body surface area (TBSA), 168
Tracheostomies, 9–16
    cuffed/uncuffed tubes, 12–13
    fenestrated tubes, 13
    indications for, 12
    inner cannulas, 13
    management of, 14–16
        airway and breathing, 14
        help and equipment, 14
        tracheostomy patency, 14–15
    patient assessment, 13–14
    physiological changes with, 12
Tranexamic acid (TXA), 227–228
Transient ischaemic attacks (TIA), 88
Transient loss of consciousness (TLoC), 83–90
    assessment for, 88–90
    management, 90
    non-syncopal, epileptic seizures, 87
    onset of, 89
    psychogenic, 88
    rare causes, 88
    syncopal, 85–87
        cardiac syncope, 87
        due to orthostatic hypotension, 86–87
        reflex syncope, 85–86
Trauma
    ankle injuries, 181–187
        examination, 185–186
        foot, anatomy and physiology, 183–185
        history of, 185
        management of, 186–187
        Ottawa ankle rules, 186, 187
        pathophysiology, 185
    conducted electrical device (CED), 175–180
        management for, 179–180
        pathophysiology of, 179
    pelvic trauma, 188–194
        associated abdominal injuries, 193
        haemorrhage, 192
        management of, 193–194
        mechanism of, 190, 192
        pelvis, anatomy of, 190, 191
        Tile's classification, 192
    thermal burns, 167–174
Traumatic pneumothorax, 19
    pathophysiology, 21–23
Tumour necrosis factor alpha (TNFα), 254
Twiddler's syndrome, 53

Index

U
Unipolar leads, 49
Upper oesophageal sphincter (UOS), 5
Urethral injuries, 193
Urinary tract infections (UTIs), 298

V
Valsalva manoeuvres, 70–71
Vascular occlusion, 58
Vaso-occlusive crisis, 60
Venous thromboembolism (VTE), 150
Ventilation (V)/perfusion (Q) mismatch, 31
Ventricular tachyarrhythmias
   incidence of, 66
Ventricular tachycardias, 69
Vertical shear (VS) fractures, 192
von Willebrand factor (vWF), 255

W
Wells score, 153
World Health Organization (WHO), 223

Z
Zone of burn injury, 171, 172